Diagnostic Imaging in Infertility

Second Edition

Diagnostic Imaging in Infertility

Second Edition

Alan C. Winfield, M.D.
Professor
Department of Radiology and Radiological Sciences
Vanderbilt University Medical Center
Nashville, Tennessee

Anne Colston Wentz, M.D.
Professor
Department of Obstetrics and Gynecology
Director
Section of Reproductive Endocrinology
Prentice Women's Hospital
Northwestern University School of Medicine
Chicago, Illinois

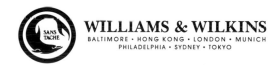
WILLIAMS & WILKINS
BALTIMORE · HONG KONG · LONDON · MUNICH
PHILADELPHIA · SYDNEY · TOKYO

Editor: Timothy H. Grayson
Managing Editor: Marjorie Kidd Keating
Copy Editor: Thomas Lehr
Designer: Wilma E. Rosenberger
Illustration Planner: Lorraine Wrzosek
Production Coordinator: Kathleen C. Millet
Cover Designer: Wilma E. Rosenberger

Accurate indications, adverse reactions, and dosage schedules for drugs are provided in this book, but it is possible that they may change. The reader is urged to
review the package information data of the manufacturers of the medications mentioned.

Printed in the United States of America

First edition, 1987

Library of Congress Cataloging-in-Publication Data

Winfield, Alan C.
    Diagnostic imaging in infertility / Alan C. Winfield, Anne Colston Wentz.—
2nd ed.
        p.   cm.
    Includes bibliographical references and index.
    ISBN 0-683-09149-2
    1. Infertility, Female—Imaging.   2. Hysterosalpingography.   3. Infertility—
Diagnosis.   I. Wentz, Anne Colston, 1940–   .   II. Title.
    [DNLM: 1. Hysterosalpingography.   2. Infertility, Female—diagnosis.   3.
Ultrasonography.   WP 570 W768d]
RG202.W56   1992
618.1′780757—dc20
DNLM/DLC
for Library of Congress   91-15342
                                                                              CIP

                                        91   92   93   94   95
                    1   2   3   4   5   6   7   8   9   10

Foreword

It is a pleasure to write a foreword to the second edition of *Diagnostic Imaging in Infertility,* which has been a valuable addition for the education of every reproductive endocrinologist and those radiologists who work as part of an infertility team. A hysterogram furnishes information unavailable from any other source that may help in the diagnosis and management of every infertility patient, whether primary, secondary, or due to repeated miscarriage problems. The congenital anomaly of a septate uterus, which causes miscarriages, can be diagnosed only by a hysterogram, and many have been completely missed by laparoscopic viewing. Other congenital anomalies, fistulae, or diverticula require this type of diagnostic procedure. One needs only to review the chapter titles—"Congenital Anomalies of the Uterus and Fallopian Tubes," "Diethylstilbestrol Exposure in Utero," "Intrauterine Synechiae"—to realize the importance of this technique.

In addition to these well-recognized applications for hysterography in gynecology, the editors have included a chapter on male infertility. This is an area that is lacking in the education of most reproductive endocrinologists. The new chapter on hysteroscopy is a welcome addition, as is the contribution on transcervical fallopian tube catheterization for management of proximal tube obstruction. Chapter 12, "Transvaginal Sonography in Gynecologic Infertility," is crucial at this time for anyone who is involved in ovulation induction, be it in anovulatory patients or in normally ovulating patients for in vitro fertilization. Chapter 13, "Transvaginal Sonography

in Normal and Abnormal Early Pregnancy," comes as a logical sequela. Those who have been interested in inducing ovulation and pregnancy are obviously eager to determine the normalcy of that pregnancy. It is important to determine this as rapidly as possible to reassure the patient in a case of a normal development or to prevent unnecessarily prolonged hope in the case of an empty sac syndrome. Patients with infertility of any etiology have a 20 to 30% miscarriage rate, most of which is associated with an empty sac. The most rapid way of identifying this abnormality is by detection of an absent fetal heart at 8 weeks.

It is important that the radiologist be aware of history, physical findings, and clinical concerns, and it is equally essential for the reproductive endocrinologist to be familiar with the best technique for demonstrating the suspected lesion in collaboration with the radiologist. The teamwork between the gynecologic specialist and the radiologist is essential, and both should be present at hysterosalpingography for appropriate evaluation and diagnosis of the problem. *Diagnostic Imaging in Infertility* has helped to reinforce these statements and therefore has improved our teaching and training in reproductive medicine. Doctors Winfield and Wentz are to be congratulated on producing its second edition.

Georgeanna Seegar Jones, M.D.
Professor
Department of Obstetrics and
*   Gynecology*
Eastern Virginia Medical School
Norfolk, Virginia

Preface

This book has been conceived to fill a need for those physicians involved in the management of the infertile couple. During the course of the diagnosis and therapy of these patients, numerous imaging techniques are needed. We have tried to bring these modalities together into one text, useful to the radiologist, gynecologist, and urologist both in the care of their patients and in the organized instruction of their students and colleagues.

It was apparent to us in the development of this text that the information included must be presented in a framework of multiple specialties. The gynecologist, urologist, and radiologist represent a team contributing to the care of the infertile patient in such a manner that the totality of their participation may well exceed the sum of the individual parts. The radiologist is more than an imager; he or she is a concerned and feeling participant in diagnosis and management. With this in mind, we hope that the chapters presenting a clinical overview of infertility are useful. Practitioners in infertility need to understand the basis of the imaging techniques and their utilization in patient management. Radiologic concepts and technical factors of importance have therefore been included.

Much more of this book is devoted to the female partner of the infertile couple, not because of any sense of relative importance but rather because the imaging techniques play a larger role in the diagnostic investigation of the female. Ultrasound has become a significant tool in the management of this special group of patients and will undoubtedly expand its usefulness in the future. Radiologic imaging of the male partner, although less frequently needed, is of tantamount im-

portance where indicated. The forthcoming role of new modalities of imaging is uncertain. There is, however, no question that imaging techniques will continue to be developed to answer the needs of our patients. As a matter of fact, the motivation to revise this text resulted from the dramatic improvements in technology since the first edition was written. Endovaginal sonography has dramatically increased our diagnostic capabilities. Magnetic resonance imaging is helpful on occasions. Interventional techniques play an increasing role in the management of our patients. These developments were of such a magnitude as to warrant the creation of this second edition.

Our collaboration has been of tremendous value in the management of our patients. The infertility evaluation is a team effort requiring coordination between several specialties. The infertility specialist assumes the leadership role in managing the diagnostic workup of the infertile couple, resulting in the development of a management plan that best serves our patients. Accordingly, over the years, we have, both individually and as a team, performed hysterosalpingograms together working with different techniques, various contrast media, and numerous methods to detail the pathology encountered. The result is this text, a personal expression of what we think is important in patient care, particularly as regards the close communication, collaboration, and cooperation among those involved in the diagnostic and therapeutic aspects of infertility. If this text can convey this concept to our colleagues and residents, it will have fulfilled our goal.

Alan C. Winfield, M.D.
Anne Colston Wentz, M.D.

Acknowledgments

A book such as this requires the input, cooperation, and efforts of many people. It is difficult to acknowledge adequately all of the help received in this task. Needless to say, major impetus has come from many of our past teachers and associates as well as the impact of a long line of patients.

Some of the illustrations found in this text were graciously offered to us by our colleagues, both in this country and abroad. Our thanks are extended to Dr. Hedi Hvricak and Dr. Howard Polluck.

Artwork was created by Bonnie Norman with skill and imagination. John Bobbitt supplied the photography with his customary devotion to excellence. We are grateful to them both.

Secretarial support, as well as unending patience, was supplied for the first edition of this book by Carolyn Cooper, Beverly A. Steele, and Vernice C. Dunlap and was received with appreciation. The Editorial Section of the Department of Radiology and Radiological Sciences at Vanderbilt University Medical Center, in the person of Holly J. Pelton, was of invaluable help. The second edition depended on the comparable contributions by Linda Pennington and Tom Ebers. We are most grateful.

George Stamathis and Carol Eckhart of Williams & Wilkins guided the development of the first edition of this text from its conception. The motivation and encouragement to develop this second edition were provided primarily by Tim Grayson. They have all reduced our burdens considerably.

Finally, we would thank Barbara and Dennis for their patience, tolerance, encouragement, and support. Their ability to share our time during the creation of this manuscript made the task a much lighter one.

A.C.W.
A.C.W.

Contributors

Arthur C. Fleischer, M.D.
Professor, Department of Radiology and
  Radiological Sciences
Associate Professor, Department of
  Obstetrics and Gynecology
Chief, Section of Ultrasound
Vanderbilt University Medical Center
Nashville, Tennessee

Carl M. Herbert III, M.D.
Director, Pacific Fertility Center
San Francisco, California

George A. Hill, M.D.
Medical Director, Program for Assisted
  Reproductive Technologies
Centennial Medical Center
Clinical Assistant Professor, Vanderbilt
  University Medical Center
Nashville, Tennessee

Donna M. Kepple, R.D.M.S.
Technical Supervisor
Department of Radiology and
  Radiological Sciences
Division of Ultrasound
Vanderbilt University Medical Center
Nashville, Tennessee

Fred K. Kirchner, Jr., M.D.
Associate Professor
Department of Urology
Vanderbilt University Medical Center
Nashville, Tennessee

Murray J. Mazer, M.D.
Associate Professor, Department of
  Radiology and Radiological Sciences
Assistant Professor, Department of
  Surgery
Vanderbilt University Medical Center
Nashville, Tennessee

Miles J. Novy, M.D.
Professor, Department of Obstetrics and
  Gynecology
Director, Reproductive Endocrinology
  and Infertility
Oregon Health Sciences University
Portland, Oregon

Amy S. Thurmond, M.D.
Assistant Professor, Department of
  Diagnostic Radiology
Director of Women's Imaging
Director of Ultrasound
Oregon Health Sciences University
Portland, Oregon

Rafael F. Valle, M.D.
Associate Professor, Department of
  Obstetrics and Gynecology
Prentice Women's Hospital
Northwestern University School of
  Medicine
Chicago, Illinois

Contents

1

Clinical Aspects of Infertility and Its Evaluation

Infertility affects an estimated 15% of couples, or about one in every seven marriages. The total number of infertile couples has increased in the past decade, due to both a larger population and an increase in sexually transmitted disease. Couples with primary infertility, or childlessness, have increased in number. The number of babies available for adoption has decreased because of the widespread use of effective methods of contraception and the availability of abortion techniques to limit unwanted pregnancy. More and more couples are seeking diagnosis of their infertility problem, and, with recent advances in therapeutic technology, they have a high expectation of a satisfactory solution. This has caused an increased demand for the services of physicians specializing in the diagnosis and management of male and female infertility (1). In response to the need, subspecialty training in reproductive endocrinology and infertility, certified by the American College of Obstetricians and Gynecologists, has been developed. However, practitioners in not just one but several specialties and disciplines must work together to improve the outcome for the infertile couple. Hysterosalpingography and ultrasonography bring the radiologist in close contact with these patients. The further evaluation of the couple requires the coordinated involvement of urologists, andrologists, geneticists, nutritionists, and many others. Cooperation and communication between the gynecologist and the radiologist are exceedingly important in the diagnostic approach to both members of the infertile couple.

Infertility is classified as either *primary*, when no pregnancy has occurred over at least a year of exposure, or *secondary*, when the couple has had a pregnancy in the past. Even if one partner has had a pregnancy, the couple must be evaluated as for primary infertility so as not to miss a diagnosis. Although the evaluation is substantially the same, the prognosis is better for subsequent pregnancies with secondary infertility.

An infertility evaluation should be instituted after no more than 1 year of unprotected intercourse, and earlier if either partner suspects that a fertility problem may exist. Approximately 25% of couples desiring pregnancy will conceive in the first month of unprotected intercourse, 60% in 6 months, 75% in 9 months, and 90% in a year. Since only an additional 5% will achieve pregnancy in the next 6 months of exposure, there is no reason to delay evaluation, particularly if the woman is over 30 years of age. Increased coital frequency will improve the chance of pregnancy: only 16% of couples having intercourse less than once a week achieved pregnancy in less than 6 months, whereas 83% of couples having intercourse four or more times a week achieved pregnancy during that time.

The infertility evaluation should be efficient and thorough. There are two goals in this investigation: (*a*) to determine the *etiology* of the couple's infertility and (*b*) to give a *prognosis* for future fertility. Until recently, even with optimal management, only 50 to 60% of couples consulting a physician or clinic for infertility could expect to achieve pregnancy. These statistics are made invalid by the rapid evolution of assisted reproductive technologies (ART), including several methods in which eggs and sperm, or embryos, are placed directly into the fallopian tubes, or embryos are placed directly into the uterus. These methods not only may circumvent some of the causes of infertility, but they may increase the number of eggs or sperm available for fertilization. Despite these advances, it is an important and basic concept that a careful evaluation to determine the reason for infertility and to provide an appropriate management plan is still needed to maximize the chances for pregnancy. The methods of diagnosis have not changed, but the likelihood of success in achieving pregnancy has increased. It must be recognized that not all couples who are infertile will have the financial, emotional, and cultural resources to undergo ART. Some patients will decide not to undergo studies essential for a thorough evaluation. The infertility workup is, after all, elective, but the limitations of an incomplete investigation should be explained. For this reason, an organized, efficient, and thorough approach is essential, both to minimize the time needed for a diagnosis to be made and to maximize the ultimate chance of pregnancy. However, a satisfactory result will be achieved only when the involved couple understands the goals of the evaluation.

The etiology of the infertility and the prognosis for future fertility are both established by taking into consideration three main areas: (*a*) the age of the woman, (*b*) the duration of infertility, and (*c*) the medical factor (or etiologic diagnosis) responsible for the infertility.

The age of the wife, not the husband, has an impact on the prognosis for infertility. The age of maximal fertility in the female is approximately 24 years, with only 1 of 60,000 births occurring past the age of 50. The fecundity or fertility capacity of a female of any particular age is difficult to analyze because there are numerous variables, but fecundity appears to decrease with increasing age. For example, at age 25, 75% of conceptions occur in less than 6 months of exposure, while after age 40 the number drops to 23%. Fecundity obviously begins to decrease minimally after the age of maximal fertility, but a significant difference is found only after age 35. Evidence from ART programs tells us that the occurrence of pregnancy in a woman 40 years old or greater is a fraction of that in the younger woman. Even more important, if a woman over 40 achieves pregnancy, she has a greater chance of spontaneous abortion; the data from in vitro fertilization cycles show that fewer than 10% of women over 40 achieve pregnancy and that if they do, they have greater than a 50% chance of miscarriage. Increased biological age of the oocytes appears to be responsible. Thus, from psychological and physiological standpoints, it is important to institute an infertility evaluation without delay in a woman over 30 years old and to understand that the prognosis for fertility decreases over time.

The length of time spent in unsuccessfully attempting pregnancy also helps to determine the prognosis for future fertility. A couple with long-term infertility clearly has something wrong and an excellent chance of having the etiologic diagnosis made. However, the longer the couple has been married without achieving pregnancy, the less the chance of pregnancy, partly because of advancing age but also because failure to conceive over many years implies a serious problem.

The third major area to be considered, crucial to prognosis, is the medical factor or etiologic diagnosis responsible for the infertility. Once the reason for infertility has been identified, then the alternatives for treatment and their chances for success can be provided to the couple. The following six factors are the most likely causes of infertility; all must be evaluated in a thorough investigation.

1. Central or ovulatory factor—Ovulation of an oocyte, which is difficult to establish, must occur. Regular menstrual cyclicity implies, but does not prove, that the ovarian processes essential to ovulation are occurring.
2. Male factor—The male partner must have sperm that can penetrate and fertilize the oocyte.
3. Mucus or cervical factor—Abnormalities of the cervix can act as a cervical barrier to fertility.
4. Endometrial-uterine factor—The lining of the uterus, the endometrium, must be properly prepared by hormone stimulation to permit implantation, and the uterine cavity must be anatomically normal to permit an early pregnancy to be maintained.
5. Tubal factor—The fallopian tube(s) must allow transport of the ovum to the uterine cavity.
6. Peritoneal factor—Pelvic adhesions, endometriosis, or other problems in the peritoneal cavity can cause a physical or mechanical block to fertility.

After the initial history and physical examination of both partners, a definite plan of evaluation, with a predictable time frame of investigation, should be established for the couple. A routine screening infertility evaluation should near completion in three or four office visits. Since two or more factors have been found to be operative in fully 35% of all infertility cases, all factors should be evaluated even if an abnormality that is found in one area appears to explain the infertility.

Five of the six factors listed above can be evaluated in one ovulatory menstrual cycle. If, by history, the wife seems to be ovulating, as judged from her description of regular menses and characteristic premenstrual symptoms, she is asked to keep a basal body temperature chart, which is useful to help with the timing and interpretation of the ensuing tests (Fig. 1.1). If the history suggests that she is not ovulatory, this diagnosis must be clarified by further gynecologic and endocrine testing to determine the cause and the correct treatment. If there are no contraindications, medications for ovulation induction may be used to re-establish an ovulatory pattern, and the evaluation proceeds.

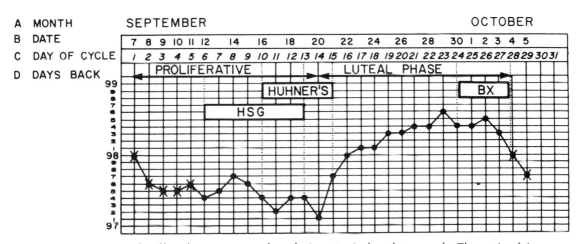

Figure 1.1. Example of basal temperature chart during a typical ovulatory cycle. The optimal times for hysterosalpingography (*HSG*), postcoital semen examination, and endometrial biopsy (*BX*) are noted. Times of active menstruation are designated by *X*.

The basic infertility workup is accomplished by scheduling a postcoital test (Huhner test) for evaluation of sperm survival in cervical mucus as close before the time of anticipated ovulation as possible. The hysterosalpingogram may be performed at the same time, if it can be established that ovulation is impending but has not yet occurred. For practical purposes, a basal body temperature that has not risen and a clear, watery cervical mucus, both observed on or before cycle day 14, suggest that ovulation is impending; if there is any question that ovulation has already occurred, it is better to defer the hysterosalpingogram until the next cycle. Before preparing the patient for hysterosalpingography, the cervical mucus is aspirated from the endocervical canal into a 1-ml syringe that is then capped and later subjected to microscopic evaluation. A semen analysis is a mandatory component in the early phase of the diagnostic investigation. The next procedure, the endometrial biopsy for evaluation of the endometrial pattern, can be accomplished in the same menstrual cycle, just before the onset of menstruation. In retrospect, if the temperature chart has a biphasic pattern characteristic of an ovulatory cycle, then five of the first six infertility factors could have been, and hopefully were, investigated in that first menstrual cycle. The ovulatory factor is evaluated by observation of a biphasic basal temperature chart and is confirmed by endometrial biopsy; the cervical mucus factor is evaluated by doing a postcoital test; the male factor by sperm count and postcoital test; the endometrial-uterine factor by the endometrial biopsy and the hysterosalpingogram; and the tubal factor by hysterosalpingography. Since the chance of pregnancy seems to increase in the 3 to 4 months after a hysterosalpingogram has been performed, it is useful to wait for three to four cycles before scheduling a diagnostic laparoscopy for evaluation of the pelvic or peritoneal factor. This time can be beneficially used to correct any abnormalities discovered in the basic infertility evaluation.

CENTRAL OR OVULATORY FACTOR

The presence or absence of ovulation can ordinarily be surmised from history. Breast tenderness, dysmenorrhea, weight gain or bloating, fatigue, and irritability are all associated more frequently with ovulatory than anovulatory cycles. The symptomatology characteristic of an ovulatory cycle is due to progesterone output in the luteal phase. Ovulation, the physical release of an oocyte from the follicle, requires formation of the stigma, an area of dissolution of the membrane of the follicle, which is induced by a complex interaction of hormones, enzymes, and prostaglandins; the follicles can produce progesterone even if the ovum is entrapped and not released, but this is a very rare finding. Absolute proof of the physical act of ovulation requires either a pregnancy or identification of the oocyte. For practical purposes, any woman not taking hormone medications, and who is having menses every 30 ± 4 days, can be considered to be presumptively ovulatory.

The basal temperature chart is a useful adjunct in the infertility evaluation (2). It cannot establish that physical ovulation is occurring, but it can aid in the scheduling and interpretation of tests. The follicular or proliferative phase of the cycle occurs between cycle day 1 (the day of menstruation) and the occurrence of ovulation, which is indirectly related to the rise in basal temperature. The luteal or secretory phase of the cycle begins after ovulation and extends to the next menses. The basal temperature is low, usually less than 97.6°F, before ovulation, and rises 0.6° to 0.8°F after ovulation under the influence of progesterone secretion, which causes a mild hyperthermia. Follicular phase shortening, late ovulation, luteal phase shortening, and delayed menses are easily ascertained from the chart. Proper timing for postcoital tests, the hysterosalpingogram, and endometrial biopsies can be decided and pregnancy diagnosed early. An elevated basal temperature on the chart suggests that ovulation may have already occurred. For example, if a hysterosalpingogram had been scheduled for cycle day 15, and the patient's basal temperature increased on day 12 and remained elevated, then the hysterosalpingogram should be cancelled to avoid performing it in the postovulatory period. The basal temperature chart should be reviewed before a hysterosalpingogram is done.

The patient should be asked to record daily temperatures only for the limited time necessary to complete the infertility evaluation. She should be instructed to take her temperature orally, at the same time each morning, before she has indulged in any activity, including getting out of bed or brushing her teeth. For women who work nights and sleep days, the temperature chart can still be valuable: the patient can take her temperature after 3 or 4 hours of uninterrupted sleep, when her temperature is likely to be at its basal level. All happenings of interest should be recorded on the chart, including late nights, alcohol consumption, sickness, intercourse, bleeding, cramping or spotting, and so forth. However, the keeping of a temperature chart should not be open-ended, and the chart itself should be used only for scheduling and interpretation of tests.

Proper treatment of a central or ovulatory factor involves first the diagnosis of why a woman is not ovulating regularly and normally. The three most important (although perhaps not the most common) diagnoses to evaluate in any amenorrheic woman are (a) pregnancy, which can be ruled out by a urine or blood pregnancy test; (b) a prolactin-producing pituitary tumor, which is diagnosed by measuring the hormone prolactin; and (c) ovarian failure or menopause, which is diagnosed by measuring follicle-stimulating hormone (FSH).

Once the causes listed above have been eliminated, the gynecologist will further pursue the diagnosis by appropriate hormonal and other testing. When the diagnosis to explain the ovulatory dysfunction has been achieved and the problem treated, menstrual cycles should become regular. If ovulatory dysfunction persists, and if there are no obvious contraindications to proceeding with ovulation induction, a plan to induce follicular development may be instituted. In patients undergoing ovulation induction, hysterosalpingography is indicated prior to treatment, to verify the presence of a normal uterus and tubes that would permit pregnancy to occur with successful ovulation stimulation. If, in the judgment of the gynecologist, an ovulatory problem is the only infertility factor, then occasionally ovulation induction will be stimulated for three or four cycles before a hysterosalpingogram is ordered. However, hysterosalpingography is indicated for all infertile women and is essential if pregnancy has not occurred within the first 3 to 4 months of ovulation induction.

Patients who are diagnosed to have ovarian failure as the cause of infertility also have an indication to undergo hysterosalpingography. Women with ovarian failure do not have oocytes and are functionally menopausal, although perhaps at a very young age. These women, however, can have implantation and maintenance of a pregnancy, if that pregnancy came from the insemination (by the husband) of eggs from an oocyte donor. By using assisted reproductive technologies, eggs from a donor may be inseminated (in vitro fertilization, IVF) and transferred either to the fallopian tubes (zygote intrafallopian transfer, ZIFT; gamete intrafallopian transfer, GIFT) or to the uterus (IVF-embryo transfer, IVF-ET) with a resultant pregnancy. Therefore, it is essential that a woman planning to undergo transfer of donor eggs or embryos be documented to have a normal uterine cavity.

MUCUS OR CERVICAL FACTOR

The cervical mucus must maintain and promote sperm survival and motility, but is only of importance for conception in the periovulatory period; therefore, the postcoital test (PCT) must be properly timed. During the follicular phase, rising estrogen levels cause the cervical mucus to become copious, watery, acellular, and conducive to sperm motility. The term "spinnbarkeit" is used to describe the ability of such mucus to be drawn out into a thread-like strand that can reach 10 to 12 cm long in the periovulatory phase. The effect of postovulatory progesterone output is to reverse all estrogen effects on the mucus, becoming thick, scant, viscous, cellular, and a barrier to sperm movement. Patients may be referred with a history of "hostile mucus" simply because the PCT was performed in the mid-luteal phase or prior to day 10 of the cycle, when the cervical mucus is physiologically inadequate to promote sperm motility. The most common explanation for "hostile mucus" is poor timing of the PCT.

The PCT is done within 24 hours of intercourse and is accomplished by aspiration of the cervical mucus, which is examined microscopically. The quantity and quality of the mucus is recorded, and an assessment is made of the number and motility of sperm present. If abnormalities are detected, it may be necessary to perform in vivo and in vitro penetration tests to identify and diagnose the cause of the mucus that is acting as a barrier to sperm.

It may be convenient for the patient to schedule both the hysterosalpingo-gram and the PCT for the same day, because both tests must be done before ovulation. The patient may be scheduled for a PCT in the gynecologist's office to be followed later by the hysterosalpingo-gram in the radiology suite. Alternatively, it is convenient to aspirate the cervical mucus immediately before performing the hysterosalpingogram. The capped syringe will maintain the mucus for examination later.

Examination of the mucus for sperm survival should give the gynecologist an indication of a mucus abnormality or a sperm problem. Mucus abnormalities, including inadequate, infected, and hostile mucus, are often not specifically treated; more frequently, the problem is simply circumvented by intrauterine insemination (IUI) using washed and prepared specimens of the husband's sperm. Sperm problems that may be detected by a PCT include total absence of sperm, too few sperm, agglutination or "sticking together" of sperm (which prevents normal progressive sperm motility), and, rarely, anatomical abnormalities such as neck defects. To evaluate mucus and sperm problems, the gynecologist may elect to perform sperm-mucus crossmatch studies, in which donor sperm and donor mucus are used in vitro to test the ability of the husband's sperm to penetrate a donor mucus, and whether the wife's mucus can be penetrated by donor sperm. The PCT is a simple indication of normality or the need to investigate either mucus or sperm further.

MALE FACTOR

Although a great deal of information about the male can be obtained from the PCT, a semen analysis is still essential. Since up to 40% of infertility diagnoses are attributed to various problems of the male partner, the quantitative measurements obtained from a sperm count, including volume, count/milliliter and total count, percentage of normal and abnormal forms, and percentage motility, are helpful in determining areas requiring further evaluation in the male. An increased number of white blood cells in the ejaculate may indicate infection. Head-to-head or tail-to-tail agglutination of sperm may suggest the presence of antisperm antibodies. The infertility specialist will be alerted to take a careful history and to guide the investigation along particular lines by abnormalities found in the routine sperm analysis. If a completely "normal" semen analysis is found, attention is then directed to evaluation of the cervical mucus to ascertain its quantity and quality. The possibility exists that the mucus may be acting as an immunological barrier to sperm penetration, particularly if other tests of sperm function have indicated their ability to swim through donor or bovine mucus. Finally, the capability of sperm to fuse with and enter a hamster oocyte may be assayed as an analogy to fertilization in the thorough evaluation of the male factor.

The need for a more thorough evaluation of the male factor may be indicated by an abnormality in either the semen analysis or the PCT. Physical examination of the male partner is important to identify such abnormalities as a varicocele or other physical problems. Infected semen may require culture or serologic testing to identify the presence of certain infectious diseases. Tests of sperm performance have been developed to provide an indication of the ability of sperm to effect fertilization.

Although no test presently used can provide definite evidence of the ability of sperm to fertilize, nevertheless some tests do give an indication of normality of certain aspects of this process. For example, for sperm to fertilize an oocyte, they must have intrinsic motility, and this can be measured by various forms of computerized semen analysis techniques. They also need an intact cell membrane,

and this can be tested by the hypo-osmotic swelling (HOS) test, a test of membrane integrity. For a sperm to fertilize a human egg, sperm must be able to fuse with and penetrate the egg cell membrane. Tests that provide some evidence of sperm's capability to accomplish this physiological task include the zona-free hamster egg penetration assay (HEPA) or sperm penetration assay (SPA). Results are provided in terms of a percentage of penetration, but for practical purposes, any positive result (greater than 0% penetration) should be viewed as positive. A modification of this test uses a specially prepared test yolk buffer for enhancement of sperm fertilization capability, with results reported as percent penetration without and with buffer treatment (e.g., 10%/20%); buffer enhancement ordinarily results in a doubling of the percentage of penetration. Another recently developed test indicates the capability of sperm to bind with the zona pellucida (or egg shell) of a specially stored human egg. The hemizona assay (HZA) is yet another test that correlates imperfectly with the capability of sperm to fertilize a human egg.

Therefore, the ultimate test of the male factor is the "ultimate fertilization test" provided by observing if a husband's sperm will fertilize his wife's egg. IVF and its variations allow us to make this determination. Under certain circumstances, it may be indicated to perform IVF earlier in the evaluation of infertility rather than later. If the result is negative, and the husband's sperm do not fertilize, then other alternatives for having a family may be explored before undergoing years of futile attempts at ovulation stimulation, intrauterine insemination, and the like.

ENDOMETRIAL-UTERINE FACTOR

Luteal phase inadequacy is a term that refers to either an inadequate output of progesterone from the corpus luteum or an inadequate endometrial response to progesterone stimulation. Its incidence in women with primary infertility is less than 5%, but it can be found with increased frequency in certain clinical settings: (a) 35% of patients undergoing the induction of ovulation with clomiphene citrate consistently manifest an inadequate endometrial development; (b) approximately 35 to 50% of patients with frequent early miscarriages have an inadequate progesterone output; (c) women over 35 are diagnosed to have endometrial inadequacy more frequently than younger women; (d) ovulating women with hyperprolactinemia are more likely to have defective corpus luteum function; and (e) women who jog or undergo strenuous athletic conditioning secrete less progesterone.

An adequate output of both estradiol and progesterone from the corpus luteum is needed to convert the proliferative endometrium into a secretory pattern, which then undergoes a predictable and reproducible change from ovulation to menstruation. In luteal phase inadequacy, an inadequate hormonal stimulation, or the inability of the endometrium to respond to hormones, results in a deranged endometrial pattern that is easily detected by taking a timed endometrial biopsy within 1 to 2 days of the expected menstrual period. The biopsy, taken from the anterior or posterior wall of the fundus or upper corpus, should produce a piece of tissue about 1.5 cm long. After fixation, microscopic sections are prepared and stained, and the histologic pattern is "dated" according to established criteria. An endometrial biopsy taken 2 days before the next period should have a histologic dating compatible with secretory day 26, because the first day of menstruation is arbitrarily called day 28. Biopsies that date early by 2 or more days lag expected development and are called "out-of-phase"; they are

suggestive of a defective progesterone output, and supplementation using progesterone suppositories is a common and successful form of therapy for this unusual cause of infertility. The site of the biopsy is rarely detected by hysterosalpingography. However, the scar may extend to the myometrium and may occasionally be observed as an indentation if a hysterosalpingogram is done in the follicular phase of the next cycle.

The uterine factor includes anatomical abnormalities of the uterus that are ordinarily detected and diagnosed by hysterosalpingography and may be important causes of infertility. Local abnormalities of the uterus, including polyps, submucous myomata, chronic endometritis, and retained products from a prior pregnancy may prevent implantation or placentation. Congenital uterine abnormalities, particularly the arcuate and bicornuate anomalies, are not ordinarily associated with impaired fertility, and only 25% of patients with a bicornuate uterus have any problems during pregnancy. The incidence of Asherman's syndrome appears to be increasing, and intrauterine synechiae may cause both secondary infertility and recurrent abortion (see Chapter 8). An unusual endometrial lesion is the deranged pattern caused by an infectious process, and culture for ureaplasma and/or chlamydia may be necessary.

Further diagnosis and treatment of any abnormalities initially detected by hysterosalpingography are ordinarily accomplished by either hysteroscopy, endometrial biopsy, or dilatation and curettage. Further discussion of these uterine abnormalities is found in Chapter 6.

TUBAL FACTOR

Hysterosalpingography provides detailed information about the uterine cavity and tubal patency. The Rubin test, in which CO_2 is introduced through the cervix, is nonspecific, is primarily only of historic interest, may give misleading information, and has technical difficulties: bilateral tubal patency and normality of the cavity cannot be readily ascertained, and tubal spasm cannot be differentiated from occlusion.

The hysterosalpingogram should be performed prior to ovulation, when the oocyte is in prophase of Meiosis I and relatively radioresistant, before resumption of meiotic maturation. No increase has been documented in the incidence of spontaneous miscarriage or congenital anomalies in patients in whom a hysterosalpingogram was performed in the cycle of conception. Importantly, all hysterograms should be performed after cessation of menses so as not to introduce blood in retrograde fashion into the peritoneal cavity, to avoid the development of endometriosis and perhaps infection.

Hysterosalpingography may be therapeutic in some women, since the incidence of conception increases during the subsequent 3 or 4 months. Although the reason for this is obscure, the observation is real. It has been suggested that hysterosalpingography may break up small intraluminal adhesions or evacuate small plugs of mucus or other desquamated material. Perhaps contrast media have a bacteriostatic effect or enhance cilial activity. A recent study has shown that both water-soluble and oil-soluble contrast media, as well as methylene blue (used at laparoscopy to indicate tubal patency), can inhibit lymphocyte proliferation in vitro (3); the peritoneal fluid of women with unexplained infertility contains increased concentrations of lymphocytes and macrophages, and cytokines generated by these cells are thought to interfere with various reproductive processes. Thus, inhibition of lymphocyte proliferation with diminished concentrations of cytokines could be another possible mechanism for tran-

siently enhanced fecundity following hysterosalpingography. Therefore, a delay before proceeding to diagnostic laparoscopy may indeed further the chance of pregnancy and avoid the need for general anesthesia and a surgical procedure. Also, the time can be used to follow up and evaluate any other problems suggested by abnormalities in the other basic tests.

PERITONEAL FACTOR

A pelvic or peritoneal cause for infertility refers to any physical or mechanical pelvic finding that can provide a barrier or block to any of the processes required for fertility. Pelvic adhesions, endometriosis, and postsurgical scarring limiting tubal mobility are the most common findings, and are not necessarily diagnosed radiographically. Hysterosalpingography tends to underdiagnose peritubal adhesions and endometriosis and to overdiagnose cornual occlusion (see Chapter 2). Endometriosis may be suspected if "convoluted oviducts," which have an appearance like corkscrews, are observed, but there are no other pathognomonic findings. Peritubal adhesions may be suspected if poor tubal mobility is seen, but this interpretation is very subjective. The introduction of contrast medium into the uterine cavity may reveal cornual spasm that may not be relieved by antispasmodics; at subsequent laparoscopy done under general anesthesia, cornual patency may be observed because the anesthesia has relaxed the spasm. Overall, when endoscopy is performed in patients in whom no other reason for infertility has been found and a thorough evaluation of the areas discussed above has been done, about 20 to 25% will be found to have intrapelvic pathology, such as endometriosis or pelvic adhesions. Therefore, diagnostic laparoscopy is an important part of the evaluation of the infertile couple (4).

PSYCHOLOGICAL ASPECTS

An additional factor, with a less obvious relation to fertility, must be considered; this is the psychogenic aspect. It is a myth that stress causes infertility; rather, it is the fact of infertility that induces stress into the lives of all infertile couples. Infertility imposes a strain on any marriage, and the anxieties and frustrations expressed by a couple with infertility are poignant. With continued failure to conceive, a woman tends to blame "poor timing" and puts such pressure on her husband to perform that ultimately the stress can lead to impotence or ejaculatory disturbances. The onset of the menstrual period becomes a time of profound depression. Recording daily temperatures can wrongly become a guide for choosing the day for intercourse, resulting in "sex-on-schedule" and a bizarre and unsatisfactory sexual relationship. The menstrual cycle becomes a vicious cycle. The unsuspecting, unaware, or insensitive hysterosalpingographer may find himself or herself in the middle of this milieu of anxiety, guilt, and emotional distress. An explanation for years of infertility may be diagnosed at hysterosalpingography and immediately precipitate a barrage of questions about etiology, treatment, and results. For these reasons, it is imperative that the hysterosalpingographer have a thorough working knowledge of the field of infertility, be cognizant of the history and previous evaluation of the patient, and have the patient's present clinic and basal temperature chart available for review. The physician involved must be sensitive to the needs of the couple. It is crucial that he or she have insight into both the infertility evaluation and the psychological and emotional distress that infertility can cause.

UNEXPLAINED INFERTILITY

What can one expect for the couple in whom a thorough infertility evalua-

tion, including diagnostic laparoscopy, has been completed without finding the etiologic reason for the infertility? Recent studies suggest that fewer than 5% of couples fail to show some etiologic factor associated with infertility; the 10 to 20% incidence of unexplained infertility quoted in the earlier literature is too high an estimate in view of the additional information made available through pelvic endoscopy, testing for immunologic causes, and improved evaluation of the male. The so-called normal infertile couple is a misnomer; these patients are obviously not normal, yet they are among the most poorly managed patients in terms of diagnosis-oriented therapy; since nothing specific was found to correct, the tendency is to try a little of every approach to help them achieve pregnancy. However, recent studies suggest that their prognosis may be better than previously thought. In one study of couples with unexplained infertility, 60% of the women found to be normal at laparoscopy conceived within 36 months (5). On the other hand, if conception has not occurred by 36 months after laparoscopy, then the couple is very unlikely to achieve pregnancy. For these couples with truly unexplained infertility, a therapeutic alternative exists: utilization of the new modalities of assisted reproduction results in an acceptable rate of pregnancy.

ASSISTED REPRODUCTIVE TECHNOLOGIES

Assisted reproductive technologies (ART) refers to a number of newly developed methods to enhance fertility. The utilization of some of these may be empiric, as in the couple who has totally unexplained infertility, or they may be the necessary solution, for example in a couple in whom the wife has obstructed fallopian tubes or the husband has a serious seminal factor with profound oligospermia. One of the simpler techniques has been the utilization of intrauterine insemination. The ejaculate from the husband, or a donor as indicated, is subjected to one of several washing, filtration, or buffering techniques, and then is introduced into the uterine cavity of the wife using a very small flexible catheter. Timing for the insemination is usually based on detection of the midcycle luteinizing hormone (LH) surge, which is now made convenient by the commercial availability of LH test kits. The only theoretical indication for intrauterine insemination is in the woman with hostile mucus; however, intrauterine insemination is now being used in cases of unexplained infertility and for fertility enhancement in general.

Ovulation stimulation is another method of assisted reproduction. Orally administered or intramuscularly injected ovulation induction agents increase the number of follicles developed in any menstrual cycle. Monitoring the follicular development is accomplished by measuring serum estradiol levels and by ultrasonographic tracking of follicle size and numbers (see Chapter 12). Ovulation is stimulated at what is deemed to be the proper time by injecting an ovulation-inducing hormone, human chorionic gonadotropin (hCG). Following ovulation stimulation, either natural intercourse or intrauterine insemination is performed. Numerous studies and investigations have indicated that all of these approaches have a variable chance at increasing pregnancy rates.

More invasive techniques of ART involve the aspiration of oocytes from ovaries that have undergone follicular stimulation as described above. Instead of intrauterine insemination, in vitro insemination using husband or donor sperm is accomplished with oocytes that have been aspirated from the ovarian follicles. Oocyte aspiration is ordinarily carried out by transvaginal ultrasound-guided follicular aspiration (see Chapter 12). The status of the woman's fallopian tubes will determine what occurs next. In the case of tubal occlusion or of significant tubal damage, in vitro culture of inseminated oocytes is carried out until fertilization and cleavage have occurred, some 18 to 24 hours following aspiration. Embryo transfer is then accomplished in the woman by the transcervical introduction of embryos into the uterine cavity. In vitro fertilization and embryo transfer (IVF-ET) is associated with pregnancy rates, depending on the woman's age, that may approach 40%, with approximately a 20% live birth rate in the best of programs. Alternatively, for the woman with normal fallopian tubes, eggs and sperm may be placed together in culture medium and almost immediately placed directly into the fallopian tubes at laparoscopy (gamete intrafallopian transfer, GIFT). A variation permits detection of fertilization by culturing eggs and sperm for 24 hours, at which time fertilization, if it is going to occur, can be observed. The fertilized egg at 24 hours has not undergone cleavage, and it is called a zygote. Transfer of zygotes to the fallopian tubes can be accomplished at laparoscopy (zygote intrafallopian transfer, ZIFT). Both ZIFT and GIFT procedures are reported to be associated with pregnancy rates in the vicinity of 30 to 40%, with live birth rates approximately 20 to 25% in the best programs.

Subsequent development in the area of ART is anticipated to introduce techniques with greater simplicity and convenience and with decreased expense for the couple involved. For example, intrafallopian transfer of eggs and sperm, or zygotes and embryos, may soon be routinely accomplished by transvaginal, transcervical, and transuterine intrafallopian cannulation under ultrasound guidance.

CONCLUSION

Success in the diagnosis and management of infertility is anticipated if an etiologic reason for the infertility is found. A systematic approach to establishing diagnosis and prognosis provides for the couple a realistic view of what to expect. If therapy is based on the discovered etiology, then the prognosis for future fertility can be determined, and the goals of an infertility evaluation will have been accomplished.

REFERENCES

1. Aral SO, Cates W Jr: The increasing concern with infertility. *JAMA* 250:2327, 1983.
2. Akin A, Elstein M: The value of the basal temperature chart in the management of infertility. *Int J Fertil* 20:122, 1975.
3. Goodman SB, Rein MS, Hill JA: Ethiodol (E), Renografin (R) and methylene blue (MB) inhibit lymphocyte proliferation: A potential mechanism for fertility enhancement in subfertile women following hysterosalpingography (HSG) and laparoscopic tubal lavage (TL). Abstract. American Fertility Society Annual Meeting, Washington, DC, October 13–18, 1990.
4. Drake TS, Grunert GM: The unsuspected pelvic factor in the infertility investigation. *Fertil Steril* 34:27, 1980.
5. Rousseau S, Lord J, Lepage Y, Van Campenhout J: The expectancy of pregnancy for "normal" infertile couples. *Fertil Steril* 40:768, 1983.

2

Techniques and Complications of Hysterosalpingography

A normal female reproductive tract is essential to fertility, and several approaches to investigation are used during the routine evaluation of the infertile couple. Healthy and patent oviducts facilitate conception, and a normal intrauterine surface without polyps, submucous myomata, septa, or scars allows the normal process of implantation to occur. An endocervical canal without diverticula, a lower segment without postoperative scars or defects, and a normal internal cervical os may be important to a successful pregnancy. The hysterosalpingogram is useful in evaluating all of these areas.

Hysterosalpingography (HSG) is indicated early in the investigation of the infertile female, particularly in those with a history of previous abdominal surgery, known episodes of pelvic inflammatory disease, prior postpartum infection or cesarean section, and/or palpable adnexal pathology compatible with hydrosalpinges or endometriosis. Hysterosalpingography has value in the evaluation of women with previous sterilization who are requesting reversal of tubal ligation and for patients prior to tubal surgery, whether or not laparoscopy has been done, because hysterosalpingography may yield information not otherwise available. Hysterosalpingography is also essential prior to utilizing assisted reproductive technologies (ART) for fertility enhancement. Ovarian stimulation with intrauterine insemination requires the presence of at least one patent fallopian tube for success. Gamete intrafallopian transfer (GIFT) and zygote intrafallopian transfer (ZIFT) (see Chapter 1) require that the tube(s) be not only patent but of normal caliber for the procedure to be successful. In vitro fertilization with embryo transfer to the uterus (IVF-ET) is done in the presence of bilateral tubal occlusion or of tubes so damaged or abnormal that a tubal transfer would be contraindicated; observation at laparoscopy of the flow of methylene blue dye from the fimbriated ends of the tubes may document tubal patency but provides no clue as to tubal anatomy. Finally, hysterosalpingography is indicated in patients who have previously undergone tubal cannulation procedures to document continued patency, since transfer attempts may induce damage or scarring in the tubal lumen (1). The appearance of the endocervical canal, the uterine cavity, and the fallopian tube lumina cannot be appreciated at laparoscopy, and some findings may be missed at hysteroscopy.

Hysterosalpingography has several advantages as a diagnostic test performed early in the investigation of infertility. It provides immediate information about serious problems such as tubal occlusion and abnormalities of the uterine cavity. General anesthesia is not required, and the procedure can be performed rapidly and is ordinarily well tolerated. On occasion, a mild analgesic is warranted (2). A prostaglandin synthetase inhibitor given an hour or so before the procedure may be of benefit. Some clinicians use a paracervical block to decrease discomfort from dilatation of the cervical os, but this is not useful to decrease pain induced by a cramping uterus and seems otherwise

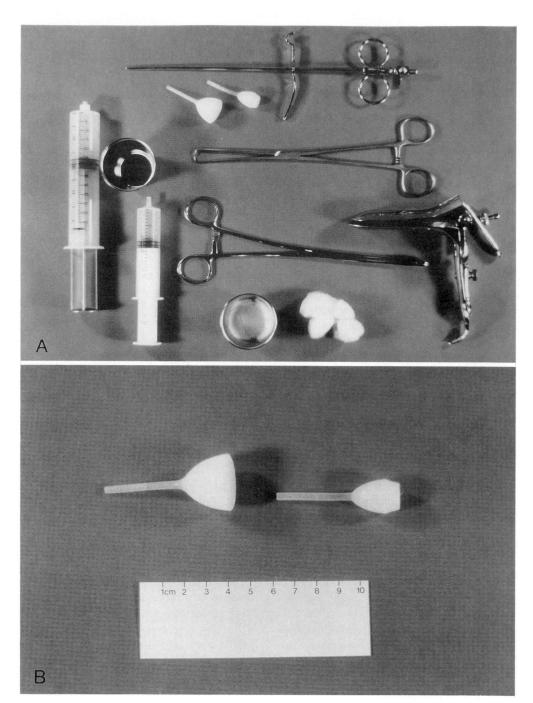

Figure 2.1.   A, Contents of hysterosalpingogram tray at Vanderbilt University Hospital. Kidde cannula and handle are the routine instrumentation. **B,** Kidde cannulas are available in two sizes. The smaller cannula is generally used. The tips may be shortened by scalpel if necessary.

unnecessary. Since so little advance preparation is required, and since hysterosalpingography is not invasive, the procedure is extremely cost effective.

Major limitations of hysterosalpingography are its inability to demonstrate
peritubal disease with consistency and to
evaluate the status of the fimbria of the
tubes. Lack of movement of the tubes
during traction may suggest fixation by
peritubal adhesions, but this observation
is neither sensitive nor specific and is
highly subjective. A convoluted, corkscrew appearance of the salpinx or
marked crowding or bunching of the tube
correlates reasonably well with peritubal
inflammatory disease (3). These findings
have been proposed to indicate pelvic endometriosis or inflammatory peritubal
disease (4). However, confirmation of
such suspicions usually requires laparoscopy, which remains the optimal technique to evaluate peritoneal abnormalities.

HYSTEROSALPINGOGRAPHIC TECHNOLOGY

Instruments for Hysterosalpingography

Various instruments have been designed and other methods adapted to the
performance of hysterosalpingography.
The most common of these include (*a*) the
Kidde cannula (Fig. 2.1); (*b*) the balloon
catheter (Fig. 2.2); (*c*) the Malmstrom
vacuum apparatus (Fig. 2.3); (*d*) the Harris Uterine Injector (Fig. 2.4); (*e*) the Fi-
kentscher and Semm portio cervix
adapter for hydroperturbation; (*f*) the
Jarcho-type cannula (Fig. 2.5); (*g*) the
Leech-Wilkinson cannula (Fig. 2.6); and
(*h*) the Cohen cannula (Fig. 2.7).

The ideal instruments for hysterosalpingography should be easily applied,
avoid uterine and cervical trauma, provide maximum delineation of the uterine
cavity, be unaccompanied by cervical

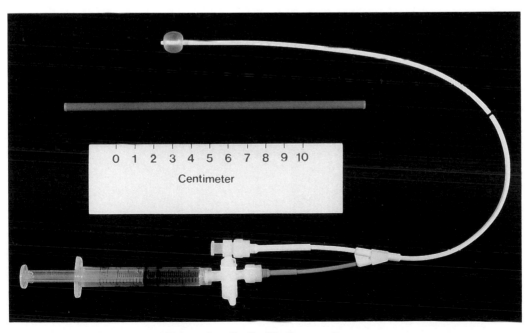

Figure 2.2. Sholkoff balloon catheter.

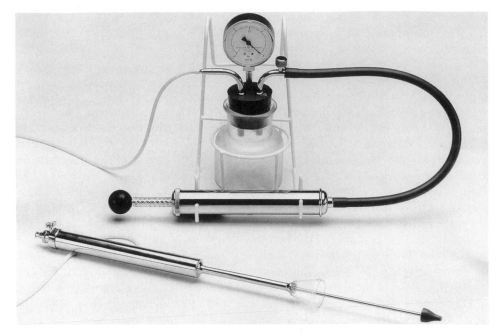

Figure 2.3. Malmstrom vacuum apparatus.

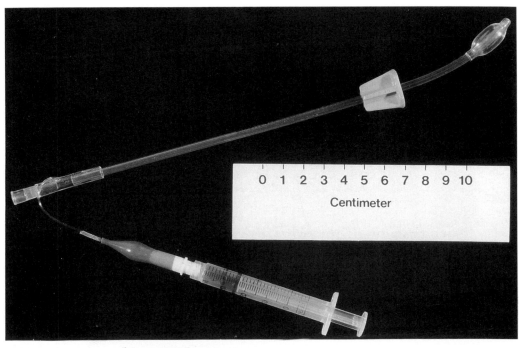

Figure 2.4. Harris Uterine Injector.

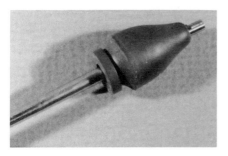
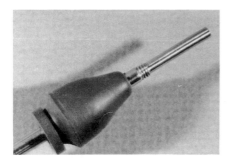
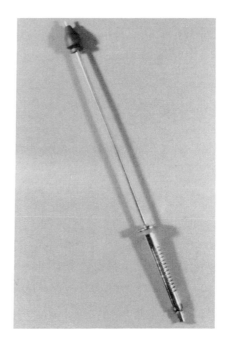

Figure 2.5. *Right,* Jarcho application device with hard rubber tip. The tip is movable. *Left upper,* Preferred position for rubber tip on metal rod. *Left lower,* Tip has moved, inappropriately exposing a long segment of metal.

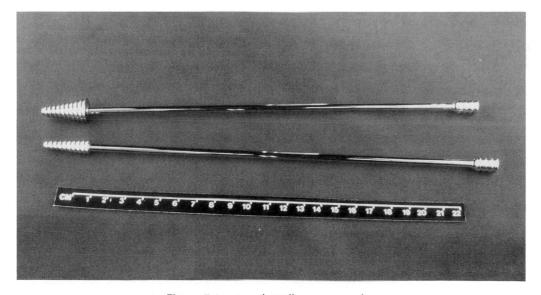

Figure 2.6. Leech-Wilkinson cannula.

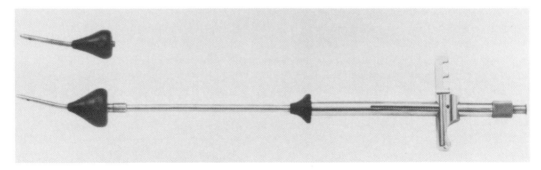

Figure 2.7.   Cohen cannula.

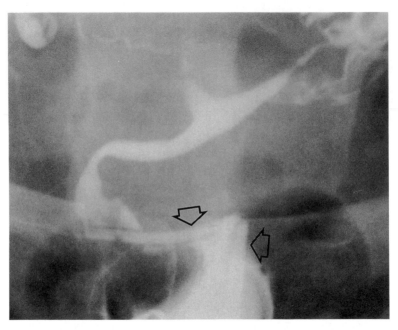

Figure 2.8.   Kidde cannula (*open arrows*) in place. Note the angulation of the cannula, permitting introduction of contrast material despite unfavorable alignment of the cervical os.

leakage, have no added discomfort due to instrumentation, and allow patient maneuverability for the performance of oblique films without dislodgment of the instrument. We have found the use of a Kidde cannula[a] to be simple, safe, rapid, and easy to teach to trainees. Its inherent flexibility permits ready positioning under most circumstances (Fig. 2.8), and

the ability to cut off or trim the cannula tip allows adapting the tip to the length of the endocervical canal.

Radiographic Instrumentation

Appropriate hysterosalpingography requires modern, well-designed radiographic equipment to produce an optimal examination yielding all pertinent information while exposing the patient to the least possible amount of radiation. It is mandatory that the examination be done

___

[a]Baxter Hospital Supplies, Norcross, GA. Uterine cannula, part no. 6605750; Kidde cannula tips, part no. 5605765.

with fluoroscopic control. Equipment design utilizing an undertable tube reduces radiation exposure to the operator. Reduction of the object-film distance, maximal collimation, a small focal spot, and a movable grid are all necessary to reduce radiation exposure and enhance patient imaging. The optimal voltage for visualization of the iodinated contrast agent should be in the 75 to 85 kVp range.

The image may be recorded on spot film, 105-mm camera film, or videotape. The modality chosen for imaging is not as important as the meticulous technique required to produce optimal radiographic images. Attempts to do hysterosalpingography without fluoroscopic observation are fraught with risk and should be discouraged.

Selection of an appropriate film-screen system is necessary. To achieve optimal imaging with reduced radiation, fast intensifying screens and moderate detail film are suggested if a cut-film technique is to be used. The rare-earth intensifying screens are of considerable value in this regard.

Fluoroscopic observation and radiographic exposures should be minimized to those necessary to complete the examination. A scout film, prior to the injection of contrast material, is advocated by some. In an uncomplicated study, this may significantly increase the radiation exposure unnecessarily, and we have not found this exposure particularly helpful. Although oblique views are sometimes of help and delayed radiographic examination is occasionally warranted, an examination satisfactorily completed with one or two exposures significantly reduces the amount of radiation. Application of traction by the tenaculum during filling and imaging of the uterus often results in improved uterine visualization (Fig. 2.9) and may avoid the necessity of oblique projections.

Importantly, radiographic equipment may change with time. It is mandatory that equipment be monitored on a regular basis for evaluation of radiation output. Radiation exposure to the pelvis should be reduced to a minimum. Radiation dosage to the gonads will vary dramatically depending on the number of radiographic exposures, duration of fluoroscopy, equipment, film-screen combination, and the like. Familiarity with the equipment and the procedure will shorten the examination and reduce the radiation exposure. Discussion of the level of gonadal radiation exposure during the procedure will be found later in the chapter.

Choice of Contrast Agents

Contrast material used for hysterosalpingography may be either water- or oil-soluble. As a matter of interest, the first contrast agent introduced to the uterine cavity was a paste-like suspension of bismuth, used by Kindfleish in 1910 in a 21-year-old woman suspected of having an ectopic pregnancy (Fig. 2.10) (5). The oil-soluble agent Lipiodol, composed of poppy seed oil with 40% iodine, was first used in hysterosalpingography in the mid-1920s and represented a satisfactory contrast agent. Concern developed over the possible effects of oil embolization to the lungs and the persistence of the iodized oil contrast material within the peritoneal cavity due to lack of reabsorption. Attention turned to the use of water-soluble agents because of their rapid absorption, improved visualization of detail in the uterine cavity and fallopian tubes, and a perceived increase in the level of safety. Nonetheless, the oil-soluble agents continued to be used, and in the 1950s, Ethiodol was introduced as an ethyl alcohol ester of poppy seed oil with 37% iodine (Fig. 2.11) (6).

Numerous agents have subsequently been developed (7). Prior to

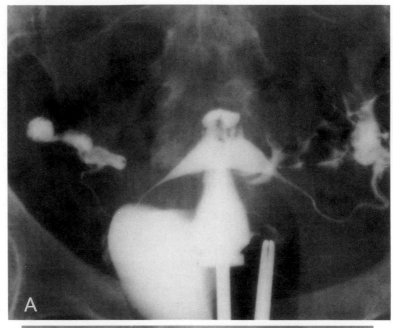

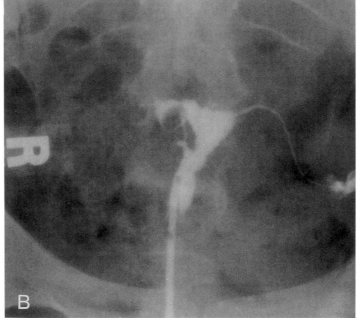

Figure 2.9.   A, Anteflexed uterus. Uterine cavity incompletely visualized. **B,** Same uterus as in **A.** Uterus deflexed by traction. Synechiae clearly noted in uterine cavity.

1981, Salpix[b] was the agent of choice of most hysterosalpingographers. When the

manufacture of this agent was discontinued, several other contrast agents were used with satisfactory results. A frequently used alternative, Sinografin,[c] had

[b]Sodium acctrizoate and polyvinyl pyroladone; Ortho Pharmaceutical Corporation, Raritan, NJ.

[c]E. R. Squibb and Sons, Inc., Princeton, NJ.

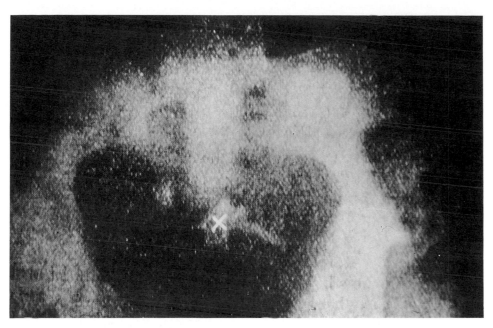

Figure 2.10. Earliest known attempt at hysterography (Rindfleisch, 1910). Bismuth suspension was introduced into the uterine cavity and radiographs were obtained. The X marks the faint visualization of the uterine cavity. (Courtesy of David B. Sping, San Francisco, CA.)

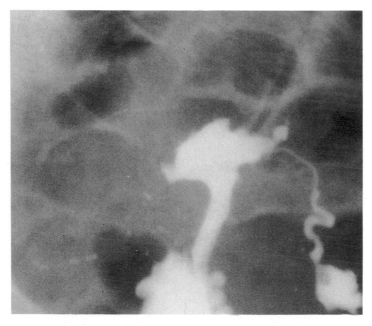

Figure 2.11. Hysterosalpingogram utilizing Ethiodol, an oil-soluble contrast agent, in a patient with uterine cavity deformities secondary to maternal exposure to diethylstilbestrol during gestation. There is less mucosal detail and a tendency toward droplet formation.

Table 2.1.   Common Contrast Agents for Hysterosalpingography

Product	Anion	Cation	Iodine	Osmolality	Viscosity (370°C CPS)
			mg/ml	mOsm/kg	
Water Soluble					
Conray 60[a]	Iothalamate	Meglumine	282	1400	4.0
Hypaque 60[b]	Diatrizoate	Meglumine	282	1415	4.1
Renografin 60[c]	Diatrizoate	Meglumine and sodium	292	1450	4.0
Sinografin[c]	Diatrizoate	Meglumine	380	1720	15.9
Renografin 76[c]	Diatrizoate	Meglumine and sodium	370	1940	8.4
Hypaque 50[b]	Diatrizoate	Sodium	300	1550	2.43
Hypaque 90[b]	Diatrizoate	Meglumine and sodium	462	2938	19.5
Hexabrix[a] (monoacidic dimer)	Ioxaglate	Meglumine and sodium	320	600	7.5
Isovue 370[c] (iopamidol)		Nonionic	370	796	9.4
Omnipaque 350[b] (iohexol)		Nonionic	350	844	10.4
Oil Soluble					
Ethiodol[d]	Iodine combined with ethyl esters of fatty acids (stabilized with poppy seed oil)		475	NA	25.8

[a]*Mallinckrodt, Inc., St. Louis, MO.*
[b]*Winthrop Pharmaceuticals, New York, NY.*
[c]*E. R. Squibb and Sons, Inc., Princeton, NJ.*
[d]*Savage Laboratories, Melville, NY.*

physical properties quite similar to Salpix but appeared to cause an increased level of postprocedure discomfort (8). Work in our laboratory suggested that methylglucamine iothalamate (Conray 60[d]) was a satisfactory agent, demonstrating reduced patient discomfort, easy injection, rapid resorption, and excellent visualization (8). Methylglucamine as the contrast cation is probably superior to the sodium salts of iothalamate or diatrizoate, causing a lesser degree of tissue reaction (9). The nonionic, low osmolar agents have been tested and, although equally satisfactory, seemed to offer no advantages. Furthermore, their significantly higher

cost is a discouraging factor. Currently, the methylglucamine salt of diatrizoate (Hypaque 60[e]) is another widely used and efficacious agent. Table 2.1 reflects many of the agents now available and commonly used for hysterosalpingography.

The optimal contrast agent should be sufficiently viscid to be introduced easily and with control. Rapid resorption is deemed an advantage. The iodine content is the most important factor for optimal visualization of the uterus and tubes. Excessively high iodine concentration may mask small filling defects or irregularities within the uterine cavity.

[d]Mallinckrodt Pharmaceutical, St. Louis, MO.

[e]Renografin-60, E. R. Squibb and Sons, Inc., Princeton, NJ.

Further, the more concentrated agents are probably more irritating to the peritoneal cavity. Concentrations of 280 to 300 mg I/ml seem quite adequate. More dilute contrast agents, on the other hand, make visualization difficult, particularly with regard to the fallopian tubes. The role of viscosity in pain production is uncertain; data in the literature conflict (7, 8). If the amount of contrast agent injected is operator-controlled by fluoroscopic observation, it seems unlikely that viscosity plays a role in pain production. It does seems likely, however, that some of the agents that increase viscosity in some preparations may act as irritants and cause increased pain. The presence of iodipamide in Sinografin may well be a case in point (8).

Oil-Soluble versus Water-Soluble Contrast Media

There are several advocates for the employment of oil-soluble contrast media (OSCM), most notably Ethiodol.[f] These investigators suggest the possibilities of less pain production and the reported incidence of increasing pregnancy rate in the several months following the performance of a hysterosalpingography with OSCM (10, 11). Our experience, as well as that of others, has not substantiated any difference in discomfort levels when methylglucamine salts of iothalamate or diatrizoate are employed (8, 12). The pain experienced during hysterosalpingography is due, in large part, to uterine cramping induced by the distention of the uterine cavity and, to a lesser degree, the application of the cervical tenaculum. Pelvic pain in the hours following hysterosalpingography is probably due to peritoneal reaction. No data are available suggesting that oil-soluble contrast media have any advantage over water-soluble

agents in this regard. Determination of the degree of pain is extremely subjective and difficult to assess. We continue to use the water-soluble agents, believing that there is no significant difference so far as pain production is concerned.

The recent work by Eisenberg et al. (9) has demonstrated delayed development of granulomatous formations on the peritoneal surfaces of guinea pigs following exposure to Ethiodol. Moore et al. have substantiated that this phenomenon occurs in the peritubal surfaces of rabbits following selective introduction of Ethiodol into the fallopian tubes (13). Although these studies employ animal models, it seems reasonable to suggest that this reaction may also occur in humans. There are several anecdotal references in the literature relating the clinical discovery of granulomatous formations containing fat-laden giant cells in patients who had previously undergone hysterosalpingography with oil-soluble agents (14). Although we do not know if these reactions found in our animal model have clinical relevance, we have to question the safety of oil-based contrast agents for use in hysterosalpingography (14).

The oil-soluble agent Lipiodol was in common usage during the 1930s and 1940s. Concern about the risk of oil embolization resulted in the increased use of the water-soluble media. Venous embolization is occasionally seen during hysterosalpingography and, although it is technique dependent, is probably even more frequent than the reported frequency of 6.3% (15). Most episodes of embolization seem to be handled with impunity by the patient with little adverse reaction (10). However, a recent report described the development of coma during hysterosalpingography, presumably the result of cerebral embolization secondary to intravasation of oil-soluble contrast material (16). We currently consider the risk of embolization

[f]Savage Laboratories, Melville, NY.

a distinct disadvantage to the use of OSCM.

Pregnancy Rates following Hysterosalpingography

Weir et al. (17) in 1957 compared the therapeutic effects of a carbon dioxide insufflation procedure (the Rubin test) and oil salpingography in patients with normal tubal patency. There was no difference pre- and postinsufflation in terms of cumulative conception rate, but the postsalpingogram rate of conception approached 30% after three ovulations, and 45% with eight cycles. As early as 1957, an increased incidence of conception occurring for the 4 and perhaps 8 months following procedures to assess tubal pregnancy was appreciated. In 1980, DeCherney and coworkers (18) established that, in the 4 months following hysterosalpingography, 13% of women in whom water-based and 29% of women in whom oil-based contrast agents had been used achieved pregnancy. Schwabe et al. (19) compared the two types of contrast media in women with unexplained infertility and found significantly higher pregnancy rates after hysterosalpingography with oil (77.8%) than with aqueous (10%) contrast medium, results similar to those reported by Cooper et al. (20) using the water-based medium Sinografin. More recently, Rasmussen and coworkers described a 21% pregnancy rate in the 6 months following Lipiodol hysterosalpingography, with almost all conceptions occurring in the first three cycles after the procedure (21). The same authors, in a later paper describing a larger sample and a control population, described confirmatory evidence (22). Acton and coworkers (23), in an extensive study describing results of 3,631 hysterosalpingograms using different contrast media, reported pregnancy rates between 20 and 40%; the therapeutic as well as diagnostic value of hysterosalpingography was discussed, and these authors thought that the use of oil-based contrast material was superior to water-soluble contrast medium.

Studies reporting pregnancy rates following hysterosalpingography obviously cannot be controlled, and this contributes to the controversy. A new line of evidence recently reported presents another mechanism by which hysterosalpingography might indeed improve the chances for fertility. Following up on a report by Boyer et al. (24) that Ethiodol inhibits phagocytosis by pelvic peritoneal macrophages, Goodman and coworkers (25) have recently shown that Ethiodol, Renografin, and methylene blue all inhibit lymphocyte proliferation, suggesting an immunologic mechanism for fertility enhancement. Since the peritoneal fluid of women with endometriosis and unexplained infertility contains increased concentrations of lymphocytes and macrophages, the cytokines generated by these cells could interfere with various reproductive processes (26, 27). Inhibition of lymphocyte proliferation could decrease concentrations of cytokines in the peritoneal environment, providing a mechanism for transiently enhancing fecundity in subfertile women following hysterosalpingography.

The bulk of evidence appears to suggest that pregnancy rates are indeed increased following hysterosalpingography. It is open to question whether or not oil-based contrast media are superior to water-soluble media in this regard and, if so, this must be balanced against the superior tubal mucosal detail and the rapid resorption from the peritoneal cavity provided by the aqueous media. "Therapeutic" hysterosalpingography with oil contrast material, if ever indicated, might be reserved for patients with a diagnosis of unexplained infertility and demonstrated tubal patency. The approach of DeCherney and coworkers (18), using water-soluble contrast medium initially to ascertain tubal normality, followed by sufficient Lipiodol to fill the tubes as a therapeutic measure, appears to be a reasonable compromise under these circumstances, but a well-controlled clinical trial seems to be in order.

Contrast Studies in Contrast Media-Reactive Persons

A history of allergy to iodine, or of a previous reaction to contrast media, is occasionally found in an infertility patient in whom hysterosalpingography is indicated. Since intravascular intravasation is common with hysterosalpingography the procedure cannot be considered risk-free. Appropriate measures should be taken before the procedure to prevent an anaphylactic or other allergic reaction.

Even with a history of reaction to iodinated contrast material, it is impossible to predict an adverse reaction with accuracy. Evidence shows that 75% of patients with past experience of such reactions will tolerate administration of contrast media with impunity (28). Nonetheless, careful consideration of the indications of the procedure should be reviewed before undertaking the administration of any contrast agent.

Accumulating data demonstrate an allergic-like basis for these adverse reactions to contrast media. Demonstration of antibody formation (29) and histamine liberation (30) during such episodes has led to the practice of premedicating with corticosteroids those patients considered at high risk for such a reaction (31). An appropriate regimen uses 150 mg/day of prednisone, or its equivalent, orally, in divided doses, the day preceding and the day of the examination (32). It is prudent to have an intravenous infusion in place and an anesthesiologist available prior to the administration of contrast material. Such precautions can permit perfor-

mance of the hysterosalpingogram with relative safety for the patient. We have, at the time of this writing, not experienced a major reaction to iodinated contrast media in our patient population.

More recent data indicate that the low osmolar (nonionic) group of contrast agents has a reduced incidence of reactions. Certainly, this seems true for the intravenous administration of contrast media (31, 33). Clinical trials (34, 35) show no specific advantages to the use of these agents, but neither can one identify any disadvantages except for the significantly increased cost. It would certainly seem logical to employ such a nonionic agent for any patient presenting with a history of previous adverse reaction to the administration of iodinated contrast material.

THE PROCEDURE OF HYSTEROSALPINGOGRAPHY

Timing of Hysterosalpingography

Hysterosalpingography is performed during the follicular or proliferative part of the cycle, after menstruation has ceased and before ovulation has occurred. This "window" between cycle days 7 and 14 is chosen to avoid potential problems. For example, if hysterosalpingography is performed after ovulation, an early fertilized oocyte might be "blown out" of the tube in a retrograde fashion, leading to the possibility of ectopic gestation. Hysterosalpingography performed late in the secretory phase might dislodge secretory endometrium that is about to break down and desquamate; this could occlude the tubal ostia or may force menstrual blood in retrograde fashion into the peritoneal cavity. This is thought to predispose to the formation of endometriosis and also may activate pelvic infection. Finally, preovulatory hysterosalpingography, when the exposed oocyte is still at a stage relatively insensitive to radiation, is preferable to radiation exposure after ovulation. The final process of oocyte maturation, beginning with the reinitiation of Meiosis I, occurs with the luteinizing hormone surge; hysterosalpingography, with its necessary radiation exposure, should be avoided after ovulation when the oocyte is in a less radiation-resistant condition, particularly since fertilization may have occurred.

It is extremely important that the hysterosalpingographer be knowledgeable in both the technique of the procedure and the history and physical findings of the patient. The examination needs to be tailored to the patient's clinical status. The patient with a history of recurrent early fetal wastage is more likely to have a uterine than a tubal abnormality, so close attention will need to be paid to the appearance of the uterine cavity and internal cervical os. A close working arrangement between the gynecologist and radiologist is needed to ensure optimal patient care and efficient utilization of time. When possible, interpretation of the films is done with both specialists in attendance.

Performing the Procedure

The availability and operability of all necessary equipment should be checked prior to beginning the hysterosalpingogram procedure. The sterile instrument tray should be inspected to ensure that necessary equipment is present and functioning appropriately. The selected cannula should be inspected for patency and filled with contrast material prior to introduction into the vagina to reduce the likelihood of introducing bubbles, a common and annoying radiographic artifact. Stopcocks and valves tend to become stiff with repeated sterilization, so operability should be verified. We have available, for possible use, vascular dilators, glucagon, appropriate small syringes and needles for intravenous administration, carbon dioxide for insufflation, and an alternate type of cannula or catheter.

Knowledge of the internal pelvic anatomy is essential before performance of hysterosalpingography. The position of the uterus, whether anteflexed or retroflexed, should be ascertained, and it is helpful to know whether or not the uterus is mobile. The absence of adnexal masses or cul-de-sac abnormalities should be verified before the procedure is performed.

Following the performance or review of a recent bimanual examination, the patient is placed in some variation of lithotomy position. The "frog leg position," with the buttocks on several folded towels and the heels resting on the table, is convenient, because stirrups are not required and the patient can move easily for oblique or other special views. Knee rests supporting the bent knee or stirrups for the heels may be employed, but depending on the equipment used, these may prevent moving the patient for oblique views. We have found rolled towels under the knees to be helpful.

Once the lithotomy position has been assumed, the perineum is visualized using an operating light, a head lamp, or even a gooseneck lamp. Good lighting is needed to see the cervix and the external cervical os and to identify possible vaginal abnormalities such as in a diethylstilbestrol-exposed patient.

The speculum used for visualization of the cervix may be metal or plastic and must be double-bladed, with or without a side opening. The disadvantage of a double-bladed metal speculum is that the speculum must be disarticulated and removed before the films are taken. The plastic speculum may remain within the vagina during the procedure. However, some patients complain that the plastic vaginal speculum is uncomfortable, and operators unfamiliar with its use may have considerable difficulty removing it from the vagina without causing uncomfortable distention. Some plastic specula have an attached light, of considerable advantage in visualizing the cervix and its environs. A side-opening bivalve speculum, a favorite of some practitioners, may be removed without being disarticulated and can be easily reinserted in the vagina should the need arise.

The cervix must be cleaned with a disinfectant. An iodine solution, not iodine soap, is entirely satisfactory, with one precaution. Excess solution should be removed with a dry swab to eliminate retrograde passage into the uterine cavity and tubes, since iodine may be a sclerosing solution.

If a postcoital test is to be performed in conjunction with the hysterosalpingogram, aspiration of cervical mucus is accomplished after the cervix has been wiped with a dry swab and before disinfectant has been applied. The cervical mucus can be aspirated using a tuberculin syringe (without needle) that can be capped for later examination of the mucus. Performance of this simple procedure before hysterosalpingography permits the two tests to be accomplished on one day, saving time and cost for patient and physician.

There is considerable debate as to whether the topical or intrauterine administration of analgesics decreases patient discomfort. We routinely use Hurricaine,[g] a 20% benzocaine spray, on the anterior lip of the cervix before applying the tenaculum, but there are no data to suggest its benefit. A recent study comparing the efficacy of cervically applied 20% benzocaine gel with intrauterine 1% or 2% lidocaine concluded that employment of analgesics compared to placebo did decrease discomfort (36). The recommended regimen is the application of 20% benzocaine gel at the start of the

[g]Bentlich Pharmaceuticals, Niles, IL.

procedure, with naproxen sodium 550 mg given orally 2 hours before.

Following cervical visualization, mucus aspiration, disinfectant preparation of the cervix, and perhaps application of a topical analgesic, the method for instillation of contrast medium is applied. If the Kidde cannula with the flexible polyethylene tip is used, a tenaculum must be placed on the anterior cervical lip. The single-tooth tenaculum is convenient, causes minimal spotting and bleeding when removed, and is associated with only a minor cramp with application. A sufficient "bite" of anterior cervical lip is essential, because a single-tooth tenaculum may tear through cervical tissue if a great deal of traction is applied. A relatively large piece of anterior lip is grasped with a single-tooth tenaculum; if less of a bite is necessary, a double or triple tenaculum is used, but bleeding and discomfort are likely to be enhanced. The Kidde cannula, which has already been filled with contrast medium and has the syringe attached, is introduced into the external os. The cannula is locked in place, the speculum is removed as necessary, and the patient is positioned for fluoroscopic observation.

We often bring the husband into the room at this time to provide support for his wife and to observe the remainder of the procedure if the couple so desires. A TV monitor is positioned so that all can view the contrast material as it outlines the uterine cavity and fallopian tubes.

Under fluoroscopic monitoring, the contrast agent is injected slowly and with even pressure. Some traction exerted by the tenaculum will deflex the uterus and may permit easier filling and improved visualization. The contrast material flows through the endocervical canal and fills the uterine cavity. About 1 to 1.5 ml of contrast medium may be introduced into the uterine cavity before significant cramping occurs. The operator may take the first radiograph at this time to record any intrauterine pathology, because the contrast medium fills this small (potential) space rapidly. The operator next watches the contrast agent begin to fill the fallopian tubes. Abnormalities are noted, and the first interval film is taken when either the first abnormality is observed or the contrast agent begins to spill from the fimbriated ends of the tubes. Excessive contrast will obscure the internal architecture of the uterine cavity and will not allow optimal delineation of tubes. We strive to reduce the total number of films taken and to perform the procedure rapidly to lessen the total radiation exposure to the patient and personnel. Once fallopian tube filling has been accomplished, it is valuable to move the uterus using the combined tenaculum and cannula. This allows evaluation of tubal mobility and may cause the fimbriated parts of the tubes to move away from the pelvic sidewall. Carbon dioxide may be introduced after the contrast material has been used. This is primarily of value when tubal patency is in doubt. Occasionally, excessive spill of contrast material from one tube may make it difficult to determine if the contralateral tube is patent. Seeing the progress of carbon dioxide passing through the tubes may resolve this question. The carbon dioxide may, on rare occasions, also enhance visualization of intrauterine abnormalities. This technique does introduce gas into the peritoneal cavity, so when the patient sits up, it may be associated with an increase in pain perceived to be in the shoulder, the result of irritation of the diaphragm by the intraperitoneal gas. Absorption of carbon dioxide occurs relatively rapidly, so the shoulder pain is self-limited and ordinarily disappears within a few hours. We have not observed significant discomfort with this addition, and occasionally find it of great diagnostic value.

When abnormalities are encountered, modifications of the technique may allow further delineation of the per-ceived abnormality. For example, the finding of intrauterine filling defects or possible synechiae may necessitate turning the patient, introducing carbon dioxide, or changing some aspect of the technique to allow a better view of the area in question. The same applies to delineating tubal abnormalities, and it may be necessary to use oblique films. The simple trick of asking the patient to cough may help disperse contrast material. Occasionally, elevating the hips or briefly assuming a sitting position may help. Flexibility of technique is useful, which is why we do not use knee rests or stirrups. Significant stenosis of the external cervical os, the so-called "pinpoint os," may impede the introduction of the cannula, tempting the use of undue pressure to force the cannula into the canal. Dilatation may be appropriate under these circumstances. We have been successful with a simple 7 or 8F angiographic dilator for both dilatation and, at times, injection of the contrast agent (Fig. 2.12); this may be adequate without the use of any other device.

Delayed films may add additional information but should not be routine. Dispersion of loculated contrast material may be identified, which indicates tubal patency that may not have been documented earlier. Uni- or bilateral tubal occlusion should almost always suggest the need for a delayed film. Cornual occlusion presents an interesting challenge. Because of the muscular arrangement in the uterine cornua, uterine contraction can result in occlusion of the tube. Although this is spasm of uterine musculature and not of the tube, it may prevent the passage of contrast material into the salpinx and give the impression of an anatomic occlusion. Before making the diagnosis of cornual occlusion, an attempt should be made to relax the spasm. The general anesthetic halothane can efficiently relax uterine musculature, but it is not usually available in the setting de-

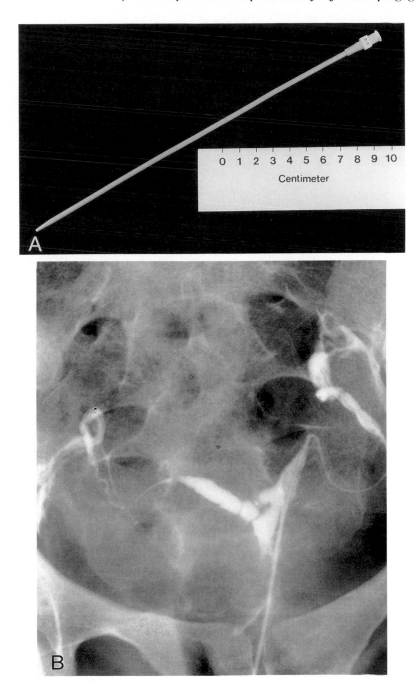

Figure 2.12. **A,** 7F Vascular dilator. **B,** Vascular dilator as cannula in patients with cervical stenosis.

sired. A number of drugs have been employed for this purpose, including atropine, nitroglycerin, various analgesics and narcotics, tranquilizers, and isoxsuprine; glucagon appears to be the most promising drug available. Glucagon has been found to be a moderately efficient agent in inducing relaxation of tubal spasm (Fig. 2.13). This straight-chain polypeptide is produced normally in the

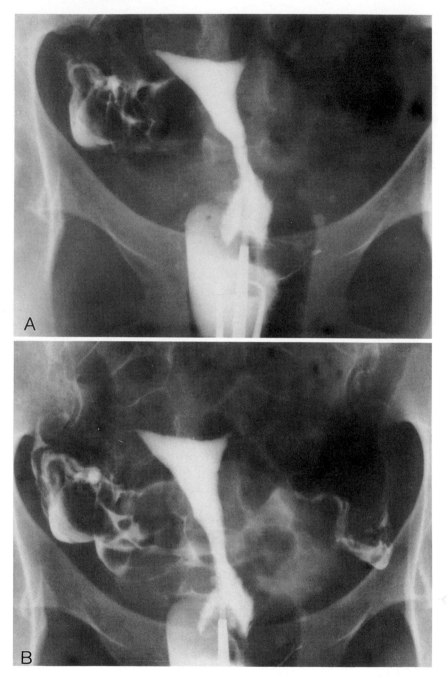

Figure 2.13. **A,** Cornual occlusion (*left*) secondary to spasm. **B,** Same examination as in **A.** Several seconds following the intravenous injection of glucagon, there is ready filling of the left fallopian tube.

pancreas, and, when intravenously administered, causes an increase in blood glucose and a relaxation of smooth muscle. One-fourth of the patients presenting with cornual occlusion were demon-strated to have patent, normally filled fallopian tubes after the intravenous administration of 1 mg of glucagon (37). Selective tubal catheterization (see Chapter 10) should resolve this issue if these simpler techniques are not successful in demonstrating a patent oviduct.

Catheter Method for Hysterosalpingography

Many operators employ a Foley catheter for hysterosalpingography, a technique that often eliminates the need for use of the tenaculum and thus avoids some associated discomfort. At the same time, it allows more maneuverability by the patient. The patient and tray setup are prepared as previously outlined. A sterile 8 or 10 French catheter is introduced into the uterine cavity with the aid of dressing forceps. If there is an element of stenosis in the cervical canal, introduction may require previous dilatation. The design of the conventional Foley catheter has been modified, with several models currently available. These catheters,[h] designed specifically for hysterosalpingog-

[h]Ackrad catheter, Ackrad Laboratories, Garwood, NJ; Sholkoff catheter, Cook Ob/Gyn, Spencer, IN.

raphy, have an increased rigidity, which permits more ready introduction of the catheter into the uterine cavity, and yet are sufficiently flexible to maintain a high level of safety and follow the flexed configuration of the uterus (see Fig. 2.2). Following distention of the balloon, which is located near the tip of the catheter, radiographic contrast material is injected. The vaginal speculum may be then removed. Turning the patient in a prone position has been advocated as a method to permit easier filling of the uterus and fallopian tubes by taking advantage of fundic and tubal dependency in this position if the uterus is anteflexed (38). Similarly, the supine position should be ideal for a woman with a retroflexed uterus. Again, the examination should be performed under fluoroscopic control and appropriate interval images obtained. Following the procedure, the balloon is deflated and the catheter removed.

The failure to visualize the endocervical canal and the lower uterine segment (Fig. 2.14) is one of the disadvantages of

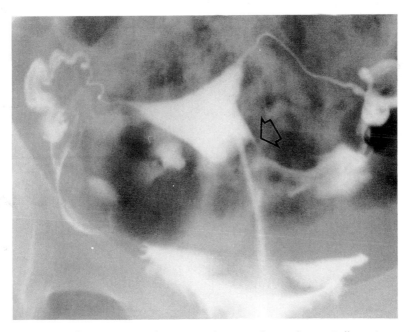

Figure 2.14. Hysterosalpingogram utilizing a pediatric Foley catheter. Balloon (*arrow*) occludes lower portion of the endometrial cavity and prevents any filling of the endocervical canal.

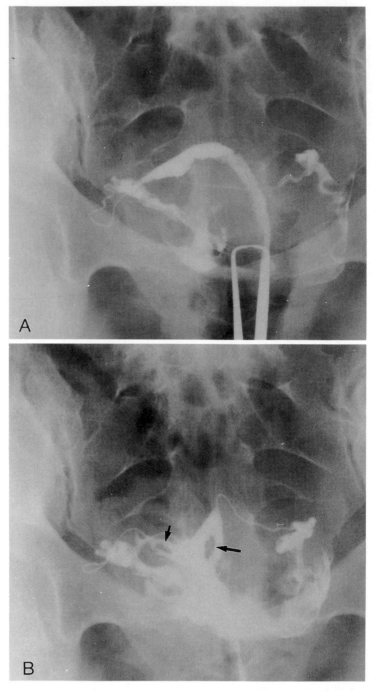

Figure 2.15. **A,** Filling of the endometrial cavity utilizing a Kidde cannula. Marked uterine flexion limits the ability to adequately visualize the uterine cavity. **B,** Same examination as in **A.** Traction applied via the tenaculum straightened the uterine cavity, permitting better visualization and allowing demonstration of two uterine synechiae (*arrows*).

the Foley catheter technique. A second disadvantage is the inability to move the uterus in the absence of a tenaculum. Traction applied during filling of the uterus straightens both the uterus and the endocervical canal and may improve visualization of the uterine cavity. This maneuver is usually not possible with the catheter technique because traction invariably pulls the Foley bulb down the canal, with considerable discomfort for the patient, or totally dislodges the catheter. Filling defects are more readily detected when using the cannula technique and traction, and one can often avoid the need for extraneous oblique radiographic projections, thus reducing radiation exposure (Fig. 2.15). Pushing the uterus up and then exerting traction may allow assessment of tubal mobility and the ability of the fimbria to move away from the pelvic side wall.

COMPLICATIONS OF HYSTEROSALPINGOGRAPHY

Some discomfort with hysterosalpingography is unavoidable. Use of a tenaculum adds one additional cramp when the tenaculum is placed on the anterior lip of the cervix. Introduction of anything into the uterine cavity causes uterine contraction and discomfort. The passage of contrast medium through the fallopian tube may be associated with some pain, which is maximized by any distention of the tube due to distal obstruction.

Mechanical complications of hysterosalpingography include uterine perforation or tubal rupture, both of which are very rare. Uterine perforation is unlikely to occur with the use of a polyethylene acorn with a flexible tip, but has been reported with metal instruments, particularly those of the Jarcho type. This cannula has a metal end with a rubber acorn fitted over the end and held in place with an adjustable-screw band. If the screw is loosened, the band could be dislodged,

allowing the metal cannula to slip farther through the rubber tip and extend into the uterine cavity. If this happened suddenly and with force, perforation could occur (see Fig. 2.5).

Traumatic elevation of the endometrium by the cannula insertion may occur, usually without significant consequence (Figs. 2.16 and 2.17).

Overdistention of a hydrosalpinx can cause tubal rupture and is accompanied by significant pain. A closed hydrosalpinx, opened by distention in this manner, can result in activation of pelvic inflammatory disease; we routinely provide antibiotic coverage in the presence of recognized tubal pathology (see Chapter 8).

Complications of hemorrhage and shock are uncommonly encountered; no large vessels are likely to be encountered. Tearing of cervical tissue with the tenaculum is unlikely to result in hemorrhage, although the friable diethylstilbestrol-exposed cervix may bleed freely. Anaphylactic shock has rarely been reported; the performance of hysterosalpingography in patients thought to be allergic to iodine-containing contrast media or to other agents used in the procedure is discussed earlier in this chapter.

Lymphatic or venous intravasation of either water-soluble or oil-based contrast medium is a dramatic event. Lymphatic intravasation with water-based contrast material results in a reticular pattern of small vessels in the broad ligament. With venous intravasation, the medium passes quickly through the uterine or ovarian veins to the lungs, delineating clearly the vascular architecture. If water-soluble contrast medium has been used, the medium is quickly dissipated, and no embolic symptoms or side effects have been reported (39). On the other hand, if embolization occurs with an oil-soluble contrast medium, the result may be detrimental to the patient. Intravasation has been reported to occur in be-

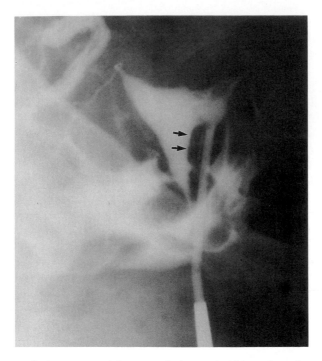

Figure 2.16.   Subintimal placement of the cannula (*arrows*). Although such occurrence is unusual and generally without incident, significant bleeding may ensue.

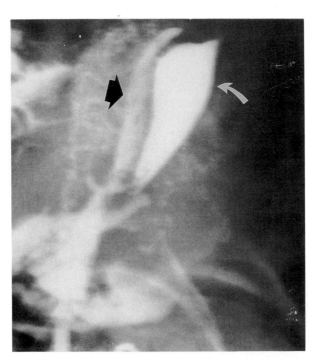

Figure 2.17.   Intramural placement of cannula has resulted in false passage and a second collection of contrast material (*black arrow*) posterior to the true uterine cavity (*white arrow*).

tween 0 and 6.3% of patients, and certain predisposing conditions may allow this to happen with increased likelihood. These include tubal disease or obstruction, recent uterine surgery, uterine malformation, synechiae, malplacement of the hysterosalpingogram cannula, and excessive injection pressure or quantity of the contrast medium. Most oil emboli are innocuous (40). However, there have been five deaths attributed to emboli after hysterosalpingography, four of which were with oil-based media (10). Two of these deaths followed major operations performed after the hysterosalpingogram, and the radiographic procedure may have only been contributory. The fifth embolus-related death was in 1959, and occurred after the use of a water-soluble contrast medium containing carboxymethylcellulose. The recent report of coma due to cerebral embolus following use of oil-soluble contrast material has already been noted (16). Six other deaths found in the world literature and attributed to hysterosalpingography have all been related to infection.

Intrauterine pregnancy, when recognized, is another major contraindication. Careful scheduling prior to the anticipated date of ovulation generally avoids this possibility. It is also helpful to verify the date of the last menstrual period and the cycle day with the patient, to look at her temperature chart to verify a low temperature, and to pay attention to the appearance of the cervical mucus. Hysterosalpingography has been performed inadvertently in the presence of an intrauterine pregnancy, but the occurrence is highly unlikely. Nonetheless, Wilson et al. (41) performed hysterosalpingograms during infertility investigations in 10 women who had apparently conceived, finding intrauterine filling defects in two; normal term infants were delivered in all 10. The concerns in the event of such an occurrence include disruption of the pregnancy, displacement

of the fertilized ovum into the peritoneal cavity, and the mutative effect of the radiation on the developing fetus.

Genetic hazards associated with hysterosalpingography are related to the irradiation encountered. The amount of ovarian radiation from a hysterosalpingogram depends on the technical equipment, the number of films obtained, the duration of fluoroscopy, the distance from the tube to the film, and the size of the patient. Using a two-film technique without fluoroscopy, Shirley (42) found that a posterior fornix dosimeter recorded a mean of 129 mrad, which increased to 1053 mrad when fluoroscopy was used. Using a different technique, Sheikh and Yussman (43) found the gonadal radiation dose to be between 75 and 550 mrad, depending almost solely on the duration of fluoroscopic time. No deleterious fetal effects from low doses of radiation received in pregnancy have been proven by epidemiologic investigations. Goldenberg and coworkers (44) evaluated the health of the infants of 26 women who had undergone hysterosalpingography during the cycle of conception; these children were all healthy and free of any congenital defects.

Another potential disadvantage of hysterosalpingography is the possibility of postprocedure infection. Reports suggest that the incidence of pelvic inflammatory disease following hysterosalpingography may be anywhere from 0.5 to 6%, depending on the technique, population base, and criteria of diagnosis. It is likely that these infectious episodes are usually due to the reactivation of pre-existing disease rather than a de novo infection, and they are more frequently seen in patients demonstrating underlying abnormal tubal inflammatory disease. When such an appearance is encountered, prophylactic antibiotic administration is appropriate (see Chapter 8). The utility of seeking serologic evidence of *Chlamydia trachomatis* infection before hysterosalpingography was tested in 118 infertile women (45). A positive correlation was found between occlusive tubal damage and serum antibodies. Suspected sepsis occurred post-hysterosalpingography in five women (4%), two of whom did not have antibodies; however, all had evidence of tubal damage, suggesting that the risk of infection is confined to women with existing tubal damage and is not predicted by serologic testing. The presence of active pelvic infection is an absolute contraindication to hysterosalpingography; peritonitis following hysterosalpingography was reported to be responsible for six of the 11 deaths in the world literature (46, 47).

ALTERNATIVE IMAGING TECHNIQUES

Alternative imaging techniques to assess tubal patency exist and may, under certain circumstances, be valuable. Richman and others (48, 49) have described sonographic techniques to observe the passage of fluid through intact fallopian tubes. Such a procedure does avoid exposure to ionizing radiation but gives no information regarding tubal anatomy or caliber. Furthermore, its accuracy in a large series is not established.

Several investigators have advocated employment of radionuclide hysterosalpingography to assess tubal patency (50–52). The technique consists of the introduction of technetium-99m–labeled microspheres at the external cervical os and subsequent detection of the tracer within the peritoneal cavity. Reported findings correlative with conventional hysterosalpingography vary widely from 49 to 80% (53). The radiation received by the ovaries is of concern. One author suggested ovarian exposure levels approximately 25 times greater than hysterosalpingography (52). Other calculations are less ominous (51), but it is clear

that the examination is not radiation-sparing. Further, the study gives no information regarding the anatomic configuration of the fallopian tubes or uterine cavity. Radionuclide hysterosalpingography has the potential to add to our knowledge of tubal physiology and may be of value in those rare instances where injection of iodinated contrast material is inappropriate, but it is clearly not an innocuous technique.

The development of magnetic resonance imaging (MRI) has expanded our abilities to visualize the uterus and adnexa. This modality, while avoiding ionizing radiation, consistently demonstrates uterine anatomy with tissue characterization not offered by other techniques. It permits recognition of many congenital anomalies and identifies and characterizes filling defects and mucosal irregularities (54). MRI currently has no role in the assessment of fallopian tube patency, and its relatively high expense must be considered a disadvantage. Nonetheless, this study may, on occasion, well serve the infertile patient.

REFERENCES

1. Haines CJ, O'Shea RT: Unilateral gamete intrafallopian transfer: The preferred method? *Fertil Steril* 51:518, 1989.
2. Owens OM, Schiff I, Kaul AF, Cramer DC, Burt RAP: Reduction of pain following hysterosalpingogram by prior analgesic administration. *Fertil Steril* 43:146, 1985.
3. Karasick S, Goldfarb AF: Peritubal adhesions in infertile women: Diagnosis with hysterosalpingography. *AJR* 152:777, 1989.
4. Cohen BM, Katz M: The significance of the convoluted oviduct in the infertile woman. *J Reprod Med* 21:31, 1978.
5. Rindfleisch W: Darstellung des Cavum uteri. *Klin Wochenschr* 17:780, 1910.
6. Palmer A: Ethiodol hysterosalpingography for the treatment of infertility. *Fertil Steril* 11:311, 1960.
7. Ekelund L, Karp W: Comparison between two radiographic contrast media for hysterosalpingography. *Acta Obstet Gynecol Scand* 60:393, 1981.

8. Winfield AC, Henderson-Slayden R, Wentr AC, Harding DR: Hysterosalpingography: Comparison of Conray 60 and Sinografin. *AJR* 138:599, 1982.

9. Eisenberg AD, Winfield AC, Page DL, Holburn GE, Schifter T, Segars JH: Peritoneal reaction resulting from iodinated contrast material: Comparative study. *Radiology* 172:149, 1989.

10. Soules MR, Spadoni LR: Oil versus aqueous media for hysterosalpingography: A continuing debate based on many opinions and few facts. *Fertil Steril* 38:1, 1982.

11. Karasick S: Oil-soluble contrast material for hysterosalpingography. *Radiology Reports* 2:205, 1990.

12. Alper MM, Garner PR, Spence JEH, Quarrington AM: Pregnancy rates after hysterosalpingography with oil and water-soluble contrast media. *Obstet Gynecol* 68:6, 1986.

13. Moore DE, Segars JH Jr, Winfield AC, Page DL, Eisenberg AD, Holburn GE: Effects of contrast agents on the fallopian tube in a rabbit model. *Radiology* 176:721, 1990.

14. Winfield AC. Water-soluble contrast material for hysterosalpingography. *Radiology Reports* 2:205, 1990.

15. Noris S: The hysterogram in the study of sterility. *Can Med Assoc J* 75:1016, 1956.

16. Dan U, Ezra D, Oelsner G, Menczer J, Gruberg L: Cerebral embolization and coma after hysterosalpingography with oil-soluble contrast medium. *Fertil Steril* 53:939, 1990.

17. Weir WC, Weir DR, Littell AS: A statistical comparison of the therapeutic value of carbon dioxide insufflation versus oil salpingography. *Am J Obstet Gynecol* 73:412, 1957.

18. DeCherney AH, Kort H, Barney JB, DeVore GR: Increased pregnancy rate with oil-soluble hysterosalpingography dye. *Fertil Steril* 33:407, 1980.

19. Schwabe MG, Shapiro SS, Haning RV Jr: Hysterosalpingography with oil contrast medium enhances fertility in patients with infertility of unknown etiology. *Fertil Steril* 40:604, 1983.

20. Cooper RA, Jabamoni R, Pieters CH: Fertility rate after hysterosalpingography with Sinografin. *AJR* 141:105, 1983.

21. Rasmussen F, Justesen P, Nielsen DT: Therapeutic value of hysterosalpingography with lipiodol ultra fluid. *Acta Radiologica* 28:3, 1987.

22. Rasmussen F, Lindequist S, Larsen C, et al: Therapeutic effect of hysterosalpingography: Oil- versus water-soluble contrast media—a randomized prospective study. *Radiology* 179:75, 1991.

23. Acton CM, Devitt JM, Ryan EA: Hysterosalpingography in infertility—An experience of 3,631 examinations. *NZ J Obstet Gynaecol* 28:127, 1988.

24. Boyer P, Territo MC, de Ziegler D, Meldrum D: Ethiodol inhibits phagocytosis by pelvic peritoneal macrophages. *Fertil Steril* 46:4, 1986.

25. Goodman SB, Rein MS, Hill JA: Ethiodol (E), Regnografin (R) and methylene blue (MB) inhibit lymphocyte proliferation: A potential mechanism for fertility enhancement in subfertile women following hysterosalpingography (HSG) and laparoscopic tubal lavage (TL). Presented at the annual meeting of the American Fertility Society, October 15–18, 1990, Washington, DC.

26. Hill JA, Faris, HM, Schiff I, Anderson DJ: Characterization of leukocyte subpopulation in the peritoneal fluid of women with endometriosis. *Fertil Steril* 50:216, 1988.

27. Hill JA, Anderson DJ: Immunological mechanisms of female infertility. *Baillieres Clin Immunol Allerg* 2:551, 1988.

28. Shehadi WH: Clinical problems and toxicity of contrast agents. *AJR* 97:762, 1966.

29. Brasch RC: Allergic reactions to contrast media: Accumulated evidence. *AJR* 134:797, 1980.

30. Lasser EC, Walters AJ, Lang JH: An experimental basis for histamine release in contrast material reactions. *Radiology* 110:49, 1974.

31. Lasser EC, Berry CC, Talner LB, et al: Pretreatment with corticosteroids to alleviate reactions to intravenous contrast material. *N Engl J Med* 317:845, 1987.

32. Zweiman B, Mishkin MM, Hildreth EA: An approach to the performance of contrast studies in contrast material-reactive persons. *Ann Intern Med* 83:159, 1975.

33. Katayama H: Report of the Japanese Committee on the Safety of Contrast Media. Presented at the 74th Annual Meeting of the Radiological Society of North America, Chicago, IL, November 1988.

34. Winfield AC, Maxson WS, Harding DR, et al: Hexabrix as a contrast agent for hysterosalpingography. *Radiology* 152:232, 1984.

35. Stiris G, Andrew E: Hysterosalpingogra-

phy with Amipaque. *Radiology* 130:795, 1979.

36. Lorino CO, Prough SG, Aksel S, et al: Pain relief in hysterosalpingography: A comparison of analgesics. *J Reprod Med* 35:533, 1990.
37. Winfield AC, Pittaway D, Maxson W, Daniell J, Wentz AC: Apparent cornual occlusion in hysterosalpingography: Reversal by glucagon. *AJR* 139:529, 1982.
38. Spring DB, Wilson RE, Arronet GH: Foley catheter hysterosalpingography: A simplified technique for investigating infertility. *Radiology* 131:543, 1979.
39. Schuitemaker NWE, Helmerhorst FM, Tjon A, et al: Late anaphylactic shock after hysterosalpingography. *Fertil Steril* 54:535, 1990.
40. Bateman BC, Nunley WC, Kitchin JD: Intravasation during hysterosalpingography using oil-base contrast media. *Fertil Steril* 34:439, 1980.
41. Wilson RV, Lee RA, Jensen PA: Inadvertent infertility investigations in pregnant women. *Fertil Steril* 17:126, 1966.
42. Shirley RL: Ovarian radiation dosage during hysterosalpingography. *Fertil Steril* 22:83, 1971.
43. Sheikh HH, Yussman MA: Radiation exposure of ovaries during hysterosalpingography. *Am J Obstet Gynecol* 124:307, 1976.
44. Goldenberg RL, White R, Magendantz HG: Pregnancy during the hysterogram cycle. *Fertil Steril* 27:1274, 1976.
45. Forsey JP, Caul EO, Paul ID, et al: *Chlamydia trachomatis*, tubal disease and the incidence of symptomatic and asymptomatic infection following hysterosalpingography. *Hum Reprod* 5:444, 1990.
46. Siegler AM: Dangers of hysterosalpingography. *Obstet Gynecol Surv* 22:284, 1967.
47. Bang J: Complications of hysterosalpingography. *Acta Obstet Gynecol Scand* 29:383, 1950.
48. Richman TS, Visconi GN, de Cherney A, et al: Fallopian tube patency assessed by ultrasound following fluid injection. *Radiology* 152:507, 1984.
49. Rasmussen F, Larsen C, Justesen P. Fallopian tube patency demonstrated at ultrasonography. *Acta Radiologica* 27:61, 1986.
50. McCalley MG, Braunstein P, Stone S, et al: Radionuclide hysterosalpingography for evaluation of fallopian tube patency. *J Nucl Med* 26:868, 1985.
51. Angtuaco TL, Boyd CM, London SN: Technetium 99-m hysterosalpingography in infertility: An accurate alternative to contrast hysterosalpingography. *Radiographics* 9:115, 1989.
52. Brundin J, Dahlborn M, Ahlberg-Ahre E, et al: Radionuclide hysterosalpingography for measurement of human oviductal function. *Int J Gynaecol Obstet* 28:53, 1989.
53. van der Weiden RMF, van Zijl J: Radiation exposure of the ovaries during hysterosalpingography. Is radionuclide hysterosalpingography justified? *Br J Obstet Gynaecol* 96:471, 1989.
54. McCarthy S: MR imaging of the uterus. *Radiology* 171:321, 1989.

3

The Normal Hysterosalpingogram

The uterus is a thick-walled, muscular organ, lying totally within the true pelvis and measuring approximately 7 × 4 × 2.5 cm in its nongravid state (Fig. 3.1). The cavity of the uterus is quite small in comparison to the overall size of the organ, primarily because of the thickness of the myometrium. In its empty state, the uterine cavity is only a potential space with anterior and posterior walls in apposition, but it is distended by the introduction of 2.0 to 3.0 ml of contrast material to create the radiographic appearance seen on a hysterosalpingogram (Fig. 3.2).

The uterine cavity can be conveniently divided into two regions. The inferior portion, the endocervical canal, extends from the cervix to the internal cervical os. The uterine body comprises the remainder of the cavity and is superior to the internal cervical os. The fundus represents the portion of the uterus above the level of the ostia of the fallopian tubes. In the adult woman of reproductive age, the uterine body is longer than the endocervical canal, while the converse is true in the child. However, radiographic measurements of the two regions are inaccurate and may vary considerably with the degree of traction used during the examination (Fig. 3.3). If one uses an elongated cannula with its tip in the uterine cavity, or the Foley catheter technique with the balloon of the catheter in the uterine cavity, the endocervical canal may not be outlined with contrast in its entirety. For these reasons, measurements of the various components of the uterus and ratio calculations of uterine body to cervix are usually not of great diagnostic value.

THE ENDOCERVICAL CANAL

The configuration of the endocervical canal, if visualized, is quite variable and strikingly different from the uterine cavity. Numerous mucosal folds, the plicae palmatae or arbor vitae, give an interdigitated frond-like appearance to the canal (Fig. 3.4). This appearance, most striking in the nulliparous uterus, is seen less commonly in multiparous women. The diameter of the endocervical canal varies considerably from patient to patient, and at times the canal may appear significantly dilated in the normal uterus (Fig. 3.5).

The course and direction of the endocervical canal are occasionally distorted and angulated and may in fact create technical problems in the introduction of a cannula because of this irregularity. Flexible tips such as the Kidde cannula are of value in this regard and are introduced more easily if significant traction is applied to the cervix. A shortened cannula may be helpful.

Dilated cervical glands may appear as diverticula-like projections of contrast in the endocervical canal (Fig. 3.6). Mesonephric remnants may produce linear filling defects that may be mistaken for endocervical synechiae or scarring (see Chapter 4). A well-defined and solitary diverticular projection in the lower uterine segment is frequently seen in patients having undergone previous lower-segment cesarean section (Fig. 3.7). Mobile filling defects, artifactual in origin, due to either the introduction of air or the displacement of cervical mucus, are occasionally seen (Fig. 3.8).

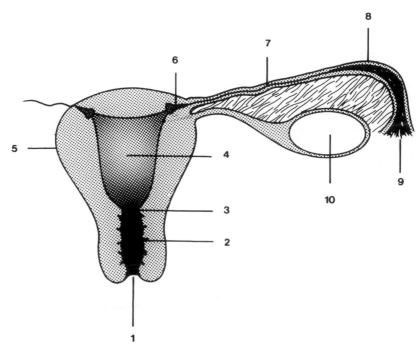

Figure 3.1. Normal uterus: *1*, external cervical os; *2*, cervical canal; *3*, internal cervical os; *4*, uterine cavity; *5*, myometrium; *6*, fallopian tube: interstitial segment; *7*, fallopian tube: isthmus; *8*, fallopian tube: ampulla; *9*, fimbria; *10*, ovary.

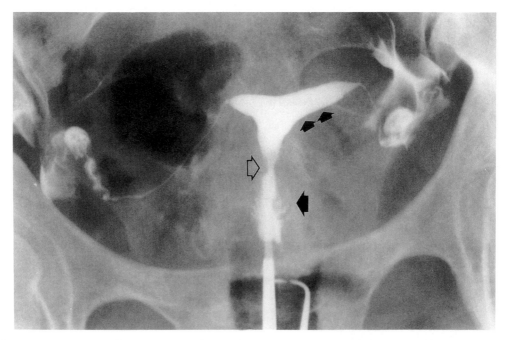

Figure 3.2. Hysterosalpingography of normal uterus. The internal cervical os (*open arrow*) is well defined. The cervical canal (*single arrow*) demonstrates coarse plicae palmatae. The uterine cavity (*double arrow*) is characterized by a relatively smooth contour.

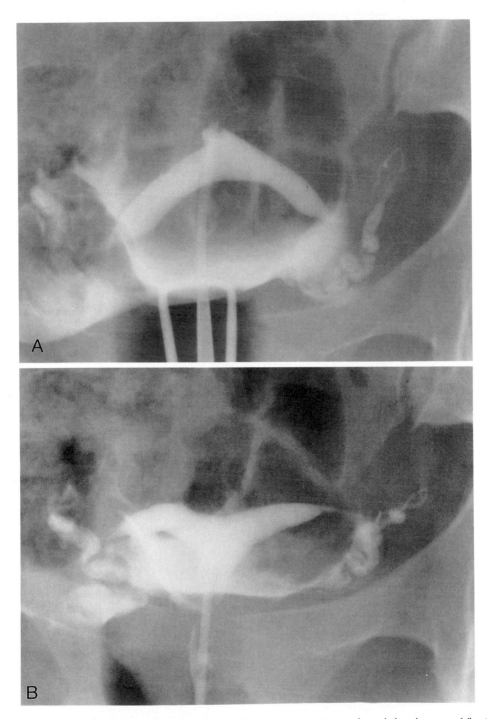

Figure 3.3. **A,** Markedly retroflexed uterus. **B,** Increasing traction reduced the degree of flexion, resulting in a differing appearance of the relationship of the uterine body and endocervical canal.

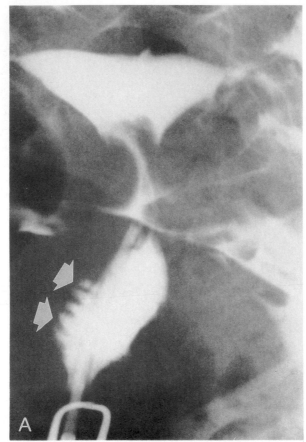

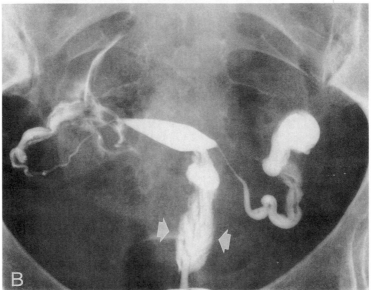

Figure 3.4. **A,** Prominent spiculated plicae palmatae are demonstrated in the cervical canal (*arrows*). Note the asymmetry. **B,** Plicae palmatae having a different pattern. A fine, fern-like, interdigitated mucosal pattern is noted throughout the cervical canal (*arrows*).

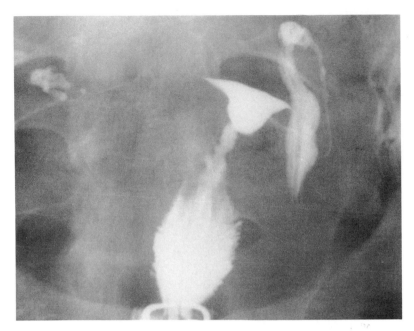

Figure 3.5. Normal uterus. Note the markedly increased diameter of the endocervical canal, a normal variant. The cervical canal is longer than the uterine body in this nulliparous patient.

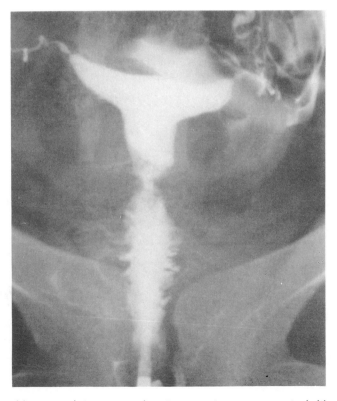

Figure 3.6. Normal hysterosalpingogram showing prominent symmetrical dilated glands in cervical canal.

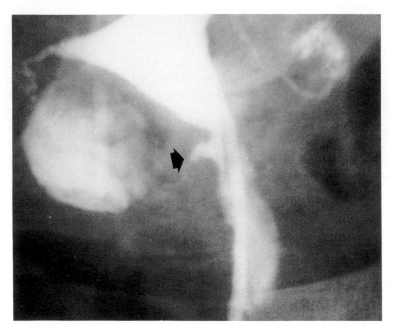

Figure 3.7. Typical pseudodiverticulum projecting from the lower uterine segment (*arrow*) in this patient with a history of previous delivery by cesarean section.

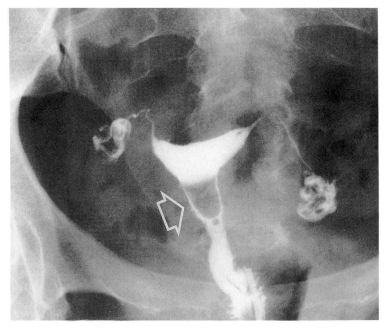

Figure 3.8. Large radiolucent filling defect (*open arrow*) caused by an air bubble introduced into the uterine cavity during hysterosalpingography.

THE INTERNAL CERVICAL OS

The region of the internal cervical os is also quite variable in its appearance. Some patients demonstrate a well-defined, markedly narrow internal os (Fig. 3.9). Others show virtually no definition of the internal os, having a gradual, funnel-shaped uterine cavity contour, which makes it impossible to identify the internal os with certainty (Fig. 3.10). Some authors have speculated that widening of the region of the os in this manner may be correlated with the clinical syndrome of "incompetent cervical os," which is responsible for recurrent second-trimester fetal wastage. In a patient who has had second-trimester fetal loss with a painless labor, this finding may be confirmatory of an incompetent os (Fig. 3.11). In a patient with primary infertility, this finding is not an indication for cerclage and has not been shown to be predictive of fetal wastage.

The diameter of the internal os may vary in the same patient during different phases of the menstrual cycle. The internal os is most narrow in the postovulatory

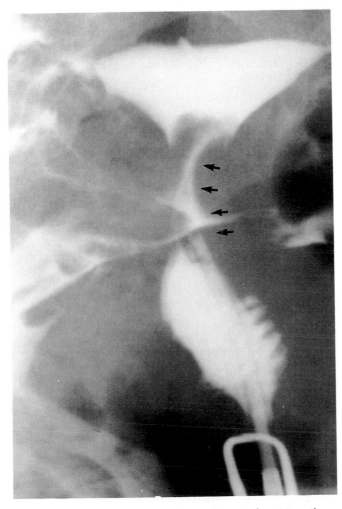

Figure 3.9. Normal variation in the region of the internal cervical os. Note the well-defined, elongated, narrow segment (*arrows*).

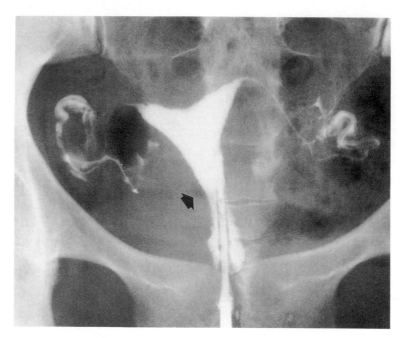

Figure 3.10.   At times the internal cervical os cannot be defined. Note the funnel-shaped transition between the uterine body and the cervical canal (*arrow*).

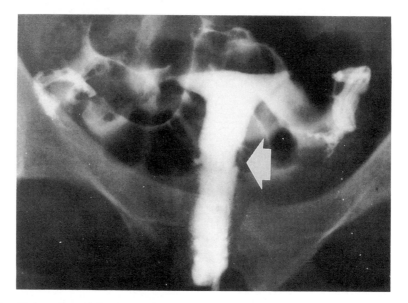

Figure 3.11.   The region of the internal os is inordinately wide (*arrow*). The significance of this is uncertain. Some speculate a relationship to the clinical syndrome of "incompetent cervical os."

phase of the cycle and achieves its maximal width during menses and the follicular phase. The apparent length of the region of the internal os can also change during the course of a single hysterosal-pingographic procedure (Fig. 3.12). This may be a reflection of asymmetric contraction of the myometrium or of variations in the degree of distension of the cavity as the quantity of injected contrast

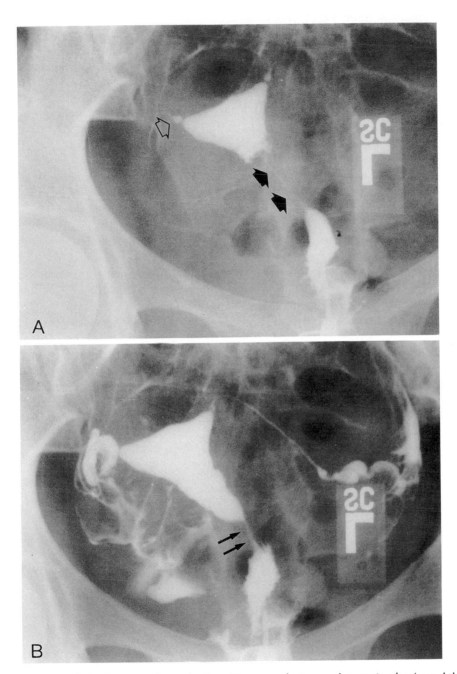

Figure 3.12. **A,** Early in the procedure, the transition zone between the uterine body and the cervical canal is markedly elongated and quite narrow (*arrows*). Note also the normal, very well defined tubal bulge at the interstitial segment of the fallopian tube (*open arrow*). **B,** With increasing amounts of contrast material, the transition zone changes contour considerably and is much shorter and slightly wider (*arrows*).

medium changes. Such alterations in appearance are unrelated to identifiable pathology and seem to have no corollary at hysteroscopic examination.

THE UTERINE CAVITY

The size and shape of the uterine body are quite variable. The alignment of the uterus, the traction applied during the procedure, the degree of flexion, and the position of the patient at the time of radiographic exposure may all alter the appearance of the shape of the uterine cavity. Such changes in the appearance are dependent on the incident angle of the radiographic beam in reference to the alignment of the uterus.

Minimal variations of the normal radiographic appearance of the uterine cavity are frequently encountered. The abnormal configuration seen in patients with maternal diethylstilbestrol (DES) exposure demonstrates a T-shaped uterine cavity with a narrowed lower uterine segment and endocervical canal and may

be confusing (see Chapter 5). The configuration of the fundus may be convex, straight, or concave, and is more fully discussed in Chapter 4 under müllerian fusion disorders (Fig. 3.13). The radiographic appearance of the contour of the fundus may appear to change with varying degrees of traction, depending on the portion of the uterine surface tangential to the x-ray beam. These relatively minimal alterations in the contour of the fundus have been postulated to play a role in infertility and fetal wastage, and their proper identity and interpretation may be clinically significant.

The appearance of the walls of the uterine cavity margin is dependent on the phase of the menstrual cycle at the time of the examination. Hysterosalpingography is optimally performed during the preovulatory phase of the menstrual cycle, when the endometrium is thickened and relatively smooth. Such timing is optimal and avoids performance of the examination after ovulation, when conception may have occurred. However, if

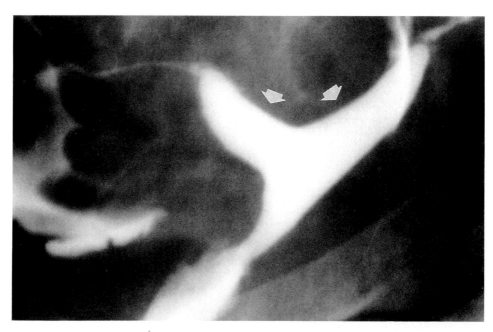

Figure 3.13.   Concave or arcuate configuration to the uterine fundus (*arrows*).

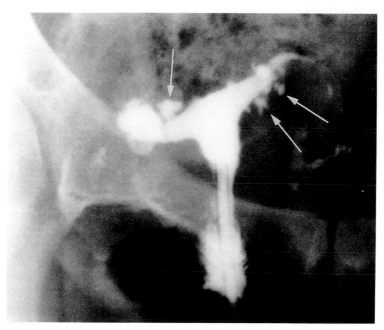

Figure 3.14. Adenomyosis. Note the coarse and irregular collections of contrast material invaginating the myometrium (*arrows*).

examined during the postovulatory secretory phase, the endometrium usually shows a more irregular contour. Such coarsely irregular margins are also noted in patients with adenomyosis. This latter entity, reflecting a benign proliferation of endometrium into the uterine musculature, results in an easily recognized radiographic pattern. The phenomenon may be local or generalized, but is typified by small collections of contrast material invaginating the myometrium and suggesting a series of palisading diverticula likened to lollipops (Figs. 3.14 and 3.15) (see Chapter 6). Another unusual but innocuous normal variation of endometrial pattern is a ridged contour, consisting of longitudinal folds involving the uterine body (Fig. 3.16). These parallel the long axis of the uterus, have no obvious corollary at hysteroscopy, and seem to have no clinical significance.

Intravasation of contrast material into the wall of the myometrium is occasionally seen (Fig. 3.17). In 593 consecutive hysterosalpingograms performed with a low-viscosity oil-based medium, intravasation into the lymphatic or venous systems occurred in 41 cases (6.9%) (1); comparable data are not available for water-based media. Embolization was documented in six patients, and there were no adverse sequelae. The most common causative factor is excessive pressure within the uterine cavity during introduction of the contrast material. This may be seen with tubal occlusion, when intracavitary pressure is markedly elevated, but may merely be a reflection of the force of injection of contrast material. If extensive synechiae are present and partially obliterate the uterine cavity, the high pressure needed to distend the potential space of the uterine cavity may also result in extravasation. Performing a hysterosalpingogram shortly after endometrial instrumentation (biopsy, dilatation, and curettage) predisposes to intravasation, as does performing the hysterosalpingogram very early in the cycle just following the cessation of menstruation. Such intravasation can be lo-

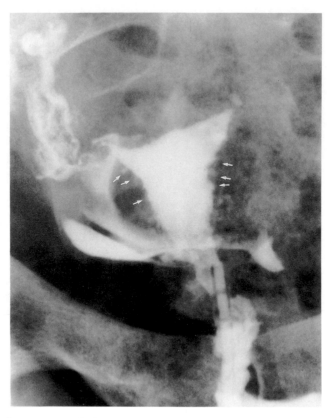

Figure 3.15. Another pattern of adenomyosis. The invaginations are small and relatively symmetrical (*arrows*).

calized or generalized (Fig. 3.18), and, when excessive, is associated with pelvic vascular filling. The deposits of contrast material in the myometrium disappear after several minutes and seem to cause no ill effects. The vascular channels, when outlined by contrast material, are transitory in their appearance, clearing in seconds as a reflection of normal blood flow. Contrast in thin, delicate lymphatic channels may also be observed; lymphatics are differentiated from blood vessels by their thinner caliber and slower emptying (Fig. 3.19).

THE FALLOPIAN TUBES

The fallopian tubes are paired structures of 10 to 12 cm in length that arise from the uterus at the fundal cornua and extend laterally. Three segments, the in-

terstitial portion, the isthmus, and the ampulla, are defined and apparently have differing functional and anatomic distinctions (Figs. 3.1 and 3.20). The interstitial segment is 1 to 2 cm in length and lies completely within the myometrium. A triangular or funnel-shaped zone of dilatation, the so-called tubal bulge, is commonly observed (Figs. 3.21 and 3.22). The junction of the interstitial and isthmic segments of the fallopian tubes is anatomically demarcated where the tube exits from the myometrium, a point not identifiable on a hysterosalpingogram. Obstruction at this point is not uncommon. Such occlusion may be anatomic or mechanical in etiology or may be due to "cornual spasm" (more properly, myometrial contraction). This resistance to filling may often be overcome by gentle, persistent pressure during induction of

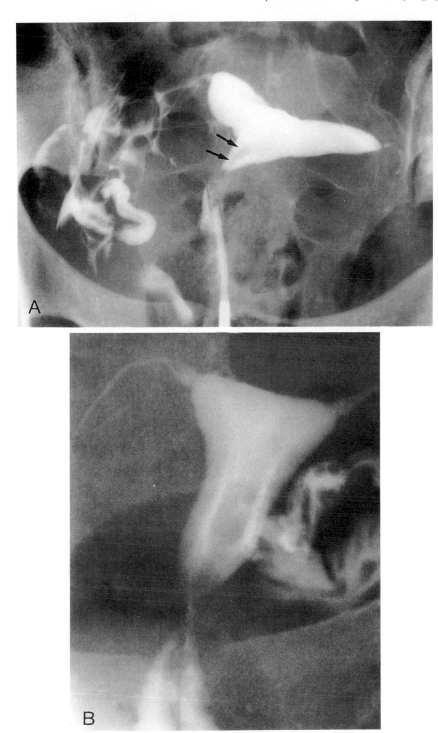

Figure 3.16.   Ridging, a normal variation. **A,** The ridged configuration is sometimes thin and delicate (*arrows*). **B,** At other times the ridged contours are rather broad and prominent. These have no apparent corollary at hysteroscopic examination.

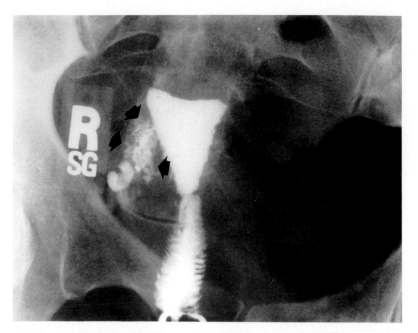

Figure 3.17. Rather large but localized area of extravasation of contrast medium into the myometrium (*arrowheads*). In this patient, the excessive pressure that resulted in the extravasation is secondary to bilateral tubal occlusion. Note also the normal variation in the appearance of the mucosal contour of the cervical canal.

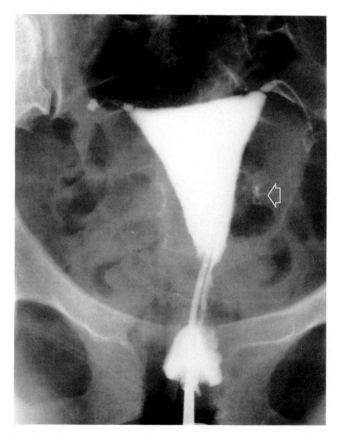

Figure 3.18. Very localized intravasation of contrast material (*open arrow*) in a patient with a previous bilateral tubal ligation.

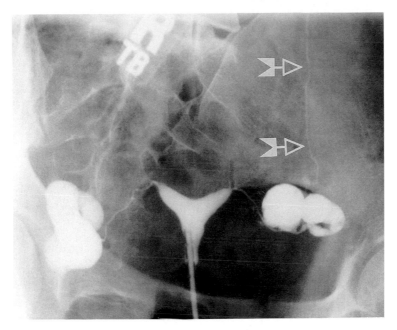

Figure 3.19. Intravasation of contrast material into lymphatic channels (*open arrows*). Note the bilateral hydrosalpinges in this patient with stigmata of chronic pelvic inflammatory disease.

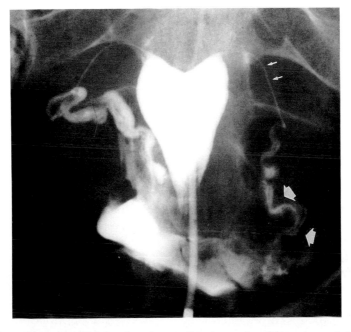

Figure 3.20. The isthmic (*small arrows*) and ampullary (*arrowheads*) portions of the fallopian tube are clearly different in appearance. Note the rugal fold in the ampullary segment of the tube.

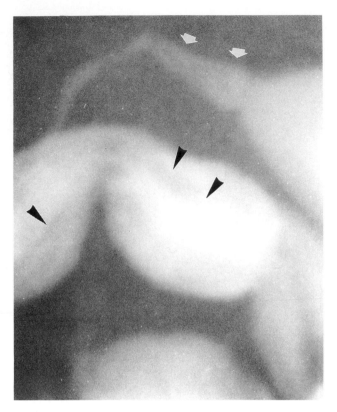

Figure 3.21.   The interstitial segment of the fallopian tube is frequently conical or triangular in shape (*arrows*). Note the rugal folds in the ampullary portion of the tube (*arrowheads*).

contrast material. Occasionally, turning the patient onto her hip seems to assist in tubal filling. If the obstruction to flow persists, the administration of antispasmodic agents may be attempted to relieve the apparent spasm. Varying degrees of success have been reported with amyl nitrate, atropine, nitroglycerin, and dihydroergotamine. Glucagon has been the most satisfactory agent in our hands, although the success rate for reversing obstruction is still only 25% (see Chapter 2).

The isthmus of the fallopian tube is tortuous, delicate, and narrow; measurements of the length of this segment are difficult on radiography because of the tortuous nature of the tube and the irregular direction of its course. The diameter of the isthmus rarely exceeds 2 mm and may be so thin as to be virtually imperceptible radiographically.

The ampulla is the widest and longest segment, with a gradual increase in diameter to an average of 5 mm. Inherent magnification may make this appear even larger on a hysterosalpingogram. Rugal folds are frequently noted and may be recognized in both normal and pathologic tubes (Figs. 3.23 and 3.24). Their presence cannot be construed as excluding inflammatory change. Numerous descriptions of peristaltic activity in the fallopian tubes are recorded, but such activity is not usually observed during the course of the examination. Conjecture as to a possible physiologic role for the isthmic-ampullary junction is beyond the scope of this text, but this zone may well have a specific function during the process of fertilization of the oocyte.

The mobility of the isthmic and ampullary portions of the tubes may be

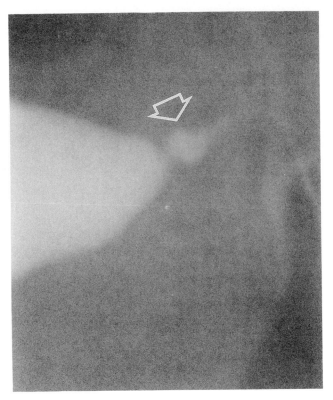

Figure 3.22. The interstitial segment of the tube at times is diamond-shaped in configuration (*open arrow*). This is a normal variation and is of no clinical significance.

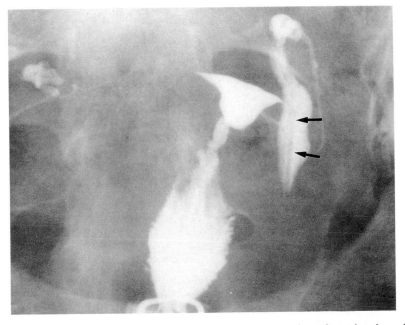

Figure 3.23. The ampullary segment of the fallopian tube is significantly wider than the isthmic portion. Rugal folds (*arrows*) are striking. This appearance is well within the limits of normal.

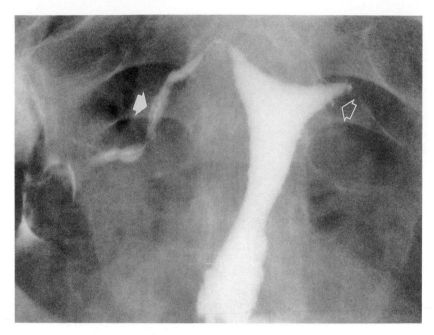

Figure 3.24.   Prominent rugal folds in the ampullary segment of the right fallopian tube (*arrow*). The left tube is occluded. Minimal adenomyosis (*open arrow*) is present.

demonstrated by varying the degree of traction on the cervix during the examination. Tubes demonstrating mobility are suggested to be free of peritubal adhesive change, but the inability to detect such mobility may simply reflect insufficient movement of the uterus.

Patency of the tube, a vital determination during hysterosalpingography, is usually readily recognized by spill of contrast material from the fimbriated end of the ampulla into the peritoneal cavity. The contrast material usually puddles along a peritoneal reflection or occasionally interjects between bowel loops. Persistence of contrast material in an immediate peritubal location may signify inflammatory adnexal disease (see Chapter 8). The free flow of contrast material deep into the pelvis and along peritoneal reflections is the common criterion of patency.

SUMMARY

The multiple appearances that may be discovered during hysterosalpingography are extensive. It is critical that these variations be recognized for what they are and not misinterpreted as abnormal structural findings. Meticulous technique and careful observations are necessary to accomplish this end.

REFERENCE

1. Nunley WC, Bateman BG, Kitchin JD, Pope TL: Intravasation during hysterosalpingography using oil-base contrast medium—a second look. *Obstet Gynecol* 70:309, 1987.

4

Congenital Anomalies of the Uterus and Fallopian Tubes

Congenital malformations of the müllerian paramesonephric system are expressed in various ways, including duplication, atresia, and complete absence of a structure. Patients with improper development of the müllerian ducts may present clinically with a variety of symptoms. Gynecologic complaints include amenorrhea, dysmenorrhea, dyspareunia, infertility, fetal wastage, and poor reproductive performance. Menstrual outflow obstruction may lead to hematometra, hematocolpos, and possibly endometriosis. Müllerian malformations may be completely asymptomatic and never detected, or they may present as surgical emergencies such as a gestation in a rudimentary uterine horn, rupture of a noncommunicating rudimentary horn, or an obstructed labor. A thorough knowledge of the embryologic development of the müllerian system is necessary for accurate diagnosis of a particular case and for planning potential surgical therapy for such diverse conditions as vaginal agenesis, imperforate hymen, uterine septa, and other anomalies. What follows is a brief summary of the embryologic development of the female genital tract (1–3).

EMBRYOLOGIC DEVELOPMENT OF THE UTERUS

The müllerian, or paramesonephric, duct system begins to develop in both sexes by 40 days of gestation and appears as a funnel-shaped opening of celomic epithelium originating near the base of the dorsal mesentery in close association with the urinary tract. The mesonephric (wolffian) duct system forms first and becomes the male reproductive tract. Normal development of the male system requires both the presence of a testis and the production of testosterone. In the male after 60 days of gestation, the embryonic testis begins to produce a müllerian inhibiting factor that causes the müllerian ducts to regress and prevents development of the female system. In the absence of the müllerian inhibiting factor the ducts continue to proliferate unimpeded, developing into paired, undifferentiated tubes that later fuse to become the primordia of the uterine corpus, cervix, and the upper portion of the vagina. In the male, failure of inhibition of the müllerian duct or failure of masculinization of the internal genitalia may allow development of the female ductal system or the formation of an ambiguous, incompletely masculinized system.

In the female, the paramesonephric or müllerian ducts develop on the lateral side of the mesonephric ridge and extend caudally parallel to the mesonephric ducts. The mesonephric duct serves as a guide for the growing müllerian duct, and any interruption of the downward growth of the mesonephric duct will result in arrested growth of the müllerian duct beyond this point. Canalization of the solid müllerian duct proceeds simultaneously with its downward growth. In the female, the wolffian ducts, for lack of stimulus, eventually persist only as microscopic islands or short segments of ductal epithelium buried in the anterolateral vaginal wall (Gartner's duct), cervix, broad ligament (epophoron), and paraovarian tissues (parophoron). At the caudal end, the paired müllerian ducts cross the wolffian ducts ventrally and medially and fuse by the eighth week with the urogenital sinus to form a solid mass, the müllerian tubercle, in the posterior wall of the urogenital sinus. The process of fusion of the two canalized müllerian ducts into the uterus starts at the caudal tip, the müllerian tubercle, and proceeds cranially up to the junction of the future round ligaments. Resorption of the fused median septum next occurs, and this may start at any level and proceed in either or both directions. This fusion of the previously paired müllerian ducts and subsequent resorption of the septum leaves a single uterovaginal canal that differentiates further into a recognizable vagina, cervix, uterine corpus, and fallopian tubes. Toward the end of the third month of embryonic life, distinct muscular and connective tissue layers can be seen in the uterus, and by the end of the sixth month the endometrium appears.

Tissue of both müllerian and urogenital sinus origin normally participates in the development of the vagina (4, 5). The müllerian tubercle, where the hymen will ultimately develop, is the site of contact between the solid tip of the fused müllerian ducts and the dorsal wall of the urogenital sinus. The mesonephric ducts, which are in the process of degeneration, enter the urogenital sinus immediately lateral to the tubercle. A solid mass of proliferating sinus cells, called the sinovaginal bulb, develops between the openings of the mesonephric ducts and the müllerian tubercle and forms a cord from the dorsal urogenital sinus wall to the solid tips of the müllerian ducts, the vaginal plate. The vaginal plate later canalizes, starting at the hymenal ring and proceeding cranially, to end at the cervix; the process is completed between the 20th and 22nd weeks.

There is still major controversy regarding the origin of the stratified squamous epithelium of the vagina. The three possible sources are the müllerian ducts, the wolffian ducts, and the urogenital sinus. Most think that the squamous epithelium of the urogenital sinus extends cranially to the level of the future external cervical os and displaces the müllerian columnar cells (5), but others have contended that the entire vaginal epithelium is of mesonephric origin (6). The major point to be understood is that müllerian anomalies affect more than just the corpus and cervix of the uterus and can involve the upper portion of the vagina as well.

The major defects can be categorized as occurring because of failure of one or more aspects of the normal embryologic development. For example, failure of initial fusion and descent of the paired caudal ends of the müllerian ducts could result in complete atresia of the uterus and upper vagina. If descent stopped on one side, a uterus unicornis would result, with a rudimentary horn on the other side. If the underlying defect was due to failure of development of the wolffian duct, then renal agenesis would be likely on the ipsilateral side. An abnormality of vertical fusion would occur with a fault in the junction between the down-growing müllerian tubercle and the up-growing derivative from the urogenital sinus; this could cause an obstructive transverse vaginal septum. A defect in lateral fusion of the two müllerian ducts could result in persistence of the two developing cords, with partial or complete duplication; total failure of fusion results in a uterus didelphys, with or without a vaginal septum. Partial fusion results in various types of bicornuate uterus with one cervix; an abnormality of resorption of the septum could explain some forms of communicating uteri. The sequence in which development occurs makes certain anatomic problems impossible and others more likely to occur.

ETIOLOGY OF VAGINAL ANOMALIES

The embryological steps in the development of the female and male genital tracts are known, but the etiology of malformations is still unclear.

Among known genetic syndromes are several in which malformations occur as part of described autosomal dominant or recessive hereditary traits. The hand-foot genital (HFG) syndrome, described by Stern et al. (7), includes genital as well as skeletal malformations and is inherited as an autosomal dominant trait; a sex-linked autosomal dominant inheritance for müllerian aplasia was proposed by Shokeir (8). Other more rare syndromes are autosomal recessive, and several family clusters with incomplete müllerian fusion have been described (9–11). Patients identified as having müllerian defects have a low frequency of affected relatives (12), which is more consistent with a multifactorial etiology.

Obviously difficult to associate with uterovaginal abnormalities, but potentially causative nonetheless, are environmental and nutritional exposures, viral disease, radiation, metabolic disturbances, medications, and hormone-induced actions. The effects of estrogen exposure on the morphogenesis and differentiation of the female genital tract explain the malformations resulting from diethylstilbestrol exposure prior to 20 weeks gestational age (2) (see Chapter 5). The formation of congenital müllerian abnormalities is influenced by polygenic, multifactorial, and familial factors (11, 12).

INCIDENCE OF UTEROVAGINAL ANOMALIES

The incidence of congenital defects of the reproductive tract varies with the population studied and the zeal and thoroughness of the investigating clinician.

Many patients with uterovaginal anomalies are never detected because they never have obstetric or gynecologic difficulties. Several retrospective surveys have estimated the prevalence of incomplete müllerian fusion as approximately 0.1 to 0.5% (13–15), although Tulandi and coworkers (16) reported an incidence in excess of 1 in 100. If manual exploration of the uterine cavity is performed at delivery, a higher prevalence of congenitally anomalous uteri will be reported, in the range of 2 to 3% (17, 18). The most common malformations include septate, bicornuate, and didelphic uteri. The unicornuate uterus is very rare (19, 20).

Concomitant malformations of uterus and urologic tract might be expected, and up to 20% of women with reproductive tract anomalies have abnormalities of the urinary tract (21, 22). Primary unilateral renal agenesis has an incidence between 1 in 600 and 1 in 1300 subjects; of female patients, 55 to 70% will be found to have associated genital anomalies (23–25). Because these patients generally present with gynecologic complaints, the association is less well known to urologists (26); nevertheless, evaluation of the urinary tract in these patients is essential. Gurin and Leiter (27) make the important point that an intravenous pyelogram (IVP) is frequently forgotten, observing that only 12 of 55 patients with abnormal müllerian development had an IVP and, inversely, only 2 of 21 women with renal anomalies had had a gynecologic evaluation. Thus, the association of müllerian duct and renal anomalies is clear, but the prevalence of the association has been inadequately evaluated (Fig. 4.1).

DIAGNOSIS OF UTEROVAGINAL ANOMALIES

The diagnosis of uterovaginal anomalies is rarely made at pelvic examination, even with a double cervix, because it is

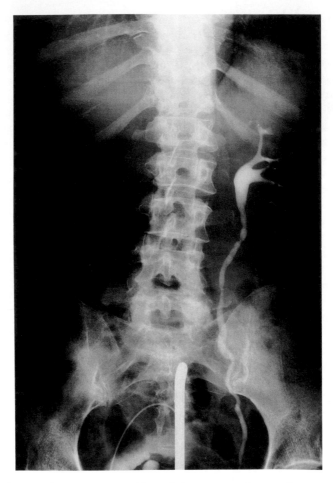

Figure 4.1. Renal agenesis, a common although inconstant abnormality associated with genital tract anomalies.

not unusual for a patient with a total vaginal septum to have intercourse on only one side of the septum. Speculum placement will be defined by the vaginal septum. Therefore, only one cervix is likely to be seen, and malformations of the uterus may be unsuspected.

Most patients with uterovaginal anomalies are detected by hysterosalpingography when the patient presents with either infertility or recurrent fetal wastage. Occasionally, abnormalities are detected by uterine exploration following delivery (17, 18). In the past, it was not crucial to differentiate between septate and bicornuate uteri, as the surgical ap-

proach to treatment was uterine unification at laparotomy, and the particular surgical technique chosen could be decided at operation. At present, these two müllerian defects are no longer repaired by the same operative approach, since a uterine septum can be removed by means of hysteroscopic metroplasty, while the bicornuate uterus must still be approached by abdominal surgery, although such correction is rarely deemed appropriate. Therefore, several other modalities for diagnosis, including ultrasonography and magnetic resonance imaging, have been added to the diagnostic armamentarium.

Hysterosalpingography

Hysterosalpingography has been the traditional method for diagnosing uterine anomalies. In distinguishing septate from bicornuate uteri, the presence of a blunt or acute angle between the uterine horns and laterally convex or straight contours of the horns, respectively, have been important criteria in establishing the correct diagnosis (28). However, regardless of the radiological diagnosis, most of these malformations are of the septate type (29), indicating that reliable differentiation can be done only by visualizing the uterine surface with laparoscopy, ultrasonography, or magnetic resonance imaging, as described below, in conjunction with examination of the uterine cavity with hysteroscopy or hysterosalpingography. Other factors that might induce errors in diagnosis by hysterosalpingography include deficient traction on the uterus (particularly if the uterus is anteflexed or retroflexed), which results in exposures that tend to normalize the fundal contour (see Chapter 2), and rotation of the uterus around the uterine plane. Reuter et al. (30) found that hysterosalpingography alone had a diagnostic accuracy of 55% in distinguishing bicornuate from septate uteri, improving to 90% when ultrasonography was included. These authors make the important point that although hysterosalpingography alone is not adequate to make the distinction between a septate and a bicornuate uterus, the measurement of the angle of divergence, if less than 75, was nonetheless diagnostic of a uterine septum.

Ultrasonography

Transvaginal or abdominal ultrasonography can provide information concerning both the external profile of the uterus and the length, width, and characteristics of a septum. Associated pelvic disease, including myomata, or ovarian cysts, as well as the location and morphology of kidneys, can also be delineated (30–32). Instillation of saline solution into the uterine cavity during ultrasonography (33) may provide additional information. Sonography performed during the luteal phase of the cycle is important in diagnosing a septum, as the endometrium is thicker and can be more clearly identified (31). Ultrasonography appears to be a useful adjunct for more precise diagnosis in cases in which hysterosalpingography has identified a uterine abnormality (see Chapter 12).

Magnetic Resonance Imaging

Magnetic resonance imaging (MRI) provides accurate details of pelvic anatomy in a precise and noninvasive way. Studies on patients known to have uterine anomalies by ultrasonography and hysterosalpingography have shown that reliable differentiation of a septate from a bicornuate uterus can be accomplished (34–36) (Fig. 4.2). Advantages of MRI are that it is not invasive, does not require hospitalization and analgesia, allows a complete and detailed exploration of the subperitoneal pelvic structures, and can be performed in patients who have previously undergone surgery or who have extensive adhesions. Its role in the clinical management of uterine abnormalities is unclear, because many of the advantages of MRI are also offered by ultrasonography at less cost.

Hysteroscopy

Hysteroscopy is a common tool for diagnosing intrauterine abnormalities (see Chapter 8) and can be performed in the outpatient setting without general anesthesia. Direct hysteroscopic visual evaluation provides useful information

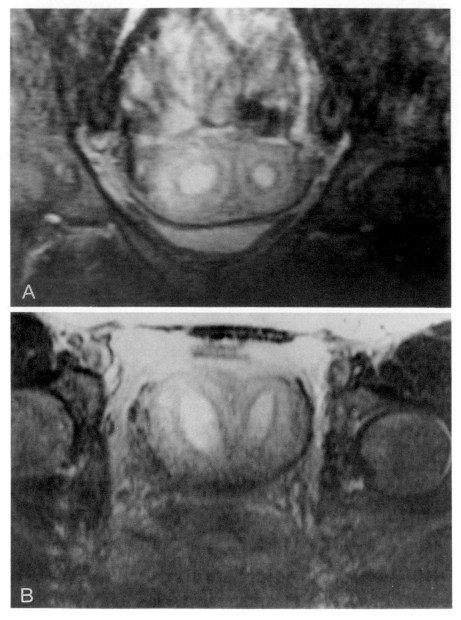

Figure 4.2. Coronal (**A**) and axial (**B**) views of bicornuate uterus using T2-weighted images. (Courtesy of H. Pollack, Philadelphia, PA.)

on the presence and configuration of a septum but does not permit differentiation of a bicornuate from a septate uterus. Hysteroscopy is ordinarily reserved for patients in whom a diagnosis has been made and in whom hysteroscopic metroplasty is to be performed.

Laparoscopy

Laparoscopy is an invasive procedure, performed under general or epidural anesthesia, that permits distinguishing bicornuate from septate uteri on the basis of the fundal contour. Laparoscopy is unreliable in diagnosing various forms of noncommunicating horns, but it is generally not required for diagnosis if the other modalities described above have been used.

CLASSIFICATION OF MÜLLERIAN ANOMALIES

Either initial failure of fusion of the müllerian duct or later failure of the resorption of the septum results in a continuum of malformations. Fusion begins caudally and extends cranially; if there is incomplete fusion, it will most likely be seen in the upper system, causing duplication of the upper uterus. However, varying patterns of separation and communication may occur (see Communicating Uteri below). Failure of lateral fusion may result in partial or complete duplication, which may be symmetrical or asymmetrical, and obstructive or nonobstructive.

Several systems of classification of müllerian malformations have been proposed. The first of these, set forth in 1907 (37), grouped malformations into symmetric (uterus didelphys, bicornis, septus) and asymmetric (uterus unicornis) types.

Symmetric malformations include those in which external division of the uterus leads to two separate uterine cavities, typified by the didelphic uterus, and those in which external separation is lacking. In the latter category, the arcuate uterus may have only a midline groove and a somewhat flattened and transversely elongated fundus; internally, a midline septum may subdivide the cavity to varying degrees (uterus subseptus or uterus septus), as exemplified in Class III, IV, and V anomalies (see below).

Most asymmetric malformations involve uterine duplication in which one uterine horn is fully developed and the other exhibits rudimentary development or is totally absent. The rudimentary horn is usually attached to the normal-appearing contralateral uterine horn by a thin fibrous band. There may be considerable disproportion between the two sides, and, if the endometrium is functional within the rudimentary horn, significant symptomatology may occur due to the obstructed (absent) outflow tract. If the rudimentary horn ends blindly, progressive accumulation of menstrual flow and hematometra gradually leads to increasing distention of the cavity. When rudimentary horns are unconnected and the endometrium is nonfunctional, there will be no clinically detectable symptoms. If the rudimentary horn connects with the normal cavity through a small channel, implantation of a viable conceptus may occur and simulate ectopic pregnancy.

Other classification systems have been described based on (a) embryologic and anatomical differences (38); (b) obstetrical functioning (39); (c) physiologic capacity differences (40); and (d) radiological differences (28). Sorenson (3) has discussed these and their advantages thoroughly.

Until recently, the most clinically relevant classification system has been one modified from Jarcho (38) but includes other abnormalities. This is the classification proposed by Buttram and Gibbons (41) (Table 4.1), who analyzed 144 cases with respect to pregnancy rates and reproductive success, and used these cases as the basis for the classification. More recently, the American Fertility Society has developed a classification system that may prove to be helpful (Fig. 4.3).

Class I: Müllerian Agenesis or Hypoplasia

Since the urogenital sinus contributes to formation of the vagina, vaginal agenesis is not exclusively a "müllerian"

Table 4.1.   Müllerian Anomalies: Classification of Buttram and Gibbons

Class I: Müllerian agenesis or hypoplasia
    A. Vaginal agenesis
    B. Cervical agenesis
    C. Fundal agenesis
    D. Tubal agenesis
    E. Combined
Class II: Unicornuate uterus
    A. With rudimentary horn
      1. With endometrial cavity
      2. Without endometrial cavity
        a. With communication with opposite horn
        b. Without   communication with opposite horn
    B. Without rudimentary horn
Class III: Uterus didelphys
Class IV: Bicornuate uterus
    A. Complete
    B. Partial
    C. Arcuate
Class V: Septate uterus
    A. Complete septum
    B. Incomplete septum
Class VI: "DES-exposed" uterus

problem; nevertheless, vaginal agenesis has been included in the Class I anomalies. Vaginal agenesis occurs in about 1 of 5000 phenotypic females, and it is difficult to clinically distinguish vaginal agenesis from a transverse vaginal septum. If the uterus and cervix are intact and only the vagina has not formed, a surgical correction can be attempted. Anastomosis has been reported with restoration of menses, but there are no documented pregnancies. The cases in which pregnancy has been reported are probably due to a vaginal septum and not to vaginal agenesis. In cervical agenesis, conception is highly unlikely because the fistulous tracts created may have contributed to the occurrence of ascending infection. Fundal agenesis has rarely been observed. Overall, a combined uterovaginal agenesis, the so-called Mayer-Rokitansky-Kuster-Hauser syndrome, is the most common Class I anomaly. Because of the

nature of the vaginal component of the deformity, hysterosalpingography plays no significant role in the diagnosis of Class I anomalies.

Class II: Unicornuate Uterus

A unicornuate configuration may result from one of several possible anomalies. Rarely, this appearance is due to agenesis of one of the müllerian pair, a true unicornuate uterus. More commonly, however, the unicornuate chamber is associated with a rudimentary horn (representing a remnant of the contralateral müllerian system) that may be either communicating or noncommunicating (Figs. 4.4 to 4.7).

Class III: Uterus Didelphys

The true didelphic uterus, reflecting complete failure of müllerian fusion, has two separate uterine cavities with a vertical septum in the proximal portion of the vagina. It is not unusual, however, for partial fusion and resorption to cause the vaginal septum to disappear (Figs. 4.8 and 4.9). As mentioned, urinary tract anomalies are common (Figs. 4.1 and 4.10). MRI has the capability to render excellent anatomic detail of this anomaly (Fig. 4.11). However, at this time, such imaging is usually not cost-effective.

Class IV: Bicornuate Uterus

A bicornuate uterus results from incomplete müllerian pair fusion. The degree of separation of the paired lumens may vary from a minimal arcuate contour at the fundus to a deep cleft with division to the level of the lower uterine segment. There is only one cervix (Figs. 4.12 to 4.15).

Class V: Septate Uterus

Fusion of the müllerian pair with failure of resorption of all or part of the

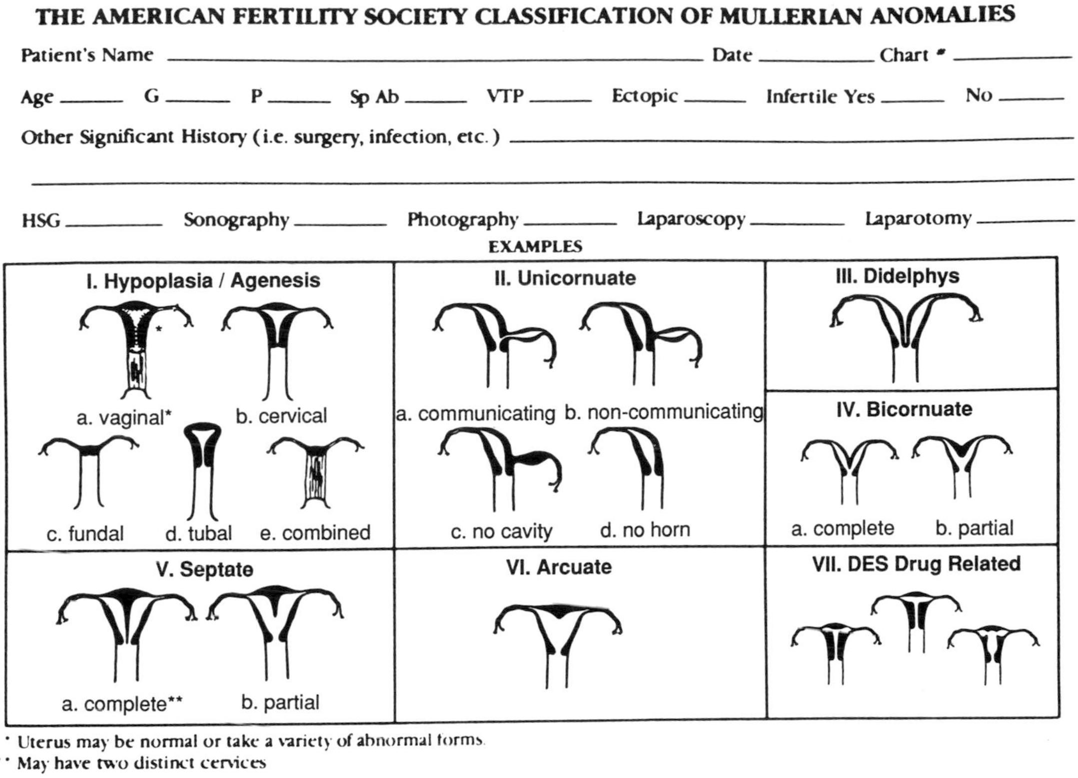

THE AMERICAN FERTILITY SOCIETY CLASSIFICATION OF MULLERIAN ANOMALIES

Patient's Name _____ Date _____ Chart # _____

Age _____ G _____ P _____ Sp Ab _____ VTP _____ Ectopic _____ Infertile Yes _____ No _____

Other Significant History (i.e. surgery, infection, etc.) _____

_____

HSG _____ Sonography _____ Photography _____ Laparoscopy _____ Laparotomy _____

EXAMPLES

I. Hypoplasia / Agenesis

a. vaginal*   b. cervical

c. fundal   d. tubal   e. combined

II. Unicornuate

a. communicating b. non-communicating

c. no cavity   d. no horn

III. Didelphys

IV. Bicornuate

a. complete   b. partial

V. Septate

a. complete**   b. partial

VI. Arcuate

VII. DES Drug Related

* Uterus may be normal or take a variety of abnormal forms.
** May have two distinct cervices

Figure 4.3. The American Fertility Society classification of müllerian anomalies.

intervening septum results in a configuration that may mimic the appearance of the bicornuate uterus on a hysterosalpingogram (Fig. 4.16). Differentiation of septate and bicornuate uteri requires laparoscopy or ultrasound examination to appreciate the presence or absence of myometrial tissue between the cornua (Fig. 4.17). Although it is noted that the cornua of the septate uterus frequently create a more acute angle than is seen with a bicornuate uterus, the range of findings of the angle of diversion as seen at hysterosalpingography makes a precise diagnosis tenuous (Figs. 4.18 to 4.20). The ability of MRI to differentiate fibrous from muscular tissue is of importance. Long TR and long TE sequences best define this anatomy. The low water content of the fibrous tissue of the septum results in a low-intensity imaging zone, whereas myometrium, because of greater fluid and thus a greater proton density, pro-

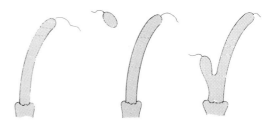

Figure 4.4. Class II anomaly. A unicornuate cavity may reflect any of the depicted configurations. The true unicornuate uterus (*left*) is most rare. Rudimentary horns of the underdeveloped müllerian duct may be either noncommunicating (*center*) or communicating (*right*).

duces a higher intensity image (Fig. 4.21).

Class VI: Diethylstilbestrol (DES) Exposed Uterus

This uterine malformation has internal luminal changes, such as a T shape, a constricting band affecting the uterine

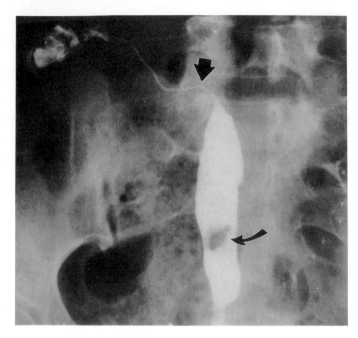

Figure 4.5. Unicornuate uterus. A single fallopian tube extends from the cornual tip (*arrow*). Note the incidental polyp in the endometrial cavity (*curved arrow*).

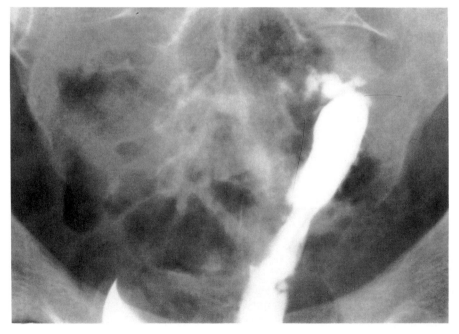

Figure 4.6. Extensive fundal synechia (see Chapter 7) can result in a configuration similar to unicornuate uterus.

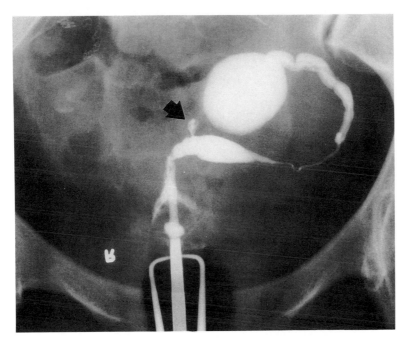

Figure 4.7. Duplication anomaly. Unicornuate uterus with a small communicating rudimentary horn (*arrow*). There is a large hydrosalpinx on the left.

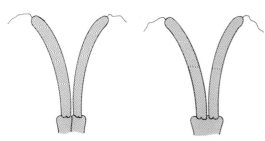

Figure 4.8. Class III anomaly. The didelphic uterus consists of two entirely separate chambers. The vagina may be partitioned in its upper portion by a vertical septum (*left*) or may be unipartite (*right*).

corpus, or a widened lower two-thirds of the uterus. These anomalies are almost entirely drug induced and are discussed in Chapter 5.

Communicating Uteri

Toaff and colleagues (42) have reviewed and classified nine types of communicating uteri, and recently, Fedele et al. (43) have described a tenth type not fitting any previous classification. These are a distinct class of uterine malformations identified by the presence of a communication between two otherwise separate uterocervical cavities. The different types of communicating uteri are induced by a teratogenic process that is active at different stages of the embryologic development. An early process would involve the development of both urinary and genital ducts and may result in the more severe anomalies of ipsilateral renal agenesis and ductal atresia. A later process could result in a failure of fusion or of complete resorption of the septum, resulting in atypically located communications, often at the level of the uterine cavity (Figs. 4.22 to 4.26).

Wolffian Duct Remnants

Residual segments of the wolffian ducts may persist in the tissue anterolateral to the vagina, adjacent to the cervix, or in the paraovarian tissues (paroöphoron). Referred to as Gartner's ducts,

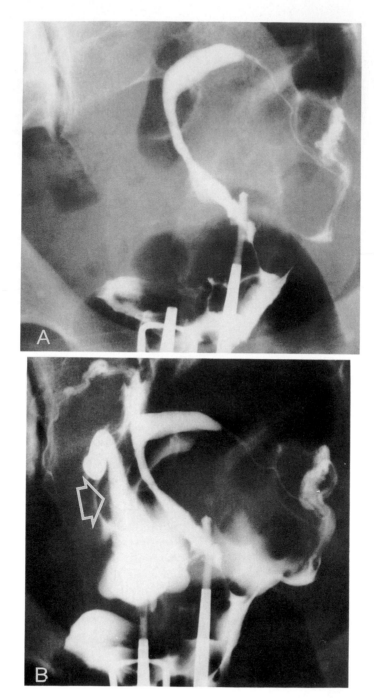

Figure 4.9.   A, Didelphic uterus with filling of only the left lumen. **B,** Second chamber is now filled (*arrow*), using a second cannula.

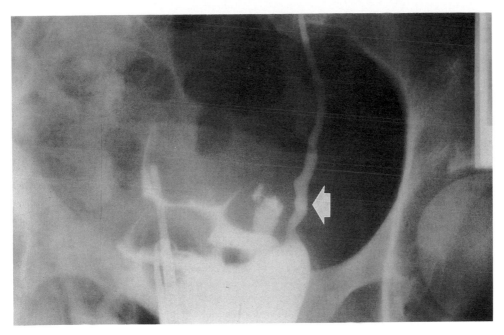

Figure 4.10. In this patient with a didelphic uterus, one also notes ectopic insertion of the left ureter into the vagina (*arrow*).

these wolffian remnants may occasionally communicate with the vagina or endometrial cavity. These duct lumens may fill with contrast material during hysterosalpingography and are identified as linear channels of contrast immediately lateral to the lateral margins of the endometrial cavity (Figs. 4.27 and 4.28) (44).

REPRODUCTIVE POTENTIAL

Pregnancy outcome for patients with congenital anomalies of the uterus obviously depends on the degree of anomaly and to a certain extent on the operative procedure employed. When uterine anomalies are grouped according to the degree of failure of normal uterine development, those with the greatest degree of abnormality seem to have the worst fetal survival. Clearly, patients fitting the Buttram and Gibbons Class I have a very low potential for fertility.

Class II, the unicornuate uterus, has a poor reproductive potential. Intrauterine growth retardation has been reported

(19, 20, 45), and the frequency of breech presentation is high. Women with a unicornuate uterus also have a high incidence of primary infertility (15 to 32%) and of spontaneous miscarriage (59%) (45, 46). A decreased blood supply from the uterine artery and the utero-ovarian artery of the abnormal side may contribute to the abnormal endometrium found in rudimentary horns in these cases (47) but does not explain the poor outcome of pregnancies implanted on the unicornuate side. Nevertheless, in a small series of five women with unicornuate uteri, three had term deliveries, one had a premature delivery with fetal survival, and one had early fetal wastage (48).

Class III, the didelphic uterus with complete failure of müllerian fusion, has high spontaneous abortion and low term delivery rates, with fetal survival from 19 to 64% (29, 46, 48, 49). In another small series of 10 women, six delivered at term and seven infants survived (48). Cervical cerclage is not useful (48, 49), nor is metroplasty indicated. Unification proce-

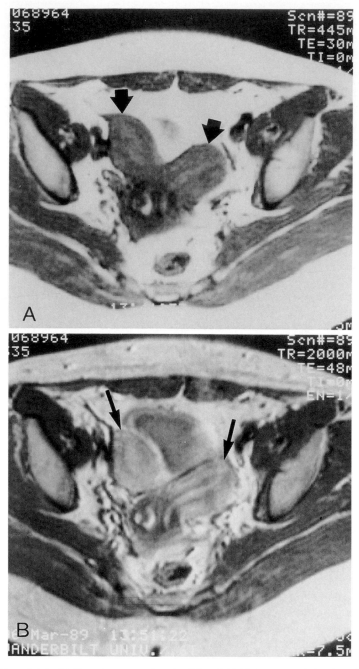

Figure 4.11. T1-weighted (**A**) and proton density (**B**) axial MR images of the female pelvis. There is a didelphic uterus, the horns of which (*arrows*) are best displayed on the T1-weighted sequence due to high contrast between pelvic fat and muscle. The proton density sequence best delineates the myometrium, junctional zone, and endometrium. (Courtesy of T. Powers, Nashville, TN.)

dures were attempted in the past (Fig. 4.29) but have been abandoned.

Class IV, the bicornuate uterus, is the most common of the anomalies. Unfortunately, the earlier literature does not distinguish the bicornuate from the septate uterus, calling both anomalies a "double uterus," so much information has been lost. Confusing and inconsistent data can be found, with fetal wastage rates of 63 to 90% (47, 50) and fetal survival of 42 to 56% (47, 50, 51) described.

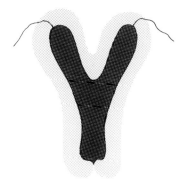

Figure 4.12.   Class IV anomaly: the bicornuate uterus.

Class V, the septate uterus, is traditionally associated with the poorest reproductive outcome, with fetal survival rates reported from 6 to 28% (29, 41, 50–53). On the other hand, Heinonen and co-workers (46) reported that uteri with complete septa have the best fetal survival rate—around 86%. In this reported series, fetal survival with the complete bicornuate uterus is about 50%, and the unicornuate about 40%. Worthen and Gonzalez (54) diagnosed and followed up (by ultrasound) seven patients with varying degrees of uterine septum. In this group, there were 17 pregnancies, 13 of which were viable. It seems likely that variable and inconsistent diagnostic criteria are responsible for all the disparate results in the septate group. In the series reported by Ludmir et al. (48), a management protocol that had worked well for didelphic and bicornuate uteri did not increase the fetal survival rate significantly.

Recent reports stress the importance of metroplasty for patients with a septate uterus (50, 51, 55). Patients with

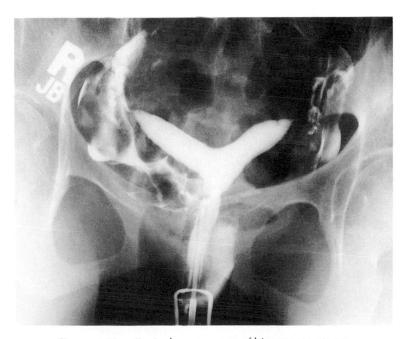

Figure 4.13.   Typical appearance of bicornuate uterus.

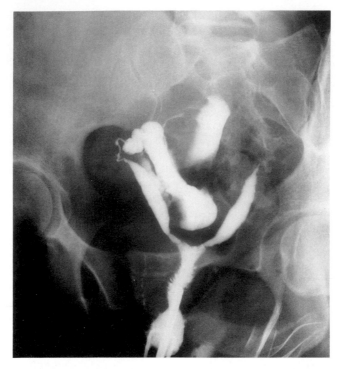

Figure 4.14.   Bicornuate uterus with a very prominent lower uterine segment. The left tube is incompletely filled. The right tube is obstructed and dilated.

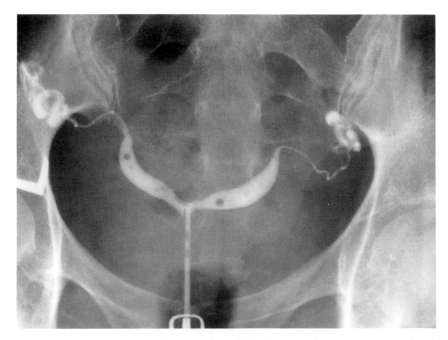

Figure 4.15.   Bicornuate uterus. Radiolucencies within the chambers represent air bubbles introduced during the procedure.

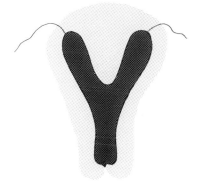

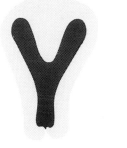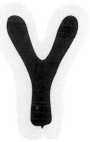

Figure 4.16. Class I anomaly: the septate uterus. The müllerian tubes have fused but there is failure of resorption of a varying amount of the septum separating the chambers.

Figure 4.17. Hysterosalpingographic appearance of septate (*left*) and bicornuate (*right*) uterus may not be differentiated. External evaluation of the uterine fundus is necessary for precise diagnosis.

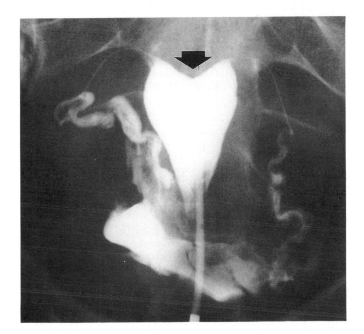

Figure 4.18. Septate uterus. There is a small septum characterized by a cleft-like defect in the fundus (*arrow*).

a septate uterus undergoing wedge metroplasty (51, 56) or Tompkins metroplasty (57) have an expectation of greater than a 75% chance of live birth. Although postoperative hysterosalpingography may show a markedly contracted or irregular uterine cavity, pregnancy rates and full-term delivery rates are excellent, and complications of pregnancy do not seem markedly greater than in the patients presenting with an infertility history.

More recently, since the advent of hysteroscopic operative techniques, metroplasty has been widely performed using hysteroscopy (58–64). The hysteroscopic approach has the advantages of less operative time, less blood loss, and a

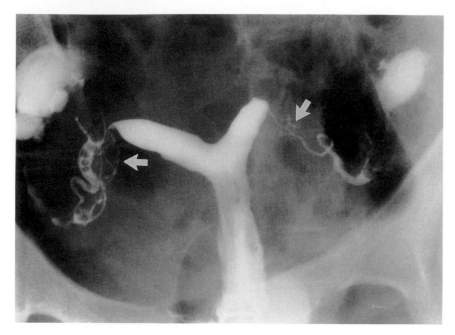

Figure 4.19. Septate uterus in a woman with bilateral hydrosalpinges and salpingitis isthmica nodosa (*arrows*).

shorter hospital stay. Hysteroscopic metroplasty may be preferable to a transabdominal procedure based on cost and morbidity considerations as well as on an anatomical and reproductive outcome (59). Importantly, hysteroscopic resection permits the option for vaginal delivery and is currently thought to be the treatment of choice in patients with uterine septa.

Whereas an operative procedure was previously reserved for patients with fetal wastage, the ease of hysteroscopic metroplasty has led to its being used in patients with only a history of primary infertility or in those in whom a septum was discovered because of instrumentation for another reason. Clearly, all pregnancies in septate uteri do not abort, and fetal survival in the presence of known but uncorrected septa may be as high as 65% (48). Furthermore, sonographic data show that the site of uterine implantation, whether on the lateral wall of the uterus or on the septum, correlated with fetal wastage (65); although the site of implantation cannot be directed, treatment of

"double uteri" with progesterone suppository supplementation seems to permit an improved pregnancy rate in an early series (52).

DIAGNOSTIC TECHNIQUES IN PATIENTS WITH CONGENITAL ABNORMALITIES

Hysterosalpingography in the patient with genital tract anomalies may require modifications of technique and meticulous care to assess the variation adequately. The limitations of differentiating septate and bicornuate uteri have been mentioned previously. The appearance of a unicornuate uterus demands particular care. Such a configuration may indeed represent a true unicornuate uterus but is much more likely to signify the presence of either an associated rudimentary horn or, even more commonly, a didelphic uterus of which only one side is filled with contrast material (Fig. 4.30). Diligent search for a second cervical os is required, particularly since

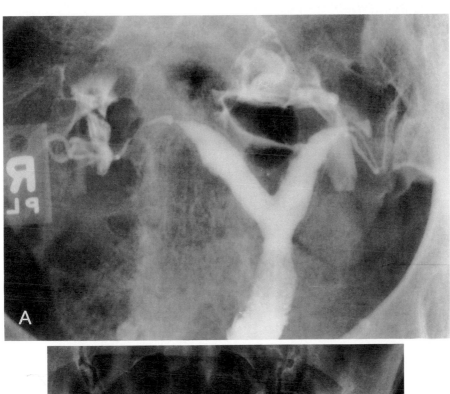

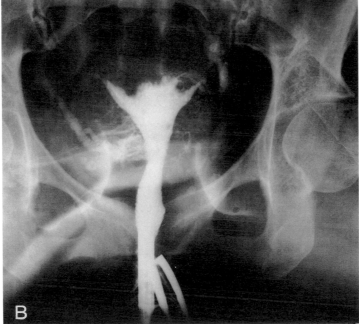

Figure 4.20. A, Septum formation. **B,** Postoperative hysterosalpingogram after metroplasty to correct the defect (see Chapter 11).

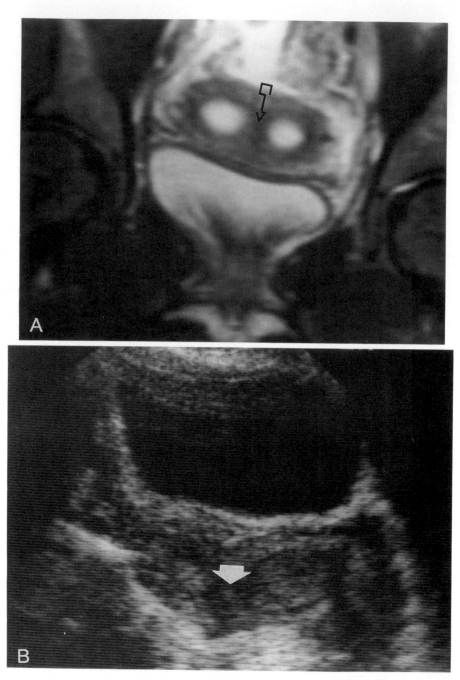

Figure 4.21. A,   Coronal MR image of septate uterus. Note the low intensity of the septum (*arrow*). **B,** Corresponding sonographic view. Septal definition (*arrow*) is less distinct. (Courtesy of H. Pollack, Philadelphia, PA.)

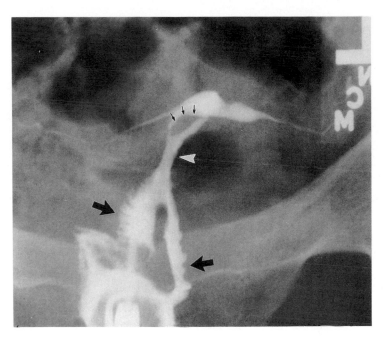

Figure 4.22. Communicating uterus. Two cervices (*arrows*) and luminal separation of the fundus (*small arrows*) with a zone of communication centrally (*arrowhead*).

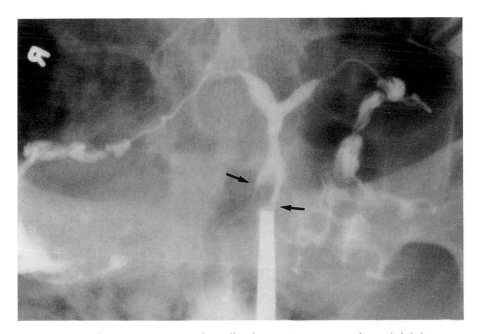

Figure 4.23. Unusual communication. Clinically, this patient presented as a didelphic uterus with two cervical ora (*arrows*). The major portion of the uterine lumen is united with a bicornuate configuration at the fundus.

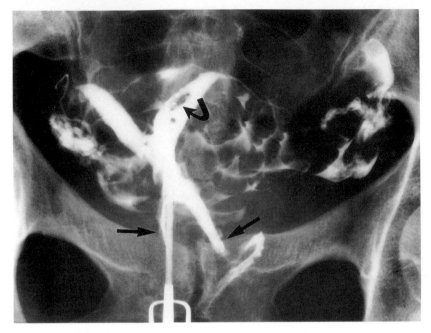

Figure 4.24.   Uterus didelphys presentation with two cervices (*arrows*). The bodies communicate and there are two distinct horns at the fundus. Laparoscopic observation demonstrated that the fundal configuration was septate rather than bicornuate. Incidental note is made of the synechia in the left uterine horn (*curved arrow*).

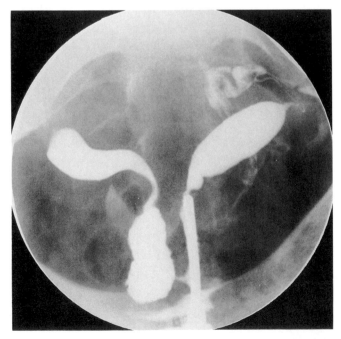

Figure 4.25.   Atypical didelphys configuration, communicating only in the cervical canal. The second cervical canal (*right*) does not open into the vagina but ends blindly.

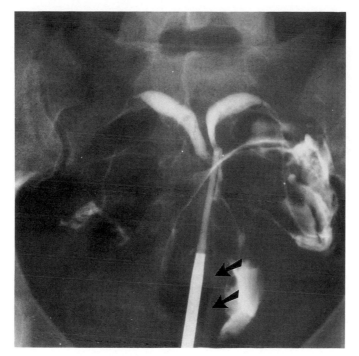

Figure 4.26. Communicating didelphic uterus. The separation between the cannula and the contrast in the vagina reflects a vaginal septum (*arrow*).

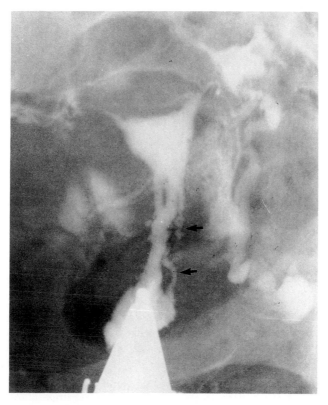

Figure 4.27. Gartner duct remnant (*arrows*). This anomaly is characterized by a line of contrast parallel to the uterine cavity. (Courtesy of L. Ekelund, Lund, Sweden.)

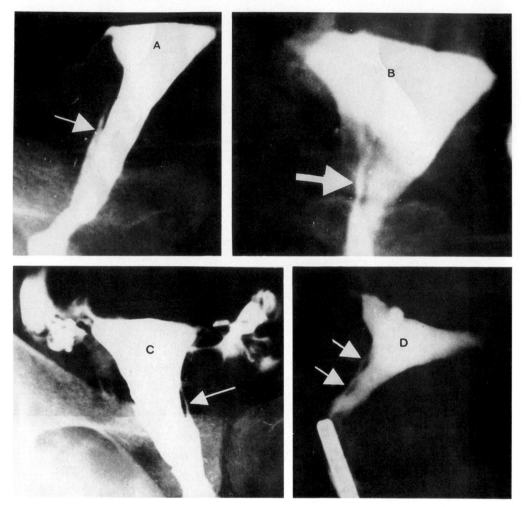

Figure 4.28.   Four examples of Gartner duct remnants characterizing their variability in appearance. (Reprinted with permission from Katz Z, Bernstein D, Lancet M: A possible causal relationship between mesonephric remnants and infertility of uterine origin. *Int J Fertil* 27:125, 1982.)

a vaginal septum may obscure this os from obvious view. Removal or replacement of the vaginal speculum may be needed.

In most of these situations, there is not a great deal of maneuvering room available for placement of instrumentation. Knowledge of previous findings is valuable to the radiographer prior to initiation of the examination. Frequently, a double cervix will appear with the external cervical openings facing the lateral vaginal walls. Under these circumstances, a flexible means of instrumentation, perhaps with the use of a flexible polyethyl-

ene acorn, one of the catheters with balloons (Sholkoff, Ackrad[a]), or a small Foley catheter, will be likely to succeed. Under certain circumstances, when the vaginal septum does not extend all the way to the cervix, it may be difficult to ascertain which cervix is which. Placing methylene blue or indigo carmine dye on the anterior lip of one cervix will allow identification of a second cervix as the vaginal

---

[a]Sholkoff catheter, Cook Ob/Gyn, Spencer, IN; Ackrad catheter, Ackrad Laboratories, Garwood, NJ.

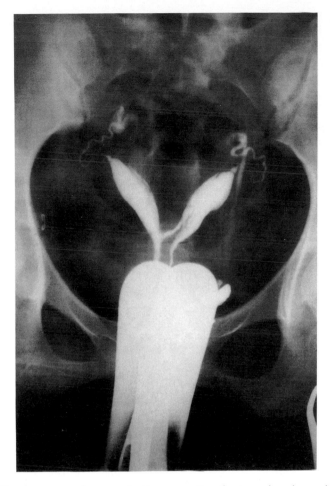

Figure 4.29. Unification procedure surgically connecting the two chambers of a didelphic uterus. This procedure has no place in the modern management of such anomalies.

septum is pressed to one or another side. The use of the Kidde cannula in conjunction with the Foley catheter is frequently helpful, because of the need of one rigid and one more flexible instrument.

Once the instrumentation has been selected, it is useful to place both within the separate cervices, and to make absolutely sure that occlusion of the external os is accomplished on both sides. Then one may elect to introduce contrast material into one side alone and to watch its progression under fluoroscopy. Having demonstrated the contours and anatomy of one side, the next side then can be injected with contrast material, and further

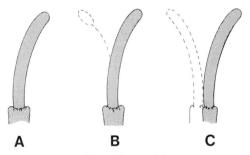

A   B   C

Figure 4.30. The radiographic appearance of a unicornuate uterus may have any of the following three explanations: **A,** True unicornuate uterus; **B,** A unicornuate uterus with a noncommunicating or "blind" horn; and **C,** Filling of only one side of a uterus didelphys. The third possibility is the most common.

information about the anatomic details can be delineated. It is not wise to introduce contrast material into both sides simultaneously, because information is lost about midline septa within the uterine cavity and sometimes about tubal patency.

On occasion, a rudimentary horn may open into the endocervical canal. The radiographer should be aware of this possibility, because the use of a short cannula is recommended in such a case unless it is impossible to get a decent fit with such a rigid apparatus. A balloon catheter may result in occlusion of the tract to the rudimentary horn. Similarly, a short cannula is helpful in the presence of a deep septum to allow filling of both cornual areas.

Clearly, ultrasonography, MRI, laparoscopy, hysteroscopy, and IVP are all valuable to complete delineation of anatomic abnormalities in patients with congenital defects. The major point is that flexibility must be maintained and plans made for delineation of the defects before the patient appears in the radiologist's office. Amassing the necessary equipment in duplicate is of importance to establishing the most information with the least time and inconvenience.

REFERENCES

1. Blandau RJ, Bergsma D: Morphogenesis and malformation of the genital system. *The National Foundation–March of Dimes Birth Defects: Original Article Series* XIII:197, Alan R. Liss, 1977.
2. Robboy SJ, Taguchi O, Cunha GR: Normal development of the human female and reproductive tract and alterations resulting from experimental exposure to diethylstilbestrol. *Hum Pathol* 13:190, 1982.
3. Sorenson SS: Minor müllerian anomalies and oligomenorrhea in infertile women: A syndrome: Gynecologic and obstetric implications. *Dan Med Bull* 36:248, 1989.
4. Ulfedler H, Robboy SJ: The embryologic development of the human vagina. *Am J Obstet Gynecol* 126:769, 1976.
5. Koff AK: Development of the vagina in the human foetus. *Contrib Embryol Carnegie Inst* 24:59, 1933.
6. Forsberg JG: Cervicovaginal epithelium: Its origin and development. *Am J Obstet Gynecol* 115:1025, 1973.
7. Stern AM, Gall JC, Perry BL, Stimson CW, Weitkamp LR, Poznanski AK: The hand-foot-uterus syndrome. *J Pediatr* 77:109, 1977.
8. Shokeir MHK: Aplasia of the müllerian system: Evidence for probable sex limited anatomical dominant inheritance. *Birth Defects* 14:147, 1978.
9. Polishuk WZ, Ron MA: Familial bicornuate and double uterus. *Am J Obstet Gynecol* 119:982, 1974.
10. Carson SA, Simpson JL, Malinak LR, Elias S, Gerbie AB, Buttram VC Jr, Sarto GE: Heritable aspects of uterine anomalies. II. Genetic analysis of müllerian aplasia. *Fertil Steril* 40:86, 1983.
11. Verp MS, Simpson JL, Elias S, Carson SA, Sarto GE, Feingold M: Heritable aspects of uterine anomalies. I. Three familial aggregates with müllerian fusion anomalies. *Fertil Steril* 40:80, 1983.
12. Elias S, Simpson JL, Carson SA, Malinak LR, Buttram VC Jr: Genetic studies in incomplete müllerian fusion. *Obstet Gynecol* 63:276, 1984.
13. Craig CFT: Congenital abnormalities of the uterus and foetal wastage. *S Afr Med J* 48:2000, 1973.
14. Semmes JP: Congenital defects of the reproductive tract: Clinical implications. *Contemp Obstet Gynecol* 5:95, 1975.
15. Rock JA, Schlaff WD: The obstetric consequences of uterovaginal anomalies. *Fertil Steril* 43:681, 1985.
16. Tulandi T, Arronet GH, McInnes RA: Arcuate and bicornuate uterine anomalies and infertility. *Fertil Steril* 34:362, 1980.
17. Greiss FC Jr, Mauzy CH: Genital anomalies in women. An evaluation of diagnosis, incidence and obstetric performance. *Am J Obstet Gynecol* 82:330, 1961.
18. Green LK, Harris RE: Uterine anomalies. Frequency of diagnosis and associated obstetric complications. *Obstet Gynecol* 47:427, 1976.
19. Williamson JG: True unicornuate uterus. A report of two pregnancies. *Int J Gynaecol Obstet* 11:233, 1973.
20. Andrews MC, Jones HW Jr: Impaired reproductive performance of the unicornuate uterus: Intrauterine growth retardation, fertility, and recurrent abortion in

five cases. *Am J Obstet Gynecol* 144:173, 1982.

21. Woolf RB, Allen WM: Concomitant malformations of the reproductive and urinary tracts. *Obstet Gynecol* 2:236, 1953.
22. Muller P: Association of genital and urinary malformations in women. *Gynecology* 165:285, 1968.
23. Anderson KA, McAninch JW: Uterus didelphia with left hematocolpos and ipsilateral and renal agenesis. *J Urol* 127:550, 1982.
24. Wiersma AF, Peterson LF, Justema EJ: Uterine anomalies associated with unilateral renal agenesis. *Obstet Gynecol* 47:654, 1976.
25. Sayer T, O'Reilly PH: Bicornuate and unicornuate uterus associated with unilateral renal aplasia and abnormal solitary kidneys: Report of 3 cases. *J Urol* 135:110, 1986.
26. Miyazaki Y, Ebisuno S, Uekado Y, Ogawa T, Senzaki A, Ohkawa T: Uterus didelphys with unilateral imperforate vagina and ipsilateral renal agenesis. *J Urol* 135:107, 1986.
27. Gurin J, Leiter E: Associated anomalies of müllerian and wolffian duct structures. *South Med J* 74:805, 1981.
28. Zanetti E, Ferrari LR, Rosi G: Classification and radiologic features of uterine malformations: Hysterosalpingographic study. *Br J Radiol* 51:161, 1978.
29. Buttram VC Jr: Müllerian anomalies and their management. *Fertil Steril* 40:159, 1983.
30. Reuter KL, Daly DC, Cohen SM: Septate versus bicornuate uteri: Errors in imaging diagnosis. *Radiology* 172:749, 1989.
31. Nicolini U, Belloti M, Bonazzi B, Zamberletti D, Candiani GB: Can ultrasound be used to screen uterine malformations? *Fertil Steril* 47:89, 1987.
32. Fedele L, Ferrazzi E, Dorta M, Vercellini P, Candiani GB: Ultrasonography in the differential diagnosis of "double" uteri. *Fertil Steril* 50:361, 1988.
33. Randolph JR, Ying YK, Maier DB, Schmidt CL, Riddick DH: Comparison of real-time ultrasonography, hysterosalpingography, and laparoscopy/hysteroscopy in the evaluation of uterine abnormalities and tubal patency. *Fertil Steril* 46:828, 1986.
34. Mintz MC, Thickman DI, Gussman D, Kressel HY: MR evaluation of uterine anomalies. *AJR* 148:287, 1987.
35. Fedele L, Dorta M, Brioschi D, Massari

C, Candiani GB: Magnetic resonance evaluation of double uteri. *Obstet Gynecol* 74:844, 1989.
36. Lerrerie GS, Wilson J, Miyazawa K: Magnetic resonance imaging of müllerian tract abnormalities. *Fertil Steril* 50:365, 1988.
37. Strassman P: Die operative Vereinigung eines doppleton Uterus. *Zentralbl J Gynak* 31:1322, 1907.
38. Jarcho J: Malformations of the uterus. *Am J Surg* 71:106, 1946.
39. Jones HW: Obstetric significance of female genital anomalies. *Obstet Gynecol* 10:113, 1957.
40. Semmens JP: Congenital anomalies of the female genital tract. Functional classification based on review of 56 personal cases and 500 reported cases. *Obstet Gynecol* 19:328, 1962.
41. Buttram VC Jr, Gibbons WE: Müllerian anomalies: A proposed classification (an analysis of 144 cases). *Fertil Steril* 32:40, 1979.
42. Toaff ME, Lev-Toaff AS, Toaff R: Communicating uteri: Review and classification with introduction of two previously unreported types. *Fertil Steril* 41:661, 1984.
43. Fedele L, Vercellini P, Marchini M, Ricciardiello O, Candiani GB: Communicating uteri: Description and classification of a new type. *Int J Fertil* 33:168, 1988.
44. Katz Z, Bernstein D, Lancet M: Possible causal relationship between mesonephric remnants and infertility of uterine origin. *Int J Fertil* 27:125, 1982.
45. Fedele L, Zamberletti D, Vercellini P, Dorta M, Candiani GB: Reproductive performance of women with unicornuate uterus. *Fertil Steril* 47:416, 1987.
46. Heinonen PK, Pystynen PP: Primary infertility and uterine anomalies. *Fertil Steril* 40:311, 1983.
47. Fedele L, Marchini M, Baglioni A, Carinelli S, Zamberletti D, Candiani GB: Endometrium of cavitary rudimentary horns in unicornuate uteri. *Obstet Gynecol* 75:437, 1990.
48. Ludmir J, Samuels P, Brooks S, Mennuti MT: Pregnancy outcome of patients with uncorrected uterine anomalies managed in a high-risk obstetric setting. *Obstet Gynecol* 75:906, 1990.
49. Fedele L, Zamberletti D, D'Alberton A, Vercellini P, Candiani GB: Gestational aspects of uterus didelphys. *J Reprod Med* 33:353, 1988.

50. Musich JR, Behrman SJ: Obstetric outcome before and after metroplasty in women with uterine anomalies. *Obstet Gynecol* 52:63, 1978.
51. Rock JA, Jones HW Jr. The clinical management of the double uterus. *Fertil Steril* 28:798, 1977.
52. Jones HW Jr, Wheeless CR: Salvage of the reproductive potential of women with anomalous development of the müllerian ducts: 1868–1968–2068. *Am J Obstet Gynecol* 104:348, 1969.
53. Zourlas PA: Surgical treatment of the malformations of the uterus. *Surg Gynecol Obstet* 141:57, 1975.
54. Worthen NJ, Gonzalez F: Septate uterus: Sonographic diagnosis and obstetric complications. *Obstet Gynecol (Suppl)* 64:34S, 1984.
55. Rasmussen PE, Pedersen OD: Metroplasty and fetal survival. *Acta Obstet Gynecol Scand* 66:117, 1987.
56. Muasher SJ, Acosta AA, Garcia JE, Rosenwaks Z, Jones HW Jr: Wedge metroplasty for the septate uterus: An update. *Fertil Steril* 42:515, 1984.
57. McShane PM, Reilly RJ, Schiff I: Pregnancy outcomes following Tompkins metroplasty. *Fertil Steril* 40:190, 1983.
58. DeCherney AH, Russell JB, Graebe RA, Polan ML: Resectoscopic management of müllerian fusion defects. *Fertil Steril* 45:726, 1986.
59. Fayez JA: Comparison between abdominal and hysteroscopic metroplasty. *Obstet Gynecol* 68:399, 1986.
60. March CM, Israel R: Hysteroscopic management of recurrent abortion caused by septate uterus. *Am J Obstet Gynecol* 156:834, 1987.
61. Perino A, Mencaglia L, Hamou J, Cittadini E: Hysteroscopy for metroplasty of uterine septa: Report of 24 cases. *Fertil Steril* 48:321, 1987.
62. Rock JA, Murphy AA, Cooper WH IV: Resectoscopic techniques for the lysis of a class V: Complete uterine septum. *Fertil Steril* 48:495, 1987.
63. Hallez JP, Netter A, Cartier R: Methodical intrauterine resection. *Am J Obstet Gynecol* 156:1080, 1987.
64. Daly DC, Maier D, Soto-Albors C: Hysteroscopic metroplasty: Six year's experience. *Obstet Gynecol* 73:201, 1989.
65. Fedele L, Dorta M, Brioschi D, Guidici MN, Candiani GB: Pregnancies in septate uteri: Outcome in relation to site of uterine implantation as determined by sonography. *AJR* 152:781, 1989.

5

Diethylstilbestrol Exposure in Utero

Both the specialist in infertility and the radiologist will encounter at hysterosalpingography the anomalies of the uterine cervix, corpus, and tubes associated with diethylstilbestrol (DES) exposure in utero. This synthetic estrogen was administered to pregnant women for almost 25 years, beginning about 1948, for the indications of recurrent miscarriage, hypertension, diabetes mellitus, threatened abortion, previous stillbirth, and/or premature labor. Usage of DES was at its peak in the early 1950s and declined abruptly after 1971, when an association was observed between the administration of DES during pregnancy and the subsequent development years later of a clear-cell adenocarcinoma of the vagina in the female offspring exposed in utero (1–3). It is estimated that at least 2 million women were exposed to DES (4). Various structural and cytologic abnormalities of the reproductive system have since been described and characterized (5–10). A brief description of normal vaginal embryogenesis is necessary to understand the development of these abnormalities (11–14).

EMBRYOLOGIC DEVELOPMENT OF THE HUMAN VAGINA

Tissue of the müllerian and wolffian ducts and the urogenital sinus are required for normal vaginal and cervical development (15). At 4 weeks of embryonic life, the paired müllerian (paramesonephric) duct system forms an invagination of celomic epithelium in the urogenital fold just lateral to the cranial end of the mesonephric ducts. As development proceeds, the paired müllerian ducts meet at the midline and then grow caudally to reach the urogenital sinus of future hymen at 7 weeks of gestational age. The paired ducts then fuse. The septum formed by the fusion disappears both caudally and cranially, resulting in the formation of a single cavity, the uterovaginal canal, lined by columnar epithelium. Beginning at about the 10th week of gestation, squamous epithelium derived from the urogenital sinus invades the distal end of the uterovaginal canal from below and extends cranially, uniformly displacing the columnar müllerian epithelium to the level of the future external cervical os. The vagina, which is initially lined by simple columnar epithelium, acquires a stratified squamous epithelium, a process that is completed by the 18th week of gestation.

Robboy (16, 17) and others (13, 18) have shown that mesenchyme in the developing cervix has inductive functions with respect to overlying epithelial cells. Epithelial cell growth and differentiations are regulated by interactions with the stroma, and the cell type produced is dependent on the stromal site at which it is located. Normal müllerian duct stroma, probably by producing a "stromal inductive factor," is capable of inducing the development of a columnar epithelium that later differentiates into the adult-type tuboendometrial lining. The squamous epithelium of urogenital sinus origin, which lines the vagina and future exocervix, is impervious to any inductive stimulus to differentiate into glandular cells and therefore remains a squamous layer of cells.

In the 14th week postovulation the cervical wall thickens, and the vaginal fornices form from the vaginal plate a week later. The muscular wall of the uterus is completely developed by 26 weeks postovulation. In the DES-exposed fetus, the estrogen causes derangement of the formation of the two mesenchymal layers. DES administered during the time of differentiation of the cervix and vagina will induce deformities (Figs. 5.1, 5.2, and 5.3). The layers fail to segregate, becoming clinically manifest in the young adult as stromal hyperplasia (ridges), hypoplasia (hypoplastic fornices), or an abnormally contoured uterine cavity (revealed by an abnormal hysterosalpingogram). The superficial stroma in the region of the future cervix splays centrifugally, causing an unusually wide zone of mucinous epithelium that surrounds the anatomic portio vaginalis and upper vagina. The DES-exposed vaginal mesenchyme impedes further upward growth of squamous cells of urogenital sinus origin. Vaginal adenosis, defined as the occurrence of columnar epithelium in the vagina, develops prenatally when the müllerian columnar epithelium of the upper vagina fails to transform its squamous epithelium, and is observed in 70 to 75% of women exposed in utero to DES (13); it is estimated that *all* women exposed have adenosis, but that detection and diagnosis are incomplete. Thus, the normal sequence of developmental events is deranged, resulting in characteristic physical, anatomic, and histologic changes. Malformations of the cervix and vagina are seen in 25 to 50% of DES-exposed daughters, the percentage varying with the time during pregnancy of exposure and with the dose and duration of administration. DES exposure in very early pregnancy and after 22 weeks gestational age is unlikely to cause structural abnormalities.

CLINICAL FINDINGS

Examination of the vagina and cervix is frequently diagnostic of DES exposure. The squamocolumnar junction is displaced caudad from its ordinary site just within the external cervical os to varying levels of the vaginal canal (Fig. 5.1). Columnar epithelium on the outer cervix and upper vagina has the appearance of a wet, mucinous, inflamed surface, which exudes mucoid material and bleeds easily (Fig. 5.2).

Structural abnormalities of the cervix and vagina are noted in such women with varying frequency and severity. Cervical hypoplasia, cervical pseudopolyps, and a transverse or circumferential ridge, the so-called cockscomb or cervical hood, have been described (Fig. 5.3). Marked cervical stenosis may occur, and a pinpoint cervical os may be difficult to cannulate with the Kidde cannula or other hysterosalpingographic equipment. The os may be completely obscured by a cervical hood that folds over like a shelf, and the whole area may be so friable that persistent probing to find the os may result in significant bleeding. Islands of reddish tissue, which are identified as vaginal adenosis, may be observed on the vaginal walls in some women.

Abnormalities of the cavity of the uterus or the fallopian tubes are found in two-thirds or more of DES-exposed

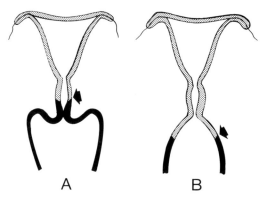

A   B

Figure 5.1. A, Diagram demonstrating the squamocolumnar junction (*arrow*) in a normal position above the external cervical os. **B,** Squamocolumnar junction (*arrow*) displaced caudally and located on the cervix or within the vagina in a patient exposed in utero to DES.

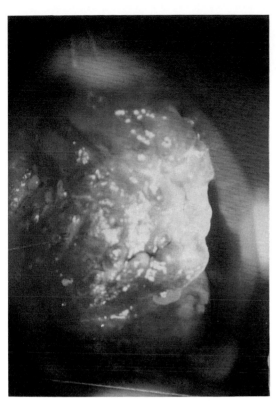

Figure 5.2. Columnar epithelium arranged in a cockscomb pattern, obscuring the external cervical os. This epithelium is extremely friable and bleeds readily on touch.

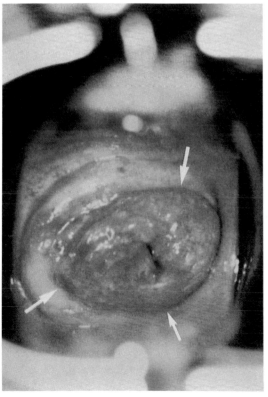

Figure 5.3. The displacement of the normal stratified squamous epithelium of the cervix by the columnar epithelium is shown. The squamocolumnar junction (*arrows*) is displaced out onto the cervix for a so-called collar. Although the external cervical os is easily visible, this area is friable and will bleed easily. (Courtesy of H. W. Jones III, M.D., Nashville, TN.)

Figure 5.4. Surgical specimen of a DES uterus, opened to show the T-shaped irregularity of the cavity.

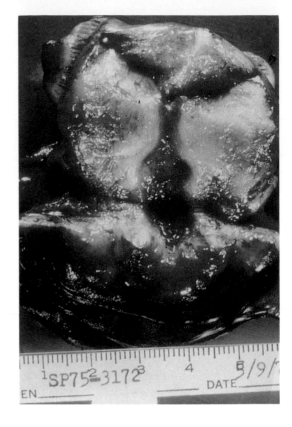

women (Fig. 5.4) (19, 20). Up to 50% of exposed women may have gross structural abnormalities of the cervix and vagina, including ridges, hoods, and cockscombs. Of those with uterine anomalies, many will have associated cervical and vaginal changes. Over three-quarters of women with cervical anomalies will be found at hysterosalpingography to have uterine defects. On the other hand, over 50% of exposed women *without* cervical anomalies had uterine abnormalities, verifying the need for hysterosalpingography in all DES-exposed women, not just those with cervical abnormalities. The occurrence of clear cell adenocarcinoma of the vagina has been noted in this population of women, and in fact directed much attention to the study of this abnormality. Fortunately, the incidence of this otherwise rare vaginal neoplasm is relatively low, 0.14 to 1.4 per 1000 exposed (2), and it remains an unusual tumor.

However, it is estimated that 100% of exposed women have vaginal adenosis.

Surprisingly, the anatomic findings in DES-exposed women may change with time and are not necessarily permanent (21, 22). Of women initially described as having a cervicovaginal hood, about one-half had a decrease in its size and one-quarter had complete disappearance of the hood over 5 years of observation. The longer the follow-up period, the greater the extent of resolution of these lesions.

FINDINGS ON HYSTEROSALPINGOGRAPHY

The upper genital tract abnormalities in the DES-exposed woman are distinctive and were observed in 376 of 632 women (59%) undergoing hysterosalpingography (19). The classic hysterosalpingographic finding is a T-shaped uterus that is characterized by a small endome-

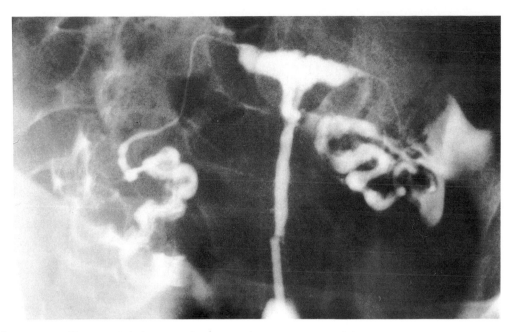

Figure 5.5. Characteristic hysterosalpingographic appearance of the uterus in a woman exposed to DES in utero. Note the T-shaped configuration, the very long endocervical canal, and the lumpy and irregular contour to the endometrial cavity.

trial cavity, shortened upper uterine segment, and narrow endocervical canal (Fig. 5.5 and Table 5.1). In addition, the endometrial cavity may be lumpy and irregular, rather than smooth and symmetrical (Figs. 5.6 through 5.11). The external configuration of the uterus at laparoscopy may remain entirely within normal limits, or there may be varying degrees of severity of malformation. The fallopian tubes may also exhibit abnormalities, but these are only observed externally at laparoscopy. A unique tubal morphologic feature consisting of a foreshortened, convoluted tube with a "withered" fimbria and pinpoint fimbrial opening has been described (9), but the fimbrial abnormality and tubal shortening cannot be distinguished at hysterosalpingography. In terms of size, the cavity of the uterus is usually compromised, and the area of the endometrial cavity, length of the upper uterine segment, and diameter of the endocervical canal are all significantly smaller in the DES-exposed group (6).

The urinary tract appears to have been spared abnormalities of development, and DES-exposed women with upper genital tract abnormalities seen on hysterosalpingograms have no increase in urinary tract abnormalities seen on intravenous pyelograms compared to a control population.

Table 5.1. Hysterosalpingographic Changes in DES-exposed Women

A T-shaped uterus with bulbous cornual extensions arising from the upper end of the uterine cavity.
Lumpy, irregular appearance of the walls of the uterine cavity.
Hypoplastic uterus.
Relatively long endocervical canal.
Narrowed lower two-thirds of the uterine cavity.
Band-like constrictions causing narrowing of the interstitial tubal segments.

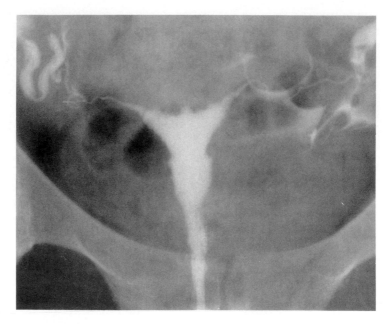

Figure 5.6.   Typical T-shaped uterus with characteristic lumpy configuration. There is considerable symmetry of contour, not an unusual characteristic.

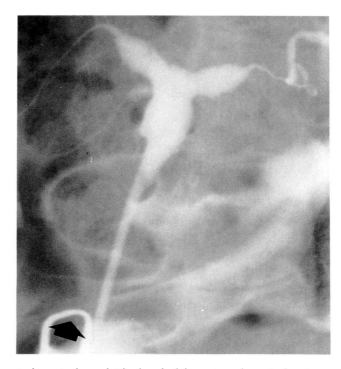

Figure 5.7.   Elongated cervical canal. The level of the external cervical os is recognized by the position of the tenaculum (*arrow*). Note the lumpiness of the endometrial cavity.

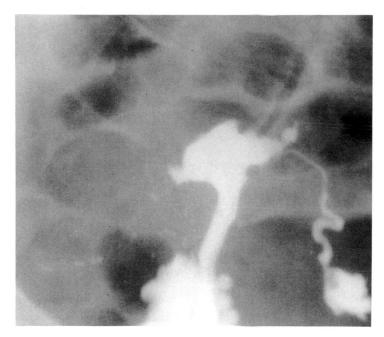

Figure 5.8. Use of oil-soluble rather than water-soluble contrast material slightly alters the sharpness of contour of the endometrial cavity. Otherwise the characteristic appearance is unchanged.

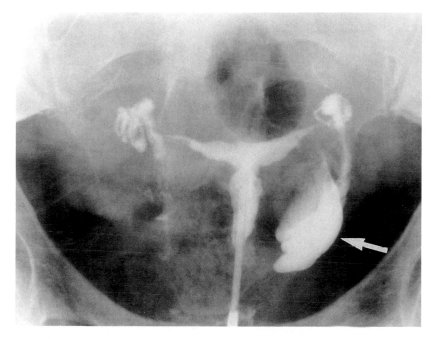

Figure 5.9. T-shaped uterine cavity. This is the typical configuration for intrauterine DES exposure. There is an unrelated coincidental hydrosalpinx on the left (*arrow*).

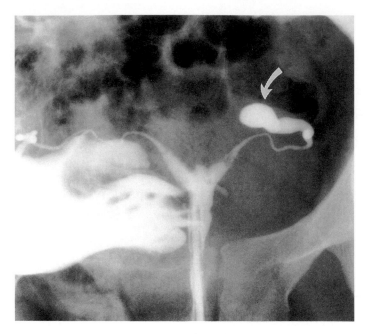

Figure 5.10. DES exposure characterized by the long endocervical canal and a lumpy configuration to the endometrial cavity. The bicornuate configuration, an anomalous variant unrelated to the diethylstilbestrol exposure, alters the characteristic T-shaped pattern. There is a coincidental hydrosalpinx on the left (*arrow*).

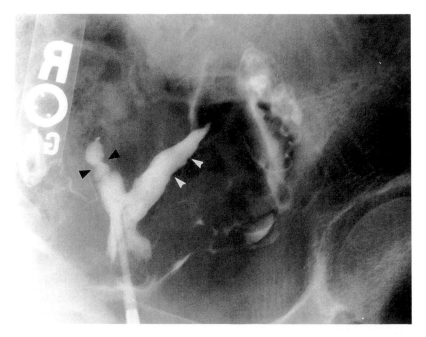

Figure 5.11. Documented history of maternal exposure to diethylstilbestrol during the first trimester of pregnancy. The only stigma of DES exposure seen on the hysterosalpingogram is the very lumpy configuration of the endometrial cavity (*arrowheads*). The bicornuate configuration is an unrelated müllerian variation.

FERTILITY OF DES-EXPOSED WOMEN

Conflicting reports have been published concerning the fertility of DES-exposed women (19, 20, 22–39). Cousins et al. (27) did not observe any differences in the incidence of pregnancy, mean number of pregnancies, or frequency of infertility problems, ectopic pregnancy, or spontaneous abortion between 71 DES-exposed women and 69 nonexposed women; the majority of other investigators dispute these findings in the early pregnancy group. On the other hand, there is general agreement that late pregnancy complications, including low birth weight, short gestation, toxemia, breech presentation, premature rupture of the membranes, and perinatal death are all increased in the group with obvious changes (39). Herbst and associates (26), studying sexually active women who did not practice contraception, found an 86% conception rate in controls versus 67% in DES daughters. Herbst also found that twice as many exposed as unexposed women had tried unsuccessfully to become pregnant for at least 1 year. Mangan et al. (33) reported that DES daughters achieved a lower percentage of desired pregnancies than did controls. Barnes et al. (28), conversely, compared 618 subjects who had prenatal exposure to DES with 618 control subjects and found that fertility measured in terms of occurrence of pregnancy did not differ between the exposed women and the controls. It is difficult to come to one conclusion concerning the fertility of DES-exposed women, because many factors must be considered. Patient populations and the intensity of DES administration vary. Use of control groups and even definitions of pregnancy differ between investigators. There is no one answer, but, clearly,

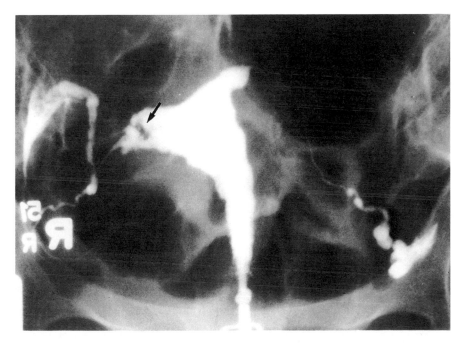

Figure 5.12. Known DES exposure in a multiparous patient. The lumpy and irregular configuration of the endometrial cavity is considered typical. The relatively normal size and overall shape of the cavity may well be a reflection of the previous pregnancies. Note the small synechia in the right cornua (*arrow*).

there is concern about the reproductive outcome in these women.

An increased risk of an unfavorable outcome of pregnancy is associated with DES exposure. Among DES-exposed women who become pregnant, 81% had at least one full-term live birth (Fig. 5.12) (28), compared to 95% for unexposed women. Spontaneous abortion, ectopic pregnancy, incompetent cervix, and premature labor occur significantly more often in the DES-exposed population than in normal controls, as discussed above.

DES-exposed women have infertility or pregnancy complications due to other causes, and DES exposure should not be an excuse to postpone or delay the definitive infertility investigation. Stillman and Miller (35, 37) reported that 50% of DES-exposed infertile women also had endometriosis, not substantially different from the 39% incidence in non–DES-exposed women, suggesting that endometriosis should be considered in the infertility evaluation and laparoscopy included for definitive diagnosis. Cervical stenosis was identified in 25% of all DES-exposed patients and could potentially provide an additional diagnosis explaining infertility. Indeed, the incidence of abnormalities unrelated to DES exposure is significant. This would suggest that, in many cases, the presence of these women in infertility groups is due to pathology other than DES exposure.

CONCLUSION

DES exposure is associated with some degree of infertility, fetal wastage, and pregnancy complications. More severe degrees of abnormality appear to be associated with a greater likelihood of reproductive dysfunction. Hysterosalpingography has an important role in elucidating the various degrees of abnormality.

REFERENCES

1. Herbst AL, Ulfelder H, Poskanzer DC: Adenocarcinoma of the vagina: Association of maternal stilbestrol therapy with tumor appearance in young women. *N Engl J Med* 284:878, 1971.
2. Herbst AL, Poskanzer DC, Robboy SJ, et al.: Prenatal exposure to stilbestrol: A prospective comparison of exposed female offspring with unexposed controls. *N Engl J Med* 292:334, 1975.
3. Burke L, Antonioli D, Rosen S: Vaginal and cervical squamous cell dysplasia in women exposed to diethylstilbestrol in utero. *Am J Obstet Gynecol* 132:537, 1978.
4. Senekjian E: Reproductive function in DES-exposed women. *The Female Patient* 13:12, 1988.
5. Kaufman RH, Binder GL, Gray PM Jr, Adam E: Upper genital tract changes associated with exposure in utero to diethylstilbestrol. *Am J Obstet Gynecol* 128:51, 1977.
6. Haney AF, Hammond CB, Soules MR, Creasman WT: Diethylstilbestrol-induced upper genital tract abnormalities. *Fertil Steril* 31:142, 1979.
7. Kaufman RH, Adam E, Grey MP, Gerthoffer E: Urinary tract changes associated with exposure in utero to diethylstilbestrol. *Obstet Gynecol* 56:330, 1980.
8. Ben-Baruch G, Menczer J, Mashiach S, Serr DM: Uterine anomalies in diethylstilbestrol-exposed women with fertility disorders. *Acta Obstet Gynecol Scand* 60:395, 1981.
9. DeCherney AH, Cholst I, Naftolin F: Structure and function of the fallopian tubes following exposure to diethylstilbestrol (DES) during gestation. *Fertil Steril* 36:741, 1981.
10. Jeffries JA, Robboy SJ, O'Brien PC, et al.: Structural anomalies of the cervix and vagina in women enrolled in the Diethylstilbestrol Adenosis (DESAD) Project. *Am J Obstet Gynecol* 148:59, 1976.
11. Prins RP, Morrow CP, Townsend DE, DiSaia PJ: Vaginal embryogenesis, estrogens, and adenosis. *Obstet Gynecol* 48:246, 1976.
12. Ulfelder H, Robboy SJ: The embryologic development of the human vagina. *Am J Obstet Gynecol* 126:769, 1976.
13. Forsberg JG: Permanent changes induced by DES at critical stages in female development: 10-year experience from

human and model systems. *Biol Res Pregnancy* 2:168, 1981.

14. Barter JF, Orr JW, Hatch KD, Shingleton HM: Diethylstilbestrol in pregnancy: An update. *South Med J* 79:1531, 1986.
15. Barber HRK: An update on DES in the field of reproduction. *Int J Fertil* 31:130, 1986.
16. Robboy SJ, Taguchi O, Cunha GR: Normal development of the human female reproductive tract and alterations resulting from experimental exposure to diethylstilbestrol. *Hum Pathol* 13:190, 1982.
17. Robboy SJ: A hypothetical mechanism of diethylstilbestrol (DES)-induced anomalies in exposed progeny. *Hum Pathol* 14:831, 1983.
18. Roberts DK, Walker NJ, Parmley TH, Horbelt DV: Interaction of epithelial and stromal cells in vaginal adenosis. *Hum Pathol* 19:855, 1988.
19. Kaufman RH, Adam E, Noller K, Irwin JF, Gray M: Upper genital tract changes and infertility in diethylstilbestrol exposed women. *Am J Obstet Gynecol* 154:1312, 1986.
20. Kaufman RH, Noller K, Adam E, Irwin J, Gray M, Jeffries JA, Hilton J: Upper genital tract abnormalities and pregnancy outcome in diethylstilbestrol-exposed progeny. *Am J Obstet Gynecol* 148:973, 1984.
21. Antonioli DA, Burke L, Friedman EA: Natural history of diethylstilbestrol-associated genital tract lesions: Cervical ectopy and cervicovaginal hood. *Am J Obstet Gynecol* 137:847, 1980.
22. Herbst AL, Hubby MM, Azizi F, Makii MM: Reproductive and gynecologic surgical experience in diethylstilbestrol-exposed daughters. *Am J Obstet Gynecol* 141:1019, 1981.
23. Siegler AM, Wang CF, Friberg J: Fertility of the diethylstilbestrol-exposed offspring. *Fertil Steril* 31:601, 1979.
24. Berger MJ, Goldstein P: Impaired reproductive performance in DES-exposed women. *Obstet Gynecol* 55:25, 1980.
25. Schmidt G, Fowler WC Jr, Talbert LM, Edelman DA: Reproductive history of women exposed to diethylstilbestrol in utero. *Fertil Steril* 33:21, 1980.
26. Herbst AL, Hubby MM, Blough RR, Azizi F: A comparison of pregnancy experience in DES-exposed and DES-unexposed daughters. *J Reprod Med* 24:62, 1980.

27. Cousins J, Karp W, Lacey C, Lucas WE: Reproductive outcome of women exposed to diethylstilbestrol in utero. *Obstet Gynecol* 56:70, 1980.
28. Barnes AB, Colton T, Gunderson J, et al.: Fertility and outcome of pregnancy in women exposed in utero to diethylstilbestrol. *N Engl J Med* 302:609, 1980.
29. Rosenfeld DL, Bronson RA: Reproductive problems in the DES-exposed female. *Obstet Gynecol* 55:453, 1980.
30. Pillsbury SG Jr: Reproductive significance of changes in the endometrial cavity associated with exposure in utero to diethylstilbestrol. *Am J Obstet Gynecol* 137:178, 1980.
31. Veridiana NP, Delke I, Rogers J, Tancer ML: Reproductive performance of DES-exposed female progeny. *Obstet Gynecol* 58:58, 1981.
32. Sandberg EC, Riffle NL, Higdon JV, Getman CE: Pregnancy outcome in women exposed to diethylstilbestrol in utero. *Am J Obstet Gynecol* 140:194, 1981.
33. Mangan CE, Borow L, Burtnett-Rubin MM, Egan V, Guintoli RL, Mikuta JJ: Pregnancy outcome in 98 women exposed to diethylstilbestrol in utero, their mothers, and unexposed siblings. *Obstet Gynecol* 59:315, 1982.
34. Mansi ML, Goldfarb AF: An analysis of pregnancy salvage in a selective DES population. *Infertility* 5:1, 1982.
35. Stillman RJ: In utero exposure to diethylstilbestrol: An adverse effect on the reproductive tract and reproductive performance in male and female offspring. *Am J Obstet Gynecol* 142:905, 1982.
36. Bibbo M, Gill WB, Azizi F, et al.: Follow-up study of male and female offspring of DES-exposed mothers. *Obstet Gynecol* 49:1, 1977.
37. Stillman RJ, Miller LRC: Diethylstilbestrol exposure in utero and endometriosis in infertile females. *Fertil Steril* 4:369, 1984.
38. Menczer J, Dulitsky M, Ben-Baruch G, Modan M: Primary infertility in women exposed to diethylstilbestrol in utero. *Br J Obstet Gynaecol* 93:503, 1986.
39. Senekjian EK, Potkul RK, Frey K, Herbst AL: Infertility among daughters either exposed or not exposed to diethylstilbestrol. *Am J Obstet Gynecol* 158:493, 1988.

6

The Uterine Cavity

The uterine cavity is a potential space, defined cephalad by the fundus and caudally by the external cervical os. Anatomically, it is readily subdivided by the internal cervical os into the endometrial cavity and the endocervical canal. Considerable normal variation in both dimensions and configuration may be encountered. Varying degrees of traction on the tenaculum during hysterosalpingography will also change these measurements. Increasing amounts of contrast media introduced into the cavity may expand it considerably. Furthermore, both uterine size and length of the cavity may vary with hormonal stimulation, correlating in a positive relationship with circulating estradiol levels. Measurements taken from radiographic films to estimate cavity size are subject to both radiologic and geometric distortion and magnification; therefore, measurements from films should not be used to define normal limits. The introduction of up to 2.0 ml of contrast medium will usually fill the uterine cavity. There is usually no significant discomfort until at least 1.5 ml has been introduced. Whether the pain is due to the volume or simply to the irritating stimulus of the contrast material, which induces uterine cramping, is unclear; almost all women will have marked cramping if 3.0 ml or more of contrast medium is introduced.

The endometrium, being soft and spongy, may be compressed by pressure from introduced contrast material, so hysterosalpingography may not differentiate abnormalities such as hyperplasia or atrophy, although the appearance of the cavity may vary with the phase of the menstrual cycle. On the other hand, if hysterosalpingography is performed late in the luteal phase of the menstrual cycle, the increased thickness of the endometrial lining of the cavity may obstruct the entrance of contrast medium into the fallopian tubes. This is yet another reason why hysterosalpingography should be performed only in the follicular part of the cycle. Further, hysterosalpingography during the secretory phase may result in an appearance of pseudo-pregnancy, as the contrast outlines a "ring" around the margin of the uterine cavity. Endometrial abnormalities can be detected only if they are of sufficient size to distort the uterine cavity or if they present as a mass displacing the contrast medium. They are visualized as either filling defects, outpouchings, or irregularities of contour.

Abnormalities of the uterine cavity that are diagnosed by hysterosalpingography include lesions of the endometrium, such as neoplasms, infoldings, and intrauterine synechiae; abnormalities of the myometrium, including submucous and intramural myomata; space-occupying masses and foreign bodies within the cavity; and congenital anomalies of müllerian development as discussed in Chapter 4.

FILLING DEFECTS

Spurious Artifacts

Intrauterine abnormalities often present as filling defects. The most common are spurious artifacts such as air bubbles or displaced cervical mucus (Fig. 6.1). Bubbles are seen as solitary or multiple round mobile defects and may be avoided, in large measure, by carefully

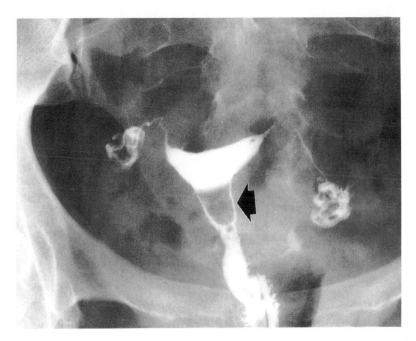

Figure 6.1. Large radiolucent filling defect (*arrow*) in the uterine cavity due to an air bubble. Subsequent films showed disappearance of this mobile lucency.

filling the introducing instrument with contrast medium prior to initiating the procedure. Fluoroscopic observation of movement of the rounded defect(s) establishes the diagnosis. Pulling back on the plunger of the syringe containing the contrast material may help dislodge a stubborn air bubble, result in motion, and allow it to be differentiated from a polyp. Rotating the patient is another trick to get an air bubble to move.

Cervical mucus pushed retrograde through the uterine cavity may also appear as a mobile filling defect. It appears as an amorphous mass, often linear in shape without clear margins or rounded contour. Blood clots, due either to preexisting bleeding or the trauma of the instrumentation, are another unlikely but possible cause of such mobile filling artifacts.

Polyps

Persistent filling defects can be caused by polyps, which give a rounded or sessile pattern (Fig. 6.2). Small polyps may be completely obscured by contrast medium, so care must be taken to inspect the configuration of the cavity as contrast material is introduced (Fig. 6.3). Polyps may be single or multiple, pedunculated or sessile, and are distinguished from synechiae by their more rounded and regular appearance (Fig. 6.4). Although their size varies, the overwhelming majority of these lesions are smaller than 1 cm in diameter. A recent case at hysterosalpingography had the appearance of multiple grape-like filling defects; at hysteroscopy, the operator likened the appearance to moguls, or humps, on a ski slope (Fig. 6.5). The appearance of multiple polyps, if of relatively uniform size, may be inseparable from polypoid hyperplasia. Perhaps they represent entities of a common spectrum. Occasionally, small filling defects, presumed to be polyps, may be seen in the fallopian tubes (Fig. 6.6) (see Chapter 9).

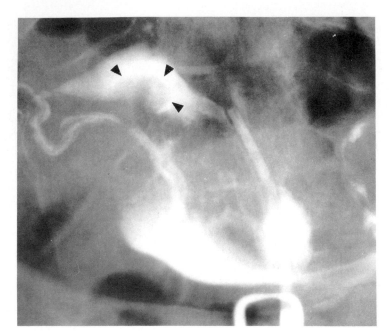

Figure 6.2. Solitary large-cell endometrial polyp (*arrowheads*).

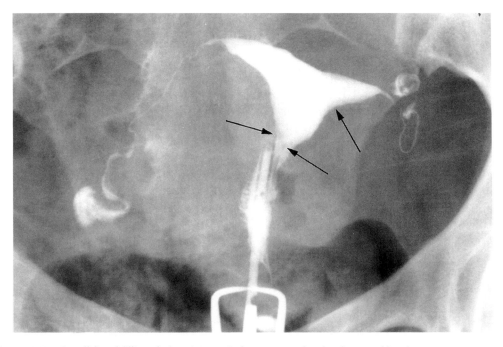

Figure 6.3. Small fixed filling defect (*arrows*) almost completely obscured by the contrast material.

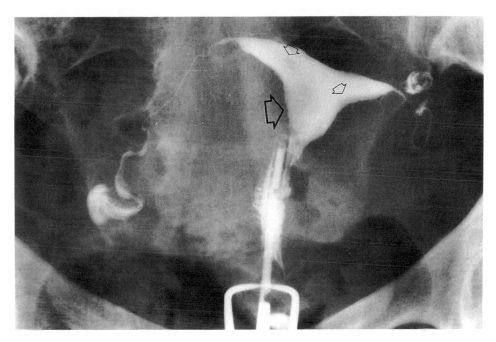

Figure 6.4. Same patient as in Figure 6.3. Reduction in the quantity of contrast material allows demonstration of multiple endometrial polyps of varying size and configuration (*arrows*).

Malignant Neoplasms

Hysterography was first used in the 1950s as a simple, reliable diagnostic technique for menopausal women with abnormal bleeding in whom the diagnosis of cervical cancer had been eliminated (1, 2). A normal uterine cavity was thought to rule out endometrial carcinoma, whereas characteristics defects allowed a presumptive diagnosis permitting hysterectomy without intervening curettage. Endometrial cancer seen on hysterography in this setting was divided into several types: (*a*) a single growth in the fundus; (*b*) multiple circumscribed growths; (*c*) surface, diffuse, or spreading growths (Fig. 6.7); (*d*) total involvement of the uterine cavity (Fig. 6.8); and (*e*) endometrial cancer coexisting with myomata.

The appearance of diagnosed endometrial cancer before and after radiation treatment was described in early studies (3, 4). In the 1970s, routine use of hysterography was recommended to identify the depth of myometrial invasion and endocervical extension of cancer (5–7), but in general the technique became replaced in the evaluation of uterine neoplasms. More recently, there has been a resurgence of interest. Stock and Gallup (8) reported the hysterographic findings in 91 patients with suspected uterine cancer and concluded that the technique was useful to differentiate between benign and malignant lesions, to diagnose endocervical involvement, to predict the depth of myometrial invasion, and to differentiate between patients at least and greatest risk to modify patient management. The possibility that such a diagnostic procedure could encourage dissemination needs to be considered and should be weighed against any perceived advantage.

Malignant neoplasms are rarely found when hysterosalpingography is performed as part of the infertility evaluation. However, it is important to know that 1 to 8% of patients with endometrial

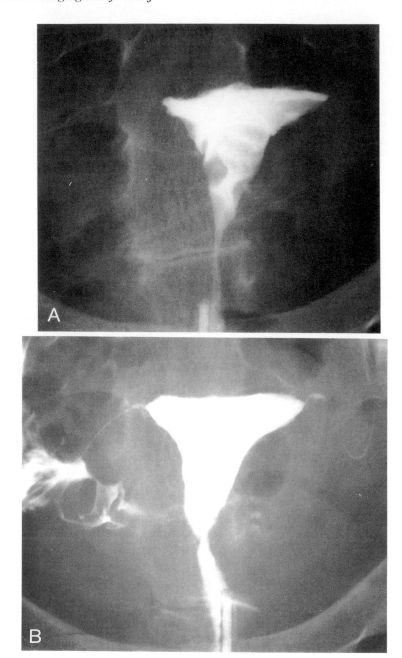

Figure 6.5.   A, Multiple endometrial polyps of varying size and configuration. **B,** Same patient after hysterography with resection and curettage.

adenocarcinoma are under the age of 40 and that these women have anovulation and infertility. Filling defects or intra-uterine adhesions found in such cases have been diagnosed to be endometrial carcinoma (9, 10).

Benign Neoplasms

Filling defects due to *myomata uteri* are usually distinctive. As myomata enlarge, they can stretch and deform the cavity into bizarre configurations, often

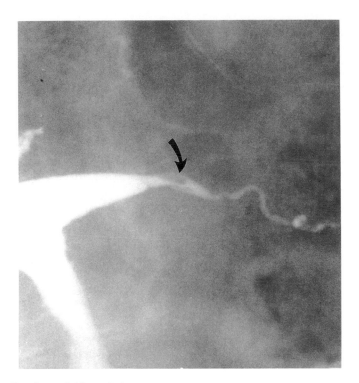

Figure 6.6. Small polypoid filling defects are occasionally seen in the proximal portion of the fallopian tubes (*arrow*).

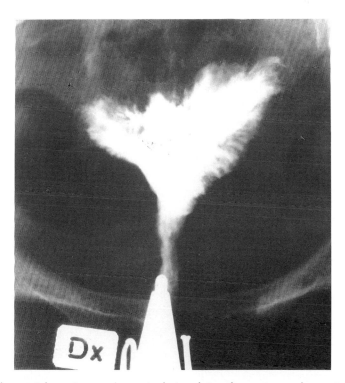

Figure 6.7. Endometrial carcinoma extensively involving the entire endometrial cavity with diffuse infiltration and irregular filling defects. (Courtesy of Leif Ekelund, Lund, Sweden.)

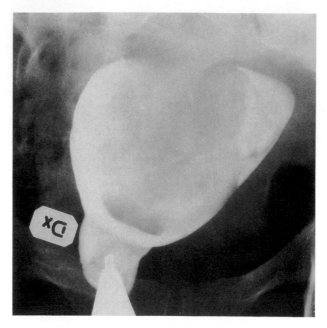

Figure 6.8.   Endometrial carcinoma presenting as a large irregular filling defect filling virtually the entire endometrial cavity. (Courtesy of Leif Ekelund, Lund, Sweden.)

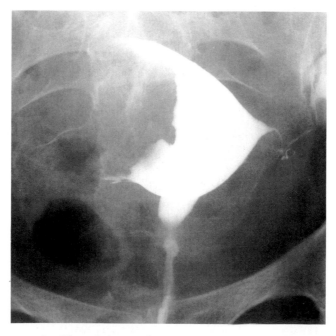

Figure 6.9.   Large irregular filling defect in the uterine cavity due to fibromyoma. In addition to deformation of the uterine cavity there is cavity enlargement and failure to fill the right fallopian tube.

eliminating usual landmarks (Figs. 6.9 and 6.10). Such distortion may induce crescentic or semilunar contours as contrast outlines the misshapen cavity (Fig. 6.11). A unique capability of myomata is to enlarge the uterine cavity markedly, probably relating to the intramural position of the tumor or tumors. On occasion, quantities of contrast material exceeding 30 ml may be introduced into the cavity without complete filling (Fig. 6.12).

A myoma located in the cornual area may cause a mechanical block and make it impossible to introduce contrast media into the fallopian tubes. Fibromyomata may demonstrate a relatively typical pattern of coarse calcifications (Fig. 6.13). A fundal location of a myomata may at times create an unusual pattern suggestive of congenital septum formation (Fig. 6.14). Large uterine myomata have variable appearances with contour distortion or asymmetric filling defects. Foci of calcifications may be present (11, 12). If degeneration and necrosis have occurred, cystic changes, best appreciated by sonography, may be noted. We have noted that local intravasation of contrast material sometimes occurs during visualization of a myoma (Fig. 6.15) (13). This may reflect such focal degeneration. Small fibroids may have the appearance of endometrial polyps, particularly if the neoplasm is pedunculated. Under these circumstances, hysteroscopy is necessary for definitive diagnosis (14).

Approaches to treatment of myomata have undergone change. Previously, symptomatic myomata have been surgically treated by hysterectomy or myomectomy, or resected at hysteroscopy. In recent years, agonist analogs of

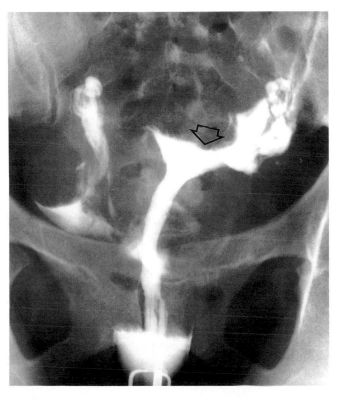

Figure 6.10. Multiple fibromyomata resulting in stretching and elongation of the cervical canal and lower uterine segment. There is minimal irregularity along the fundus (*arrow*) secondary to a myoma in this location.

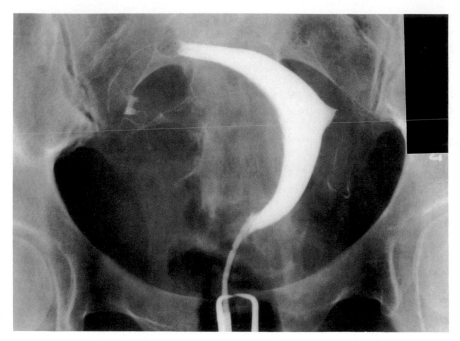

Figure 6.11. Markedly enlarged uterine cavity distorted by a large fibromyomata along the right lateral margin of the endometrial cavity. The resultant cavity is crescentic in contour.

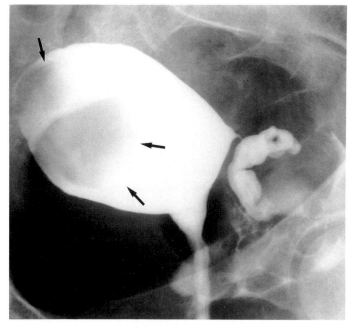

Figure 6.12. Marked stretching of the endometrial cavity by fibromyomata. More than 30 ml of contrast medium was introduced into the cavity. The large filling defect (*arrows*) is the result of indentation of the lumen by the large myoma.

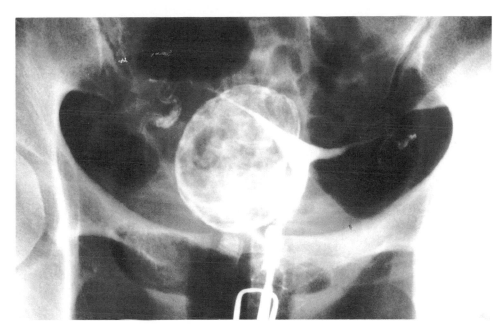

Figure 6.13. Large calcified fibromyomata indenting and deforming the endometrial cavity. This coarse, calcified pattern is relatively typical for fibromyomata.

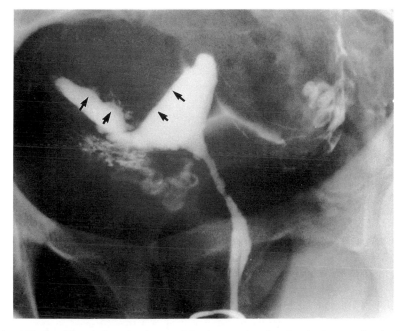

Figure 6.14. Wedge-like deformity (*arrows*) in the uterine fundus is the result of a large solitary myoma. The configuration is somewhat suggestive of congenital septum formation.

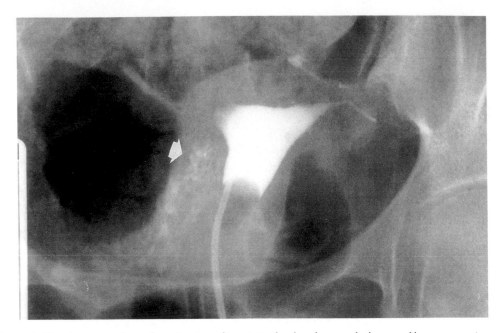

Figure 6.15.   Intravasation of contrast medium into the focal area of a known fibromyoma (*arrow*).

gonadotropin-releasing hormone have been used to cause shrinkage of myomata, decreased uterine volume, restoration of tubal patency (15) and decreased uterine bleeding, either as primary treatment alone or as a preoperative adjunct to myomectomy (16, 17). Post-treatment hysterosalpingography is useful under either circumstance to evaluate the uterine cavity and tubal patency. The size of the cavity decreased 5 to 18% in 19 of 20 patients over 8 weeks of treatment (18).

Pregnancy

Although hysterosalpingography is usually done only in the follicular part of the cycle, some patients may not be taking basal temperature charts and may mistake spotting in early pregnancy for a menstrual period. For this reason, inadvertent hysterosalpingography in the presence of pregnancy occasionally occurs. A pregnancy may have the appearance of a sessile polyp or, at later stages, appear as a large filling defect (Fig. 6.16).

Isaacs (19) has reported a characteristic but most unusual pattern, a double outline sign, caused by infiltration of contrast media into the decidua. As previously stated, this may be mimicked by a normal study during the secretory phase (Fig. 6.17).

The question of both traumatic and radiation injury to the pregnancy then arises. Miscarriage due to the instrumentation may result, with the usual bleeding and cramping. However, if the pregnancy continues, one must determine the appropriate course of action. Is termination of pregnancy warranted because of the radiation incurred during the hysterosalpingogram? Some have suggested that radiation exposure of more than 10 rads to the fetus in the first 6 weeks of pregnancy warrants therapeutic abortion (20). Current opinion, on the other hand, estimates that risk of congenital anomalies increases only from 1 to 3% following radiation exposure of up to 15 rads in the first trimester (21). As mentioned in Chapter 2, estimates of gonadal radiation dosage vary but certainly seem less than

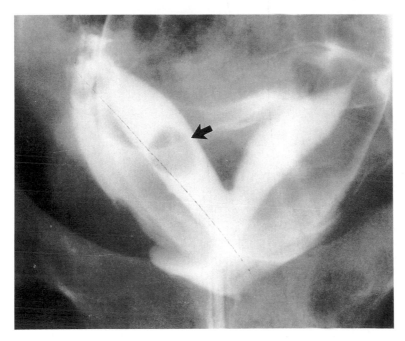

Figure 6.16. Bicornuate uterus with a discrete large filling defect in the right horn, subsequently demonstrated to be an intrauterine pregnancy.

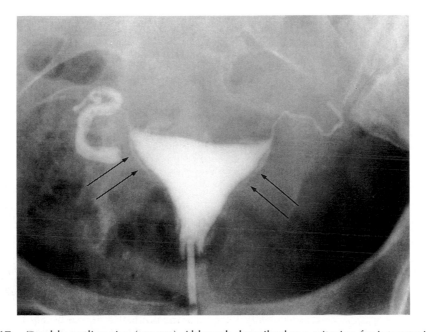

Figure 6.17. Double outline sign (*arrows*). Although described as a criterion for intrauterine pregnancy, this may also occur in the normal uterus during the secretory phase.

1 rad. The survey published by the American College of Radiology suggests average ovarian radiation exposure to be 590 mrad (22). It seems reasonable to review this slight risk with the couple prior to any course of action. Such risk factors may well be acceptable to the involved couple.

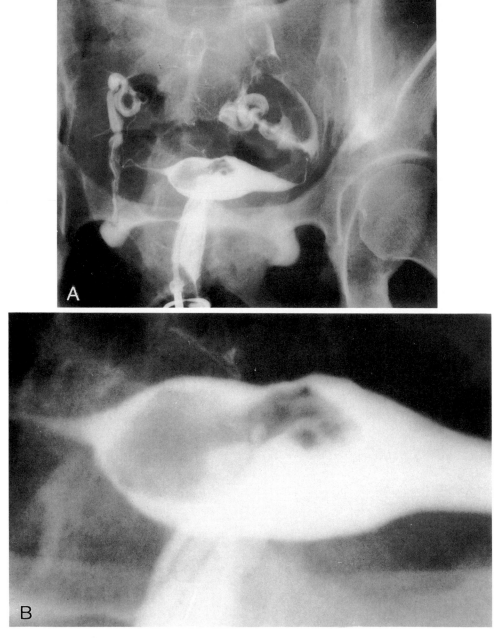

Figure 6.18.   A, Large polypoid-like filling defect near the fundus of the uterus. Hysteroscopy and resection demonstrated retained products of conception. **B,** Magnification view.

Retained Products of Conception

Retained products of conception following fetal loss are a relatively common cause of intrauterine filling defects. These may be of any size and shape but are frequently irregular in contour and of significant size (Fig. 6.18). Their appearance may suggest malignant neoplasm (Fig. 6.19).

Foreign Bodies

Defects resulting from introduced foreign bodies are occasionally encountered. Unusual elongated or irregular filling defects can tax the diagnostic ingenuity of the observer. History of previous placement of an intrauterine contraceptive device (IUD) is important. Inability to visualize the "tail" or string of the device, resulting in a "lost" IUD, occasionally requires hysterosalpingography, although careful ultrasound examination usually suffices. Elongation of the uterine cavity during pregnancy may result in such displacement of the string of the IUD into the uterine cavity (23).

The IUD, or a fragment of it, may become embedded in the wall of the myometrium, resulting in partial perforation of the uterus, or, progressively, may extrude completely from the uterine cavity and reside in the peritoneal cavity (24). Ultrasonography and hysterography are complementary tools in these situations and are generally diagnostic. Although an unsuspected IUD is not often

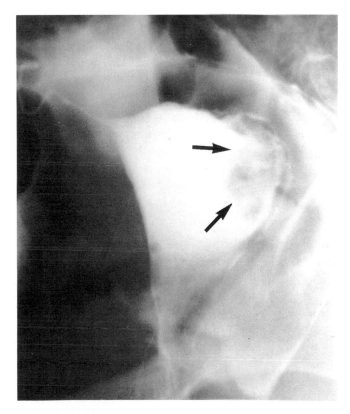

Figure 6.19. Large irregular filling defect in the left uterine cornua (*arrows*) representing retained products of conception.

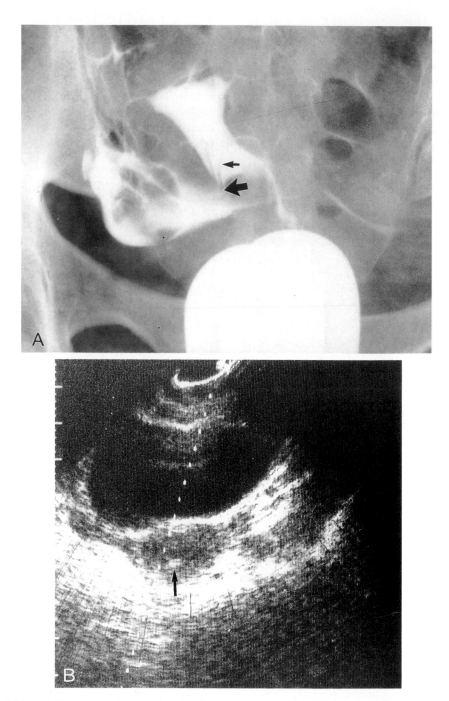

Figure 6.20.   A, Partial uterine perforation by a Cu-7 IUD. Much of the IUD remains within the uterine cavity (*small arrow*), although the inferior portion of the device extends beyond the lumen and into the myometrium near the lower uterine segment (*lower arrow*). **B,** Ultrasound reveals a low position of the IUD but cannot establish the diagnosis of partial perforation. (Courtesy of W. Stern, New York, NY.)

seen nowadays, incomplete removal of an IUD has been reported (Figs. 6.20 and 6.21) (25).

Post-Abortion Fetal Parts

Finally, prolonged intrauterine retention of fetal parts after spontaneous or induced abortion may cause infertility, leading to the performance of a hysterosalpingogram. Dawood and Jarrett (26) were unable to distinguish the hysterosalpingographic appearance of fetal bones from synechiae, but calcification may occur, making a more obvious and readily diagnosed finding. Fetal bones tend to have a linear appearance. Intrauterine synechiae, or scars, are one of the

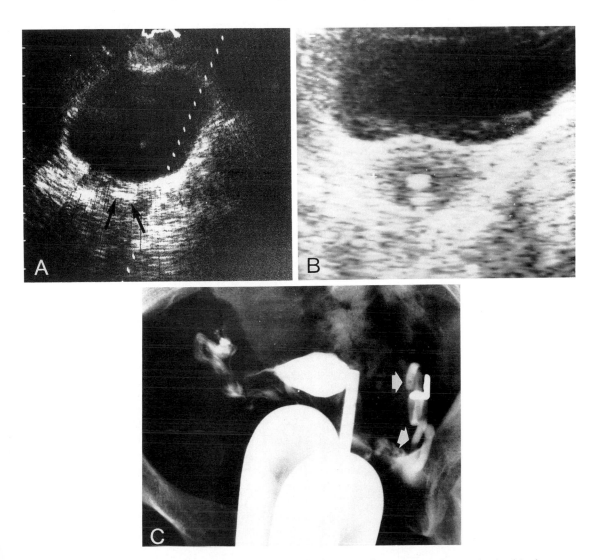

Figure 6.21.   A, Lippes Loop IUD (*arrows*) identified remote from the uterine cavity in this demonstration of complete perforation. The IUD lies in the cul-de-sac. **B,** Ultrasound fails to detect the IUD within the uterine cavity. **C,** IUD (*arrows*) identified free in the cul-de-sac, separated from the uterus. (Reprinted with permission from Rosenblatt R, Zakin D, Stern W, Kutcher R: Uterine perforation and embedding by intrauterine device: Evaluation by US and hysterography. *Radiology* 157:765, 1985.)

more common of the filling defects. The usually distinctive angular, irregular appearance is characteristic, but occasionally these are sources of diagnostic confusion. The frequency and importance of these synechiae warrant their being discussed separately (Chapter 7). Although a history of secondary infertility and pregnancy wastage is usually obtained (27), other etiologies, including metaplasia and heteroplasia, have been proposed (28).

MARGINAL IRREGULARITIES

Adenomyoma and Adenomyosis

An adenomyoma is a benign tumor composed of smooth muscle and endometrial glands and separated from normal myometrium by a pseudocapsule similar to that of leiomyomata. Patients present with abnormal uterine bleeding and, at hysterosalpingography, have a characteristic network of multiple interconnected channels in a circumscribed area within the myometrium (Fig. 6.22). An adenomyoma can be removed surgically as easily as can a leiomyoma (29).

Adenomyosis is a process in which endometrial glands are found within the myometrium, and may occur in patients with external endometriosis. Adenomyosis is a diagnosis made only by a pathologic examination of the uterus and cannot definitely be made by hysterosalpingography, dilatation and curettage, diagnostic laparoscopy, or any other surgical procedure. A clinical hint suggesting adenomyosis is an enlarged uterus and cavity, presumably due to the thickened and boggy myometrium, and a history of irregular bleeding and spotting. At hysterosalpingography, the presence of adenomyosis may be suggested by the appearance of "lollipops," diverticular-like projections from the uterine cavity into the walls of the uterus (Fig. 6.23). The spicular projections end in small sacs that are thought to be endometrial glands extending into the myometrium and dis-

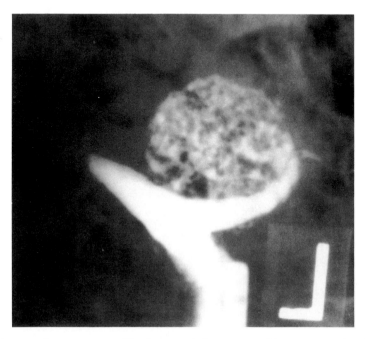

Figure 6.22.   Large adenomyoma with characteristic pattern of interconnecting interstices outlined with contrast. (Courtesy of Glenn E. Hofmann, New York, NY.)

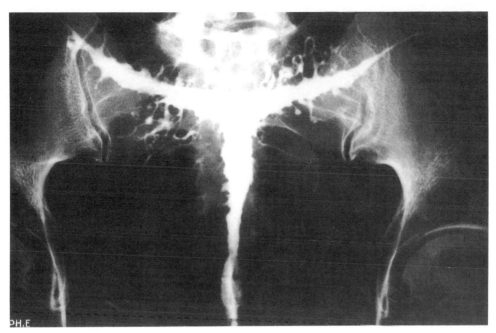

Figure 6.23. Adenomyosis. Marked and total involvement of an enlarged uterus.

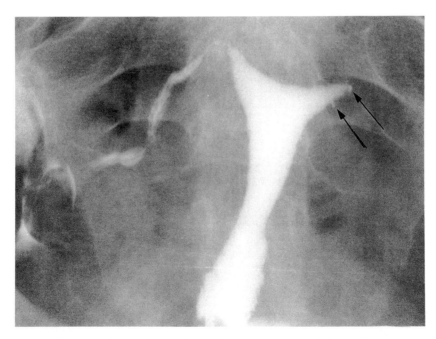

Figure 6.24. Small marginal irregularities (*arrows*) suggesting tiny "lollipops" in a patient with histologically proven adenomyosis.

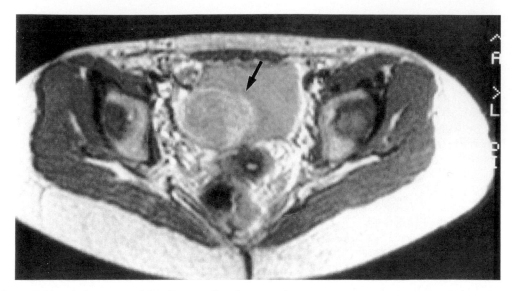

Figure 6.25. Leiomyoma. MRI (T2-weighted image) demonstrates a sharply defined mass with an area of increased signal intensity (*arrow*). (Courtesy of Thomas Powers, Nashville, TN.)

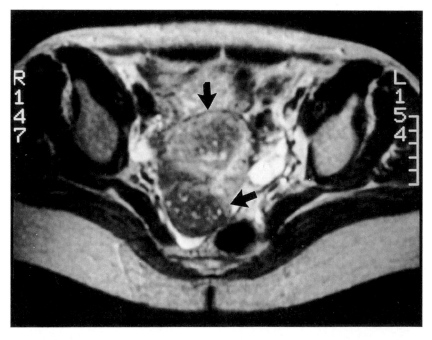

Figure 6.26. MRI (T2-weighted image) in the axial plane reveals focal adenomyosis characterized as low-intensity masses with irregular margins and multiple high-intensity foci (*arrows*). (Courtesy of Hedy Hricak, San Francisco, CA.)

metrium and distended with contrast medium. The involvement may be extensive (Fig. 6.23) or may be localized and of minimal magnitude (Fig. 6.24).

Magnetic resonance imaging is an effective, although not foolproof, technique to differentiate leiomyomas from adenomyosis within the myometrium. T1-weighted images demonstrate masses of low to medium signal intensity, while T2-weighted images have increased signal intensity within the mass (Fig. 6.25). Adenomyomas or focal adenomyosis, on the other hand, are generally not demonstrated well on T1-weighted images. Using T2-weighted technique, adenomyomas are seen as ill-defined or low-signal-intensity masses within the myometrium, demonstrating indistinct margins and high-intensity foci (Fig. 6.26). Finally, generalized adenomyosis, not generally perceived on T1-weighted images, presents as diffuse thickening of the junctional zone on T2-weighted images only (30, 31).

Postsurgical Abnormalities

Abnormalities of the uterine cavity secondary to previous surgery are discussed more thoroughly in Chapter 11. Contour irregularity, saccular dilatations, and defects simulating neoplasms may present. The most common of these alterations are secondary to previous cesarean section, with an abnormal uterine cavity observed in 36% of patients undergoing a low-segment cesarean section (32). Most such deformities are clinically insignificant, but larger defects may dictate elective cesarean section in the event of pregnancy.

REFERENCES

1. Beclére C: L'hysterigraphie dans le diagnostic des lesions intrauterines et des metrirragics fonctionelles. *Bull Soc Obstet Gynecol* 22:815, 1933.
2. Norman O: Hysterosalpingography in cancer of the corpus of the uterus. *Acta Radiol* 34 (suppl 79):1, 1950.
3. Norman O: Hysterographically visualized radionecrosis following intrauterine radiation of cancer of the corpus of the uterus. *Acta Radiol* 37:96, 1952.
4. Beclére C, Fayolle G: *L'Hystero-salpingographie.* Paris, Masson et Cie, 1966.
5. Schwartz PE, Kohorn EL, Knowlton AH, Morris JM: Routine use of hysterography in endometrial carcinoma and postmenopausal carcinoma. *Obstet Gynecol* 45:378, 1975.
6. Anderson B, Marchant DJ, Munzenrider JE, Moore JP, Mitchell GW: Routine noninvasive hysterography in the evaluation and treatment of endometrial carcinoma. *Gynecol Oncol* 4:354, 1976.
7. Tak WK, Anderson B, Vardi JR, Beecham JB, Marchant DJ: Myometrial invasion and hysterography in endometrial carcinoma. *Obstet Gynecol* 50:159, 1977.
8. Stock RS, Gallup DG: Hysterography in patients with suspected uterine cancer: Radiographic and histologic correlations and clinical implications. *Obstet Gynecol* 69:872, 1987.
9. Aksel S, Wentz AC, Jones GS: Anovulatory infertility associated with adenocarcinoma and adenomatous hyperplasia of the endometrium. *Obstet Gynecol* 43:386, 1974.
10. Menczer J, Frenkel Y, Serr D: Hysterosalpingography in young infertile patients with unsuspected endometrial adenocarcinoma. *Am J Obstet Gynecol* 3:352, 1980.
11. Dudiak CM, Turner DA, Patel SK, Archie JT, Silver B, Norusis N: Uterine leiomyomas in the infertile patient: Preoperative localization with MR imaging versus US and hysterosalpingography. *Radiology* 167:627, 1988.
12. Baltarowich OH, Kurtz AB, Pennell RG, Neddleman L, Vilaro MM, Goldberg BB: Pitfalls in the sonographic diagnosis of uterine fibroids. *AJR* 151:725, 1988.
13. Green WJ, Fendley SM, Wintzell EC, Green AE Jr, Lorino CO, Rodning CB: Cystic degeneration of a large uterine leiomyoma: Radiologic and surgical analyses. *Invest Radiol* 24:626, 1989.
14. McCarthy S: MR imaging of the uterus. *Radiology* 171:321, 1989.
15. Gardner RL, Shaw RW: Cornual fibroids: A conservative approach to restoring

tubal patency using a gonadotropin-releasing hormone agonist (goserelin) with successful pregnancy. *Fertil Steril* 52:332, 1989.

16. Kessel B, Liu J, Mortola J, Berga S, Yen SSC: Treatment of uterine fibroids with agonist analogs of gonadotropin-releasing hormone. *Fertil Steril* 49:538, 1988.

17. Schlaff WD, Zerhouni EA, Huth JAM, Chen J, Damewood MD, Rock JA: A placebo-controlled trial of a depot gonadotropin-releasing hormone analogue (Leuprolide) in the treatment of uterine leiomyomata. *Obstet Gynecol* 74:856, 1989.

18. Donnez J, Schrurs B, Gillerot S, Sandow J, Clerckx F: Treatment of uterine fibroids with implants of gonadotropin-releasing hormone agonist: Assessment by hysterography. *Fertil Steril* 51:947, 1989.

19. Isaacs I: Hysterographic double-outlined uterine cavity: A sign of unsuspected pregnancy. *AJR* 131:305, 1978.

20. Hammer-Jacobsen E: Therapeutic abortion on account of x-ray examination during pregnancy. *Dan Med Bull* 6:112, 1959.

21. Swartz HM, Reichling BA: Hazards of radiation exposure for pregnant women. *JAMA* 239:1907, 1978.

22. *Medical Radiation: A Guide to Good Practice.* American College of Radiology, Washington, DC, 1985.

23. Guha-Ray DK: Translocation of the intrauterine contraceptive device: Study of thirty-one cases. *Fertil Steril* 28:9, 1977.

24. Rosenblatt R, Zakin D, Stern W, Kutcher R: Uterine perforation and embedding by intrauterine device: Evaluation by US and hysterography. *Radiology* 157:765, 1985.

25. Rowe T, McComb P: Unknown intrauterine devices and infertility. *Fertil Steril* 47:1038, 1987.

26. Dawood MY, Jarrett JC II: Prolonged intrauterine retention of fetal bones after abortion causing infertility. *Am J Obstet Gynecol* 143:715, 1982.

27. Taylor PJ, Hamou J, Mencaglia L: Hysteroscopic detection of heterotopic intrauterine bone formation. *J Reprod Med* 33:337, 1988.

28. Wetzels LCG, Essed GGM, Haan JD, van de Kar AJF, Willebrand D: Endometrial ossification: Unilateral manifestation in a septate uterus. *Gynecol Obstet Invest* 14:47, 1982.

29. Hofmann GE, Acosta AA, Gaddy NE: Hysterosalpingographic diagnosis of uterine adenomyoma. *Obstet Gynecol* 73:885, 1989.

30. Mark AS, Hricak H, Heinrichs LW, Hendrickson MR, Winkler ML, Bachica JA, Stickler JE: Adenomyosis and leiomyoma: Differential diagnosis with MR imaging. *Radiology* 163:527, 1987.

31. Togashi K, Ozasa H, Konishi I, Itoh H, Nichimura K, Fujisawa I, Noma S, Sagoh T, Minami S, Yamashita K, Nakano Y, Konishi J, Mori T: Enlarged uterus: Differentiation between adenomyosis and leiomyoma with MR imaging. *Radiology* 171:531, 1989.

32. Durkan JP: Hysterography after cesarean section. *Obstet Gynecol* 24:836, 1964.

7

Hysteroscopy in the Evaluation of Infertility

Rafael F. Valle

Uterine factors affecting successful reproduction constitute only about 10% of all infertility problems. These uterine factors are intrauterine adhesions, uterine leiomyomas significantly distorting the anatomy of the uterus, uterine anomalies (particularly the septate uterus), and chronic endometritis. In this chapter the structural abnormalities amenable to hysteroscopic evaluation are discussed. Although the uterus itself seldom interferes with fertility, it can be the source of reproductive failure and early pregnancy losses.

Reproductive failure includes infertility and repeated pregnancy wastage, and both are of importance, particularly because of their significant impact on reproduction and the inability to conceive or to carry the early pregnancy to a successful completion with a live baby at term. Therefore, some conditions not causing infertility directly but associated with reproductive failure are addressed in this chapter (1, 2).

The uterus has been evaluated in a variety of manners to obtain information on the uterine cavity and surrounding uterine walls. Tactile appraisal, blind exploration with forceps or curettes, and x-rays used after instilling radiopaque material to demonstrate filling defects have been used by gynecologists for the detection of intrauterine pathology (3–5). Ultrasonic evaluation has been most helpful in determining the symmetry and contour of the uterus to confirm or rule out intrauterine anomalies, submucous leiomyomas, or endometrial polyps. Being a noninvasive method of examination, it has been found useful in the evaluation of the uterus, particularly in early pregnancy. Because of the limitations of these various methods, hysteroscopy has been added recently for diagnosis and treatment of a variety of intrauterine conditions (6–9).

Appropriate instruments specifically designed for uterine visualization, the availability of fiberoptics (which now permit safe delivery of a high-intensity light through endoscopes), and the appropriate use of distending media (such as dextran 32% in dextrose 10%, CO_2 gas, and dextrose 5% in water or in saline) to obtain panoramic visualization of the uterine cavity have provided an efficient, relatively simple, and safe technique for hysteroscopy. Hysteroscopy has been facilitated as an office procedure, with the addition of small-caliber endoscopes. Furthermore, because of the simplicity and ease of the procedure, it is applicable as a screening method for patients with abnormal uterine bleeding or questionable hysterograms and for patients with suspected intrauterine pathology (Table 7.1).

Although hysteroscopy has revealed a significant rate of abnormal findings in selected infertility patients, the routine use of hysteroscopy in the evaluation of the infertile patient does not seem justified, particularly in view of the low incidence of uterine factors affecting infertility and the low prevalence of these

Table 7.1.   Indications for Hysteroscopy for Infertility

Abnormal hysterogram
Abnormal uterine bleeding
Suspected intrauterine pathology
Uterine anomalies
Unexplained infertility
Pregnancy wastage
Planned intrauterine surgery
 Polyps
 Submucous leiomyomas
 Uterine septa
 Intrauterine adhesions
 Misplaced or embedded foreign bodies
 Tubal cannulation

factors in infertile patients. When associated factors that may be responsible for the infertility are present, hysteroscopy offers a valuable adjunct in their evaluation and treatment (1, 2, 4) (Tables 7.2 and 7.3, Figs. 7.1 to 7.5).

ABNORMAL HYSTEROSALPINGOGRAM

Hysterosalpingography, although useful for intrauterine evaluation, may produce false-positive results because of transient distortion of the uterine cavity by blood, mucus, debris, and air bubbles. Errors in technique, selection of the contrast agent used, and interpretation of findings may also contribute to failure. The ability to observe the inside of the uterus can confirm or rectify an abnormal shadow seen on the hysterogram and adds to the feasibility of obtaining biopsies of pathologic lesions.

It is undeniable that a hysterosalpingogram, performed adequately with water-soluble contrast medium injected fractionally and selectively into the uterine cavity, with observation under image intensification fluoroscopy, can give invaluable information concerning the

Table 7.2.   Abnormality Rate at Hysteroscopy (Primary or Secondary Infertility)[a]

Author	No. of Patients	Abnormalities
		%
Cohen and Dmowski	34	43.7
Mohr and Lindemann	167	59.3
Rosenfeld	110	19
Taylor and Cumming	75	44.1
Valle	142	62

[a]From Valle RF, Sciarra JJ: Current status of hysteroscopy in gynecologic practice. Fertil Steril 32:619, 1979. Reproduced with permission of the publisher, The American Fertility Society.

Table 7.3.   Uterine Factors in Infertility (Estimated Prevalance and Contribution to Infertility)[a]

Condition	Prevalence	Infertility
	%	%
Uterine anomalies	0.1 — 3.3	<1.0
Uterine leiomyomas	15.0 — 20.0	3.0 — 4.0
Intrauterine adhesions	3.7 — 23.4	4.0
Chronic endometritis	0.3 — 4.8	2.0 — 9.0

[a]Reprinted with permission from Valle RF: Clinical management of uterine factors in infertile patients. Semin Reprod Endocrinol 3:149, 1985.

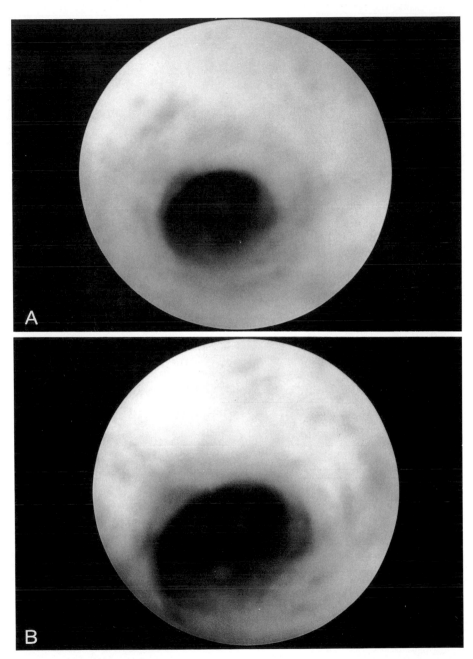

Figure 7.1.   Normal hysteroscopic examination. **A,** Visualization of the endocervical canal, close to the ectocervix. **B,** Hysteroscope being advanced under direct view. **C,** Plicae palmatae of the endocervical canal. **D,** Hysteroscopic view of the internal cervical os with the uterine cavity in background. **E,** Panoramic view of the uterine cavity, showing the right tubal opening. Endometrium, early proliferative phase.

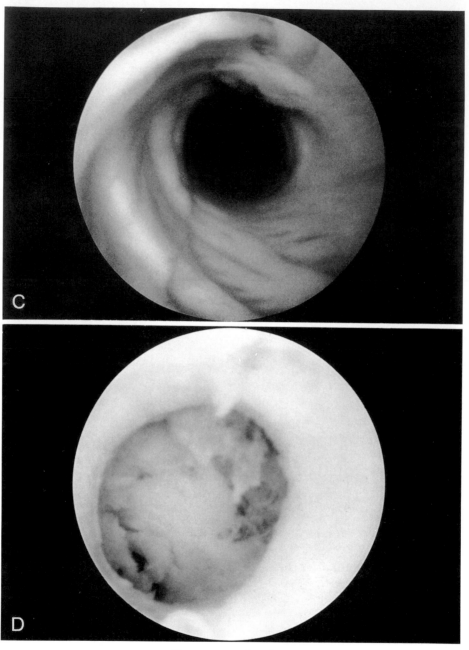

Figure 7.1.   C and **D.**

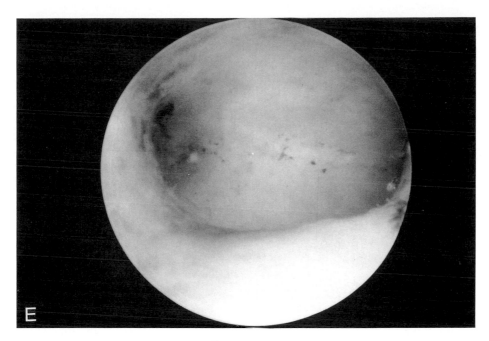

Figure 7.1.   E.

uterine cavity. When interpreting this technique dynamically, the rate of false-positives is low. Nonetheless, because interpretation must often be achieved from static films taken serially, misinterpretation may occur. A hysteroscopic confirmation of abnormal hysterographic findings has been found to be in the range of 43 to 68% in studies comparing these two techniques (10, 11) (Table 7.4).

The abnormal hysterogram is the main indication for hysteroscopy in the infertile patient. The radiographic image may be clarified, and recognized lesions can be biopsied and removed transcervically under hysteroscopic control. Polyps, submucous leiomyomas, uterine septa, and intrauterine adhesions may be diagnosed and treated. Hysteroscopy does not exclude the value of a hysterosalpingogram; rather, it complements its findings and adds to its accuracy. The hysterosalpingogram offers more areas of examination than hysteroscopy, and it also allows appraisal of the fallopian tubes and their architecture, intratubal defects, ep-

ithelial lining and diverticula, and tubal patency (12–16) (Table 7.5).

EVALUATION AND TREATMENT OF INTRAUTERINE ADHESIONS

Hysteroscopy is the best method for evaluation and treatment of intrauterine adhesions. Blind division of intrauterine adhesions by curettage has proved unsatisfactory; the addition of hysteroscopy has facilitated diagnosis and precision in dissecting and dividing adhesions without injury to the surrounding endometrium. Although extensive connective tissue adhesions have been difficult to treat, even with hysteroscopy, the visual approach to the division of these adhesions has improved treatment and has decreased the risk of uterine damage, incomplete treatment, and potential creation of new adhesions. Hysteroscopy has offered the opportunity to delineate the extent of uterine cavity occlusion and the type of adhesions present, providing an

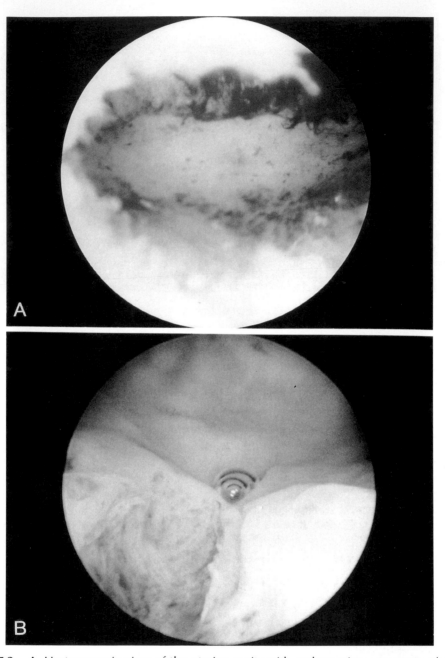

Figure 7.2.   A, Hysteroscopic view of the uterine cavity with endometrium, secretory phase. **B,** Closer view of the secretory endometrium showing the openings of the glands.

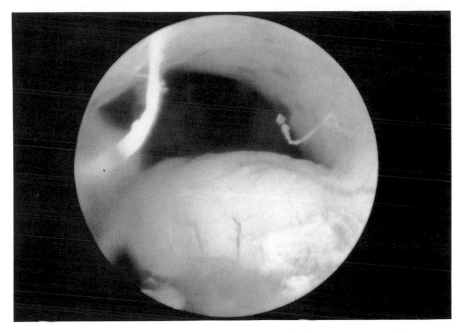

Figure 7.3. Submucous leiomyoma projecting into the lower portion of the uterus.

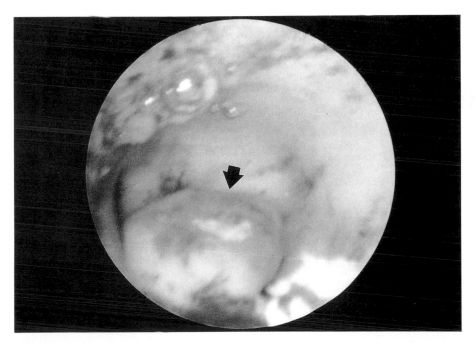

Figure 7.4. Sessile endometrial polyp arising from the posterior uterine wall (*arrow*).

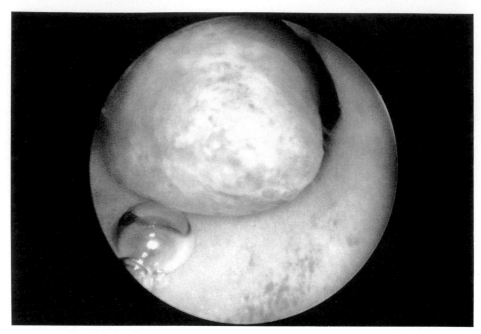

Figure 7.5.   Right fundal endometrial polyp. Note the small bubbles in the left lower pole of the polyp from distending medium.

Table 7.4.   Hysteroscopic Confirmation of Hysterographic Abnormal Findings[a]

Author	No. of Patients with Abnormal Hysterograms	Confirmed by Hysteroscopy (%)
Edstrom and Fernstrom	30	53.3
Englund et al.	21	50
Gribb	14	43
Levine and Neuwirth	11	60
Norment	50	60
Porto and Serment	76	58
Sugimoto and Nishimura	206	65
Taylor and Cumming	68[b]	55.5
Valle	63	68.3
Varangot et al.[c]	71	55

[a]*From Valle RF, Sciarra JJ: Current status of hysteroscopy in gynecologic practice. Fertil Steril 32:619, 1979. Reproduced with permission of the publisher, The American Fertility Society.*
[b]*Normal hysterograms; only 30 confirmed.*
[c]*Contact hysteroscopy.*

accurate appraisal of the severity of this condition and offering a useful prognostic index for the outcome of therapy (17, 18).

The degree of intrauterine involvement, as shown by hysterosalpingography, and the extent and type of intrauter-ine adhesions found at hysteroscopy are the most useful prognostic factors in the evaluation and treatment of patients with intrauterine adhesions.

The hysteroscopic treatment of intrauterine adhesions has resulted in the restoration of normal menstruation in

Table 7.5.   Comparison of Hysteroscopy and Hysterosalpingography

Hysteroscopy	Hysterosalpingography
Direct visualization of uterine cavity	Indirect visualization (contrast medium's shadow)
Diagnosis and specification of intrauterine lesions	Recognition and presumptive diagnosis
Possibility of targeted biopsies and surgical therapy	No possibility
Localization of abnormalities (polyps, myomas, malformations, adhesions, carcinoma, and precursors)	Localization of abnormalities is less precise
Direct access to tubal lumen (biochemical or biophysical studies, selective chromopertubation)	No direct access (indirect study, possible spasm)
No evaluation of fallopian tubes possible	Evaluation of tubal lumen, patency, epithelial folds, and abnormalities
Requires special instrumentation, experience, more expensive	Simple instrumentation, easy to perform, less expensive

over 90% of the patients treated. However, the reproductive outcome seems to correlate with the severity of the condition. Of patients who have achieved pregnancy, over 80% have carried the pregnancy to term. Nonetheless, the more extensive, dense, and old the adhesions are (especially if they are connective tissue adhesions), the worse the prognosis is.

The outcome of therapy seems to correlate well with the severity and extent of the adhesions. Three stages of intrauterine adhesions may be defined. *Mild adhesions* are filmy adhesions (endometrial) that produce partial or complete uterine cavity occlusion. *Moderate adhesions* are fibromuscular adhesions that are characteristically thick and are still covered with endometrium that may bleed on division. *Severe adhesions* are composed of connective tissue only, lack any endometrial lining, and are not likely to bleed on division; these adhesions partially or totally occlude the uterine cavity. This classification is based on the degree of intrauterine involvement shown by hysterosalpingography and the extent and type of adhesions found at hysteroscopy (Figs. 7.6 to 7.11).

When intrauterine adhesions cause infertility, usually it is due to tubal occlu-

sion or extensive uterine cavity occlusion, and the reproductive outcome of these patients is lower than it is in patients with pregnancy wastage, with a lower cumulative pregnancy rate for patients with severe intrauterine adhesions compared to women with mild or moderate adhesions. Valle and Sciarra (18) showed a pregnancy rate of 59.2% in 81 infertile patients treated hysteroscopically for intrauterine adhesions, with a term pregnancy rate of 60.4%. However, the spontaneous abortion rate reached 35.4%.

Increased awareness of the entity of intrauterine adhesions following postpartum and post-abortal curettage or any trauma to the uterine cavity may contribute to early diagnosis; best results are achieved when adhesions are mild and filmy. The modern management and treatment of intrauterine adhesions should include hysteroscopy as the most accurate method in diagnosis and treatment (19, 20).

UTERINE SEPTA: EVALUATION AND TREATMENT

In the evaluation of patients with pregnancy wastage, hysteroscopy may be

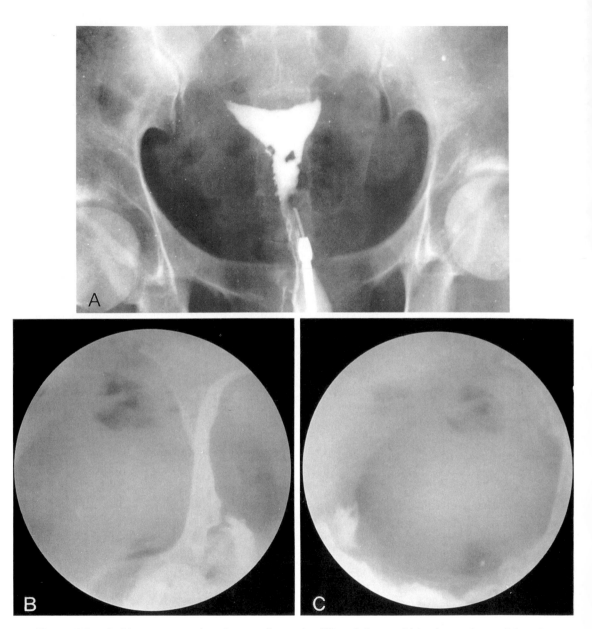

Figure 7.6.   A, Hysterogram showing small angular filling defects within the endometrial cavity, typical for synechiae. **B,** Hysteroscopic view showing filmy adhesion. **C,** Uterine cavity after division of adhesion.

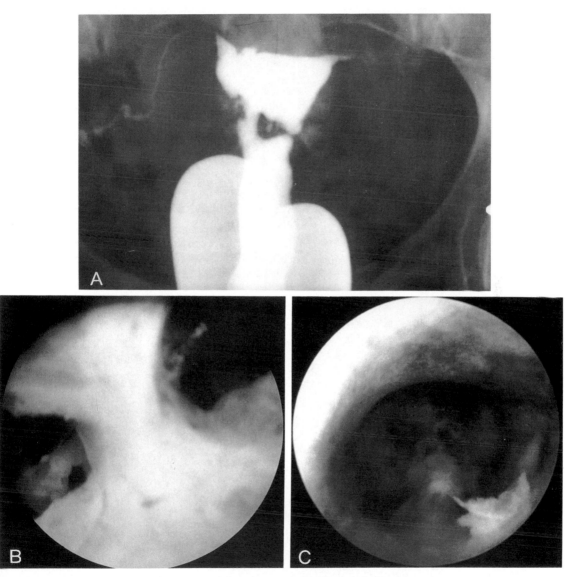

Figure 7.7. **A,** Hysterosalpingogram showing irregular filling defects in the uterine cavity. **B,** Central thick adhesion found by hysteroscopy. **C,** Normal uterine cavity following hysteroscopic division of adhesion.

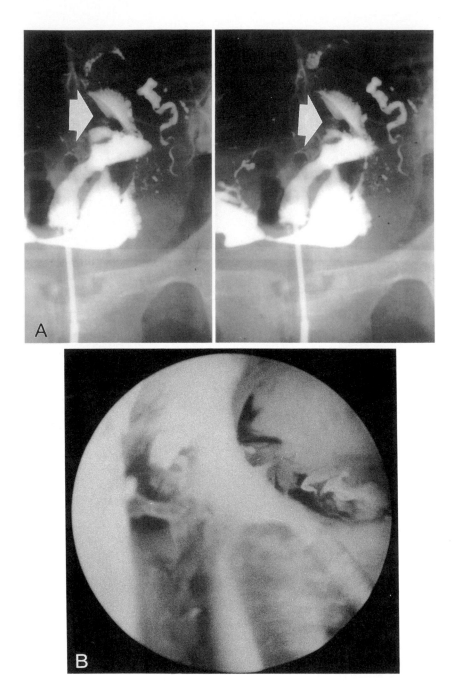

Figure 7.8.   A, Hysterosalpingogram showing angular filling defect at right cornual cone (*arrow*). **B,** Hysteroscopy revealing right cornual cone adhesion and tip of scissors in place. **C,** Hysteroscopic division of adhesion. **D,** Uterine cavity symmetry, reestablished following hysteroscopic division of adhesion.

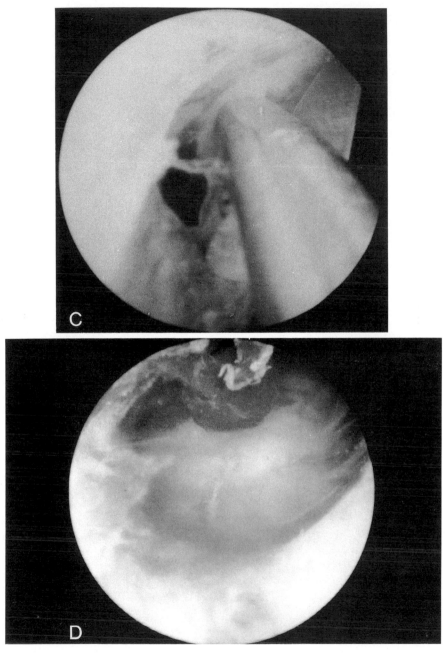

Figure 7.8. C and D.

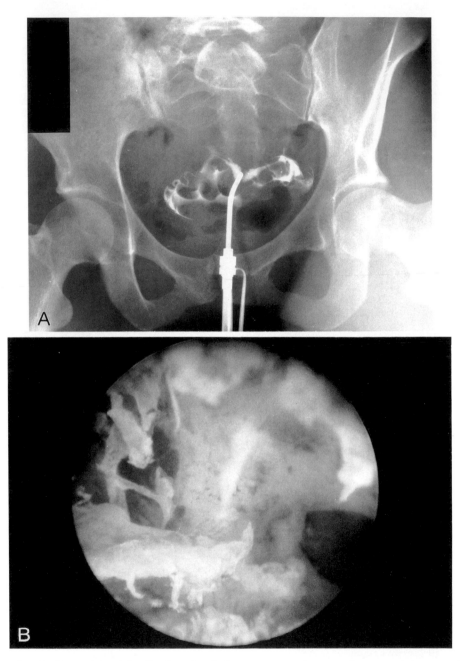

Figure 7.9.   **A,** Central fundal adhesion simulating a septum shown at hysterosalpingography. **B,** Hysteroscopic view of adhesion before division.

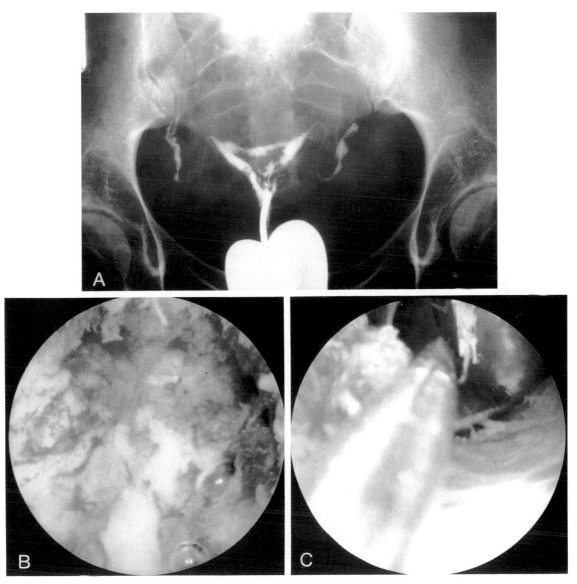

Figure 7.10.   **A,** Hysterosalpingogram showing extensive adhesions occluding a large portion of the uterine cavity. **B,** Hysteroscopic division of adhesions. **C,** Uterine cavity with remaining stumps from divided adhesions.

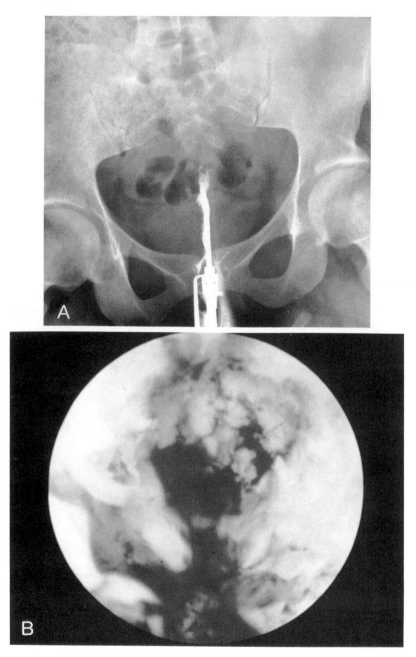

Figure 7.11.   A, Complete uterine cavity occlusion at hysterosalpingography. **B,** Small uterine cavity following hysteroscopic division of adhesions, with thick residual stumps from divided adhesions.

complementary to the hysterosalpingogram in providing visualization of the endocervical canal and the internal cervical os, and observation of the sphincter-like action mechanism of this latter area. It can also provide visual appraisal of uterine anomalies with direct visualization of their extension, the resultant distortion of the uterine architecture, and their direct treatment by division through hysteroscopy. The hysteroscopic division of uterine septa, as originally reported by Edstrom (11) in 1974, has been refined; as the experience and follow-up have accumulated, the results have proved the effectiveness and superiority of this approach over any other procedure performed by laparotomy and bisection of the uterine corpus. This ambulatory procedure has become the treatment of choice for a symptomatic septate uterus, sparing the patient a laparotomy, hysterotomy, prolonged hospitalization, increased morbidity, and a cesarean section (20, 21) (Figs. 7.12 and 7.13).

UNEXPLAINED INFERTILITY

Although the incidence of unexplained infertility may be low (3 to 4%), the evaluation of these patients requires a meticulous examination of all factors

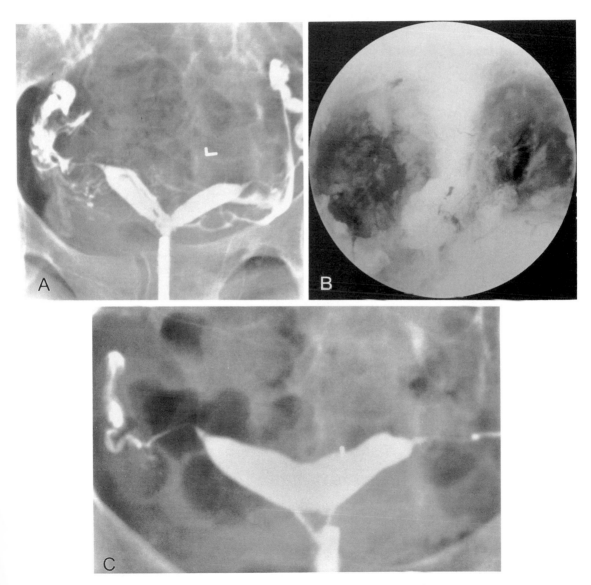

Figure 7.12. **A,** Hysterosalpingogram showing divided uterine cavity of a septate uterus. **B,** Hysteroscopic view of the uterine septum. **C,** Hysterogram following hysteroscopic treatment of the uterine septum, showing a unified uterine cavity.

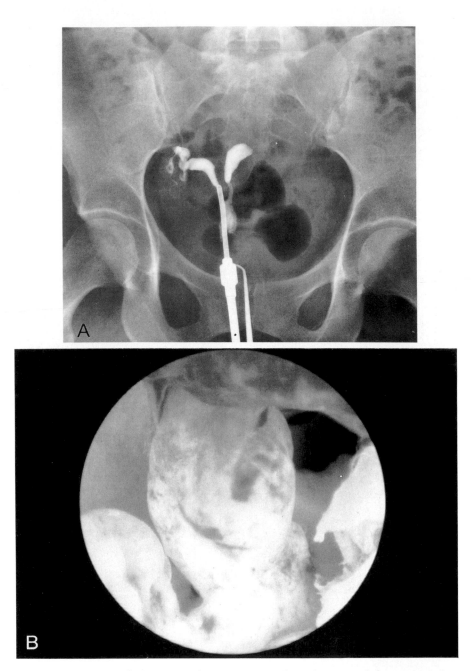

Figure 7.13.   A, Hysterosalpingogram showing a complete division of the cavity of a septate uterus. **B,** Hysteroscopic view of the long uterine septum at its nadir, showing two horns. **C,** Hysteroscopic division of the septum. **D,** Postoperative hysterogram demonstrating a unified uterine cavity.

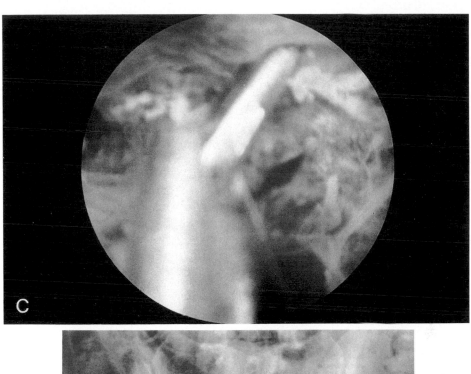

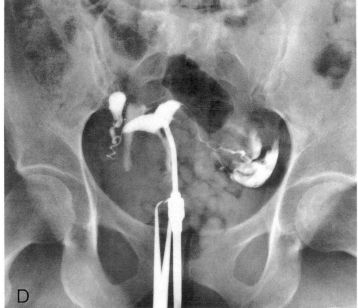

Figure 7.13.   C and **D.**

that could explain the infertility. Endometrial lesions such as small polyps or adhesions at the uterotubal cones, which may not be detectable by hysterosalpingography, can be delineated and treated by hysteroscopy, even though these defects may not seem to be the cause of infertility. A combined approach of laparoscopy and hysteroscopy is most useful in these situations to evaluate with precision any tubal-peritoneal, cervical, and uterine lesion that may explain the infertility. The actual yield of significant intrauterine pathology found at hysteroscopy in these patients is relatively low; however, the assurance that the uterine cavity is normal can only be provided by direct visualization (22–24).

Topographic changes of the endometrium during the proliferative and secretory phases of the menstrual cycle can now be determined, particularly with optics permitting magnification. Eventually, maturation of the endometrium and the absence of dystrophy may be correlated with receptivity to the early embryo for implantation, thus benefiting women having problems with embryo transfers, despite normal hormonal support (25–28) (Fig. 7.14).

ABNORMAL UTERINE BLEEDING

Although most patients with abnormal uterine bleeding and infertility have ovulatory dysfunctions, when this condition is treated and the symptomatology persists, evaluation of the uterine cavity becomes necessary. The addition of hysteroscopy in the evaluation of patients with abnormal uterine bleeding has contributed to the accurate diagnosis and treatment of pathologic intrauterine conditions that may be missed by endometrial biopsy or curettage, such as submucous leiomyomas, endometrial polyps, and focal pathologic lesions, including endometrial hyperplasia or carcinoma of the endometrium. Additional pathologic

findings may include focal areas of osseous metaplasia and forgotten foreign bodies (8, 19, 29, 30) (Figs. 7.15 to 7.23). Because diagnostic hysteroscopy requires only a small-caliber endoscope (< 4 mm OD), cervical dilatation is not required, and the examination can be performed simply in an office setting. The small-caliber outer diameter endoscope simplifies the examination and permits safe investigation of the uterine cavity. Nonetheless, it carries some limitations, as no instrument can be passed throughout a small endoscope, and only one medium, CO_2 gas insufflation, seems adequate to distend the uterine cavity. There are advantages, however: the examination can be performed in a simpler, faster, and cleaner way, decreasing the need for anesthesia and analgesia. Patients with normal findings at diagnostic hysteroscopy in the office are spared additional manipulation or biopsy. Patients with abnormal uterine bleeding in whom the uterine cavity is found to be normal may nonetheless have some irregular desquamation of the endometrial lining. At the completion of hysteroscopic examination, a 4-mm soft plastic cannula can be introduced and a suction biopsy performed for histologic confirmation (31–33).

TUBAL CANNULATION

The hysteroscopic access to the uterotubal junctions introduced an excellent platform for intratubal direct studies by cannulation. In 1972, Quinones et al. (34) demonstrated the potential of tubal cannulation for delivery of sclerosing substances to obtain tubal sterilization and for evaluation of the intratubal milieu. Further refinement in manufacturing of smaller and softer catheters as well as flexible wire-guides less than 0.5 mm in diameter permitted a less traumatic method of introducing catheters into the fallopian tube. A significant number of patients with cornual occlusion did not

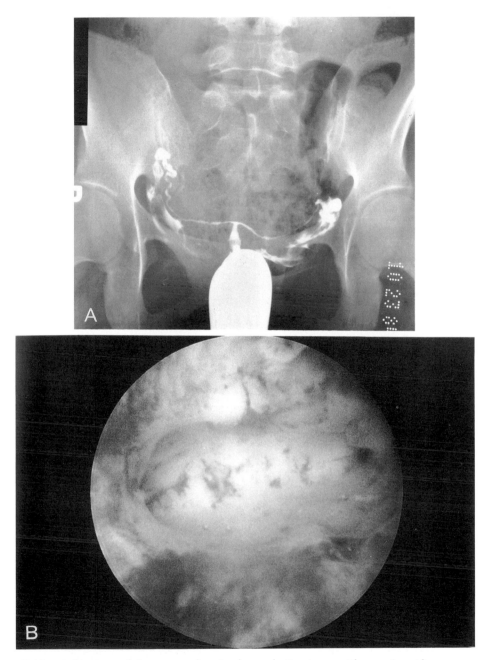

Figure 7.14.   **A,** Hysterosalpingogram showing hypoplastic uterus with prominent lower segment. **B,** Hysteroscopy demonstrating a small uterine cavity.

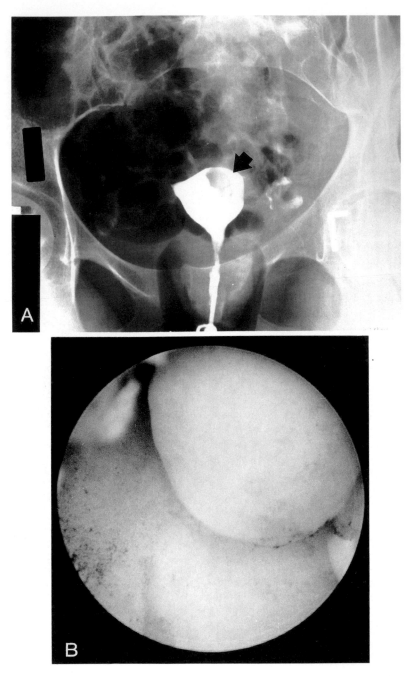

Figure 7.15.   A, Large filling defect (*arrow*) at the left uterotubal cone. **B,** Large endometrial polyp seen at hysteroscopy.

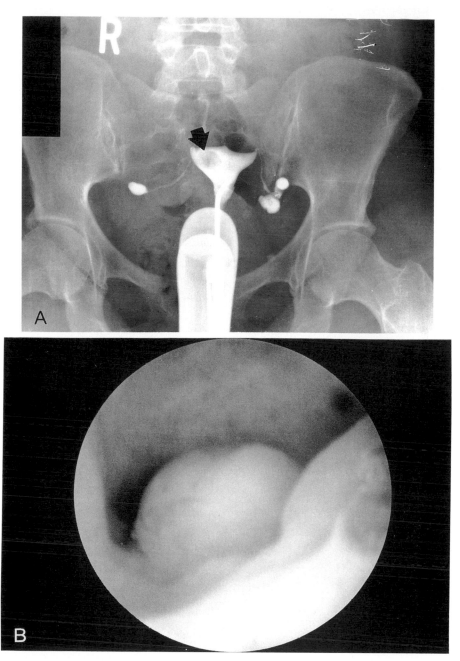

Figure 7.16. **A,** Filling defect on the right uterine cornual cone (*arrow*) in a patient evaluated for tubal reversal. **B,** Hysteroscopy demonstrating an endometrial polyp.

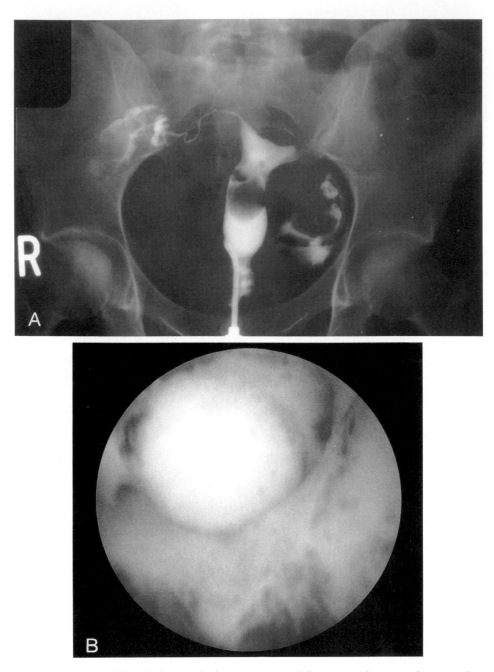

Figure 7.17.   A, Large filling defect in the lower portion of the uterus shown on hysterosalpingography. **B,** Hysteroscopy demonstrating a submucous leiomyoma with a thick pedicle. **C,** Hysteroscopic removal of the myoma. **D,** Myoma after transcervical removal.

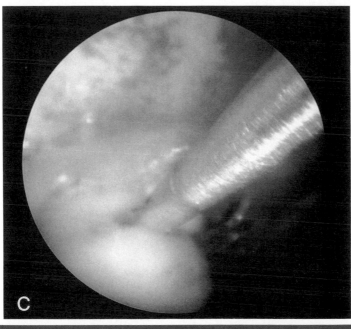

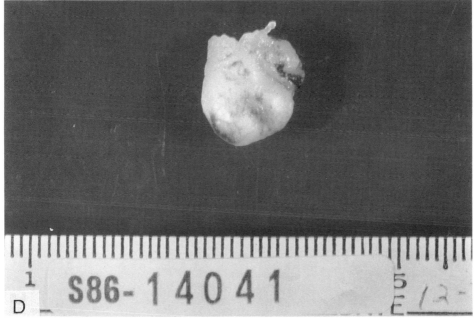

Figure 7.17. C and D.

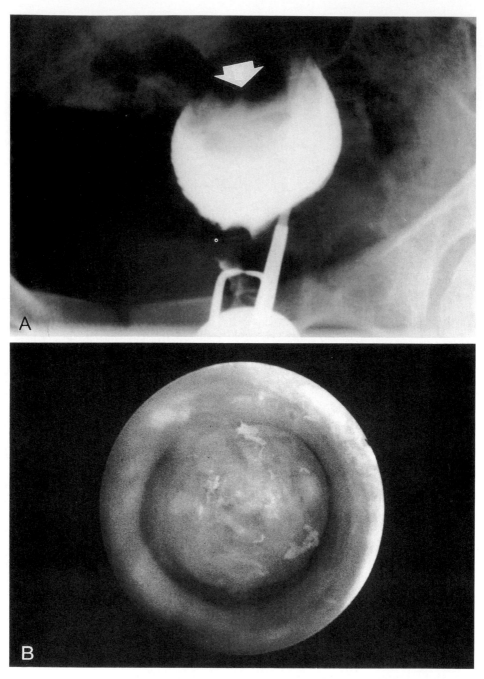

Figure 7.18.   A, Hysterogram showing enlargement of the uterine cavity and marked dilatation by a fundal mass (*arrow*). **B,** Hysteroscopic examination demonstrating a large fundal submucous myoma.

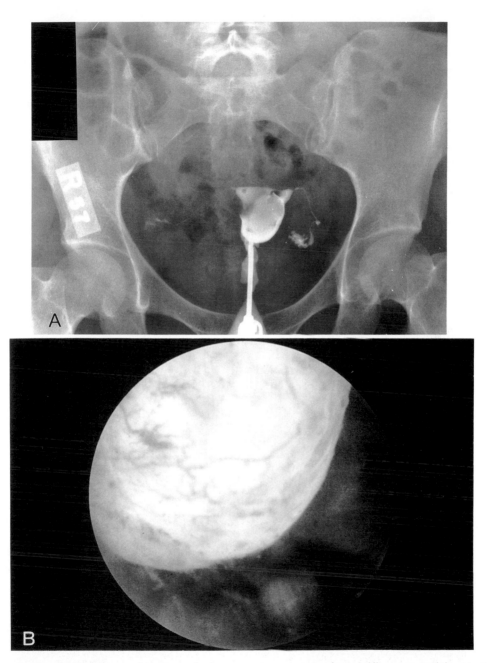

Figure 7.19. **A,** Hysterographic view of a large space-occupying lesion filling most of the uterine cavity. **B,** Hysteroscopy demonstrating a large submucous myoma before its removal. **C,** Postoperative hysterogram, 3 months after treatment, showing marked reduction in the size of the uterine cavity.

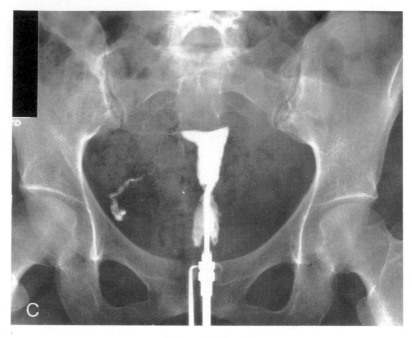

Figure 7.19.   C.

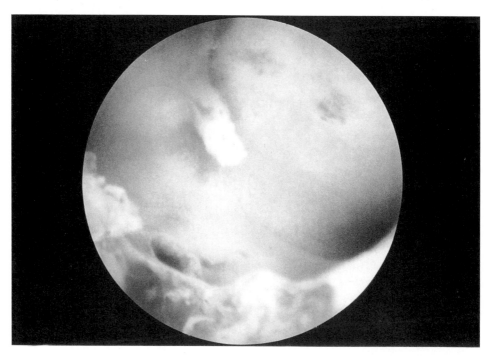

Figure 7.20.   Hysteroscopic view of fetal bones (remnants of previous abortion) encrusted in the uterine wall.

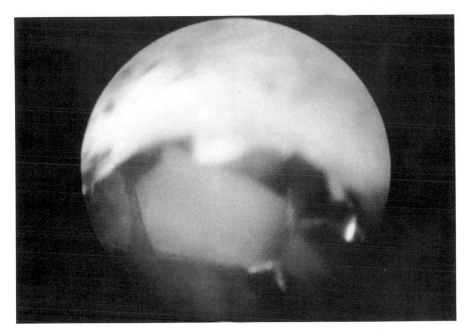

Figure 7.21. Foreign body being removed from the uterine cavity under hysteroscopic control.

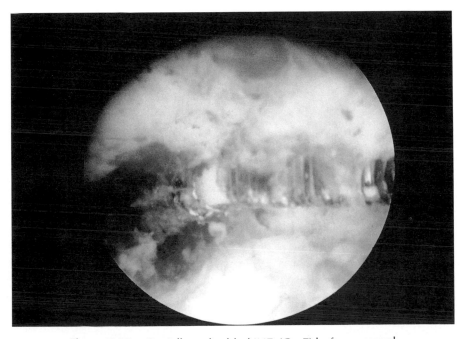

Figure 7.22. Partially embedded IUD (Cu-7) before removal.

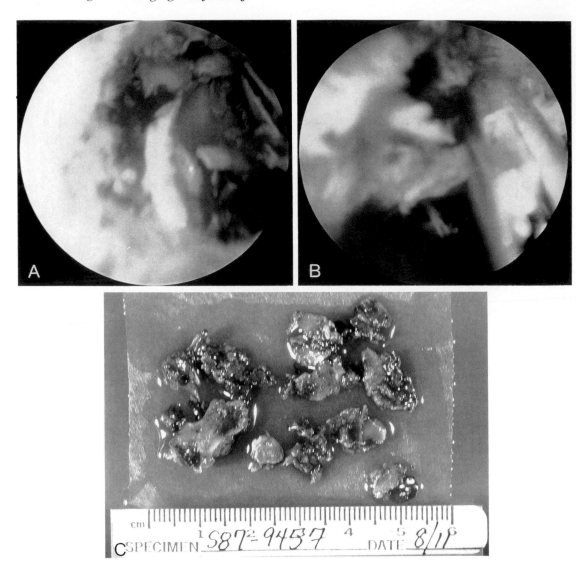

Figure 7.23. **A,** Osseous metaplasia covering the right lateral uterine wall. **B,** Removal of fragments of osseous metaplasia under hysteroscopic control. **C,** Multiple fragments of osseous metaplasia after hysteroscopic removal.

not demonstrate pathology at this area when subjected to laparotomy and microsurgery of the tubal cornual regions, but rather were found to have amorphous material that was easily dislodged. It was logical to extend selective tubal chromopertubation to actual tubal cannulation. The approach was initiated by the radiologist using fluoroscopy and then extended to hysteroscopy. The hysteroscopic tubal cannulation has proved to be an excellent diagnostic and therapeutic adjunct in these situations. Furthermore, it not only offers the alternative of demonstrating true occlusion under laparoscopy (therefore eliminating patients with tubal spasm) but also serves as an adjunct for therapeutic laparoscopy, should additional pathology such as tubal or pelvic adhesions, partial tubal occlusions, or distortions be found. The preliminary reports are encouraging, not only with regard to effectiveness in treating tubal occlusion but also because the reproductive outcome seems to compare well to, and in some instances to surpass, previous microsurgical tubal occlusion treatment. Furthermore, when these techniques fail, they probably represent true tubal occlusion by fibrosis, thereby selecting pa-

tients who may benefit from tubal microsurgery (35) (Fig. 7.24).

The role of hysteroscopy for hysteroscopic selective tubal insemination and tubal transfer of gametes and embryos is being explored and tested in selected patients as an outpatient method that offers a direct and clear view of the tubal os-

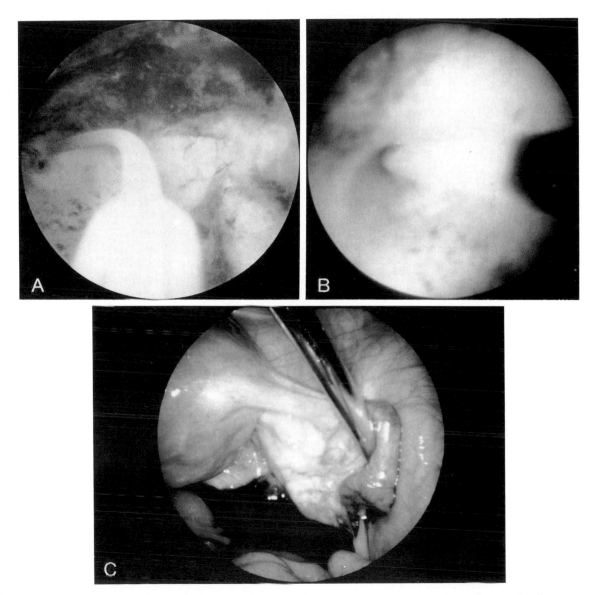

Figure 7.24.   A, Hysteroscopic tubal cannulation in progress. **B,** The cannula in place and indigo carmine being injected. **C,** Patency of the fallopian tube demonstrated at laparoscopy, following tubal cannulation.

tium, ensuring intratubal placement and the accurate delivery of the gametes or embryos. Furthermore, it offers a good appraisal of the depth that the catheter must be inserted prior to intratubal delivery of gametes and embryos (36).

The technique of tubal cannulation has opened the way to introduce flexible mini-endoscopes for intratubal visualization. In its infancy, due to technological drawbacks to achieve good resolution and visualization with these small fibers while attempting to distend the intratubal lumen, tubaloscopy is nonetheless progressing slowly but steadily and may in the future be of use in the clinical setting.

TIMING OF HYSTEROSCOPY

Although best performed within 5 days after the completion of menstruation, when the endometrium is thin, hysteroscopy for the evaluation of infertility is frequently performed in the secretory phase in combination with laparoscopy. If special care is taken to avoid abrasion of the endometrium or unnecessary manipulations, the uterine cavity can be studied without difficulty. Therapeutic hysteroscopy should be performed in the immediate postmenstrual period. When hysteroscopy in combination with laparoscopy is performed in the luteal phase, laparoscopy is performed first, before any cervical or intrauterine manipulation is done (37). Once the laparoscope is in place, hysteroscopy is performed. Uterine or tubal pathology may be detected during laparoscopy. In patients with equivocal cornual occlusions, a selective chromopertubation can be performed by hysteroscopy by cannulating the first 4 to 5 mm of the fallopian tube. Because this area is usually patent, indigo carmine can be injected directly at this level, and the obstruction or spasm will be overcome. Should this fail, tubal cannulation can be performed. Laparoscopy followed by

hysteroscopy offers an excellent way to examine the genital tract and rule out or treat cervical, uterine, and tubal peritoneal factors affecting fertility.

CONCLUSIONS

The addition of visual appraisal of the uterine cavity offers invaluable information in diagnosis and supplements the hysterosalpingogram in the overall evaluation of the infertile patient. When intrauterine factors may be responsible for infertility, hysteroscopy provides a valuable aid in their evaluation. It offers an excellent approach for treatment of many conditions that in the past required laparotomy and bisection of the uterine corpus, which might otherwise predispose these patients to secondary pelvic adhesions, impaired fertility, or even a cesarean section should pregnancy occur and be carried to viability.

The main indication of hysteroscopy in infertile patients is the abnormal or ambiguous hysterogram. Hysteroscopy is, therefore, complementary to hysterosalpingography. Used in conjunction, these two techniques add accuracy and precision in the evaluation of infertility.

REFERENCES

1. Wallach EE: Evaluation and management of uterine causes of infertility. *Clin Obstet Gynecol* 22:43, 1979.
2. Valle RF: Clinical management of uterine factors in infertile patients. *Semin Reprod Endocrinol* 3:149, 1985.
3. Slezak P, Tillinger KG: Hysterographic defects of polypoid filling defects in the uterine cavity. *Radiology* 115:78, 1975.
4. Slezak P, Tillinger KG: The incidence and clinical importance of hysterographic evidence of cavities in the uterine wall. *Radiology* 118:581, 1976.
5. Nickerson CW: Infertility and uterine contour. *Am J Obstet Gynecol* 129:268, 1977.
6. Mohr J, Lindemann HJ: Hysteroscopy in the infertile patient. *J Reprod Med* 19:161, 1977.

7. Valle RF: Hysteroscopy: diagnostic and therapeutic applications. *J Reprod Med* 20:115, 1978.

8. Valle RF: Hysteroscopy in the evaluation of female infertility. *Am J Obstet Gynecol* 137:425, 1980.

9. Valle RF: How endoscopy aids the infertility work-up. *Contemp Obstet Gynecol* 3:191, 1984.

10. Siegler AM: Hysterosalpingography. *Fertil Steril* 40:139, 1983.

11. Valle RF, Sciarra JJ: Current status of hysteroscopy in gynecologic practice. *Fertil Steril* 32:619, 1979.

12. Siegler AM: Hysterography and hysteroscopy in infertile patients. *J Reprod Med* 18:148, 1977.

13. Kessler I, Lancet M: Hysterography and hysteroscopy: a comparison. *Fertil Steril* 46:709, 1986.

14. Fayez JA, Mutie G, Schneider PJ: The diagnostic value of hysterosalpingography and hysteroscopy in infertility investigation. *Am J Obstet Gynecol* 156:558, 1987.

15. Taylor PJ: Correlations in infertility: symptomatology, hysterosalpingography, laparoscopy, and hysteroscopy. *J Reprod Med* 18:339, 1977.

16. Snowden EU, Jarrett JC, Dawood MY: Comparison of diagnostic accuracy of laparoscopy, hysteroscopy, and hysterosalpingography in evaluation of female infertility. *Fertil Steril* 41:709, 1984.

17. Klein SM, Garcia CR: Asherman's syndrome: a critical and current review. *Fertil Steril* 24:722, 1973.

18. Valle RJ, Sciarra JJ: Intrauterine adhesions: hysteroscopic diagnosis, classification, treatment, and reproductive outcome. *Am J Obstet Gynecol* 158:1459, 1988.

19. Valle RJ: Therapeutic hysteroscopy in infertility. *Int J Fertil* 29:143, 1984.

20. Siegler AM, Valle RF: Therapeutic hysteroscopic procedures. *Fertil Steril* 50:685, 1988.

21. Hassiakos DK, Zourlas PA: Transcervical division of uterine septa. *Obstet Gynecol Surv* 45:165, 1990.

22. Drake T, Tredway D, Buchanan D, Takaki N, Daane T: Unexplained infertility: a reappraisal. *Obstet Gynecol* 50:644, 1977.

23. Moghissi KS, Wallach EE: Unexplained infertility. *Fertil Steril* 39:5, 1983.

24. Vancaillie T, Schmidt EH: The uterotubal junction: a proposal for classifying its morphology as assessed with hysteroscopy. *J Reprod Med* 33:624, 1988.

25. Menken FC: Endoscopic observations of endocrine processes and hormone changes. In: Albrecht FR, Sanchez JR, Willowitzer H (eds). *Simposio Esteroids Sexuals.* Museo Nacional, Bogota, Columbia, June 26, 1968. Berlin: Saladruck, 1969, pp 276–281.

26. Vancaillie T, DeMuylder E: Hysteroscopic evaluation of hormonal influence on the endometrium. In: Van der Pas H, Van Herendael BJ, Van Lith DAF, Keith LG (eds). *Hysteroscopy: Proceedings of the First European Symposium on Hysteroscopy.* A.Z. Jan Palfijn O.C.M.W., Antwerp, Belgium, September 2–3, 1982. Boston: MTP Press Limited, 1983, pp 101–103.

27. Sorensen SS: Hysteroscopic evaluation and endocrinological aspects of women with müllerian anomalies and oligomenorrhea. *Int J Fertil* 32:445, 1987.

28. Bordt J, Belkien L, Vancaillie T, Stening C, Schneider HPG: Ergebnisse diagnostischer Hysteroskopien in einem IVT/ET–Programm. *Geburtsh Frauenheilk* 44:813, 1984.

29. Valle RF: Hysteroscopic removal of submucous leiomyomas. *J Gynecol Surg* 6:89, 1990.

30. Taylor PJ, Hamou J, Mencaglia L: Hysteroscopic detection of heterotopic intrauterine bone formation. *J Reprod Med* 33:337, 1988.

31. Scarselli G, Tantini C, Mencaglia L, Chelo E, Gargiulo A: Microhysteroscopy and infertility. In: Van der Pas H, Van Herendael BJ, Van Lith DAF, Keith LG (eds). *Hysteroscopy: Proceedings of the First European Symposium on Hysteroscopy.* A.Z. Jan Palfijn O.C.M.W., Antwerp, Belgium, September 2–3, 1982. Boston: MTP Press Limited, 1983, pp 151–154.

32. Van Herendael BJ: Hysteroscopy in subfertility. In: Van der Pas H, Van Herendael BJ, Van Lith DAF, Keith LG (eds). *Hysteroscopy: Proceedings of the First European Symposium on Hysteroscopy.* A.Z. Jan Palfijn O.C.M.W., Antwerp, Belgium, September 2–3, 1982. Boston: MTP Press Limited, 1983, pp 155–157.

33. March CM: Hysteroscopy as an aid to diagnosis in female infertility. *Clin Obstet Gynecol* 26:302, 1983.

34. Quinones-Guerrero R, Alvarado-Duran A, Aznar-Ramos R: Tubal catheterization: applications of new technique. *Am J Obstet Gynecol* 114:674, 1972.

35. Novy MJ, Thurmond AS, Patton P, Uchida BT, Rosch J: Diagnosis of cornual obstruction by transcervical fallopian tube cannulation. *Fertil Steril* 50:434, 1988.

36. Valle RF: Future growth and development of hysteroscopy. *Obstet Gynecol Clin North Am* 15:111, 1988.

37. Taylor PJ, Leader A: Laparoscopy combined with hysteroscopy in the management of the ovulatory infertile female. *Int J Fertil* 28:59, 1983.

8

Intrauterine Synechiae

Intrauterine scarring first appeared in the medical literature in 1894 when Fritsch reported a 25-year-old who developed amenorrhea following a curettage performed 3 weeks postpartum (1). By 1946, when Asherman described the condition that now bears his name, the literature already contained 61 cases. Asherman described a variable syndrome of intrauterine adhesion formation with scarring and obliteration of the potential space of the uterine cavity, resulting clinically in hypo- or amenorrhea (2, 3). At the time, the most common etiologic factor was thought to be genital tuberculosis; it has since been shown that other causative factors are much more prevalent.

The incidence of intrauterine synechiae is unknown and there is no general agreement as to its prevalence or its impact on fertility. This uncertainty is multifactorial and reflects differences in the experience of investigators, the use of induced abortion throughout the world, the incidence of genital tuberculosis in varied localities, the techniques used to evaluate the infertile couple, and the criteria used to diagnose synechiae. It is possible that a significant incidence exists in asymptomatic women who do not seek medical care.

However, there is a general consensus as to the major etiologic factors responsible for the development of these synechiae. Asherman's syndrome, or endometrial sclerosis, occurs when intrauterine adhesions form and obliterate, either partially or completely, the uterine cavity, cervical canal, internal cervical os, or one or both tubal ostia. The major predisposing factors are pregnancy, trauma, and infection, and synechiae are almost always iatrogenic in origin. From a practical standpoint, formation of adhesions should be suspected in any patient who has undergone (*a*) curettage following pregnancy, (*b*) induced abortion (Fig. 8.1), or (*c*) any uterine surgery (including cesarean section) in the presence of pregnancy. In a reported series of 187 patients, 179 (96%) were related to curettage because of a pregnancy-related state (4). However, pregnancy is not essential for the development of synechiae. Trauma without pregnancy, i.e., dilatation and curettage (D&C), can predispose to the condition (5), and, furthermore, the presence of infection seems to increase the likelihood of synechiae formation. Rabau and David (5) maintained that infection, frequently low grade or subclinical, is almost always associated with scarring. However, other investigators report no evidence of infection (6–9), and still others have been unable to document evidence of inflammatory cells or endometritis in the surgical specimens obtained in patients with synechiae (10, 11).

Asherman's syndrome offers a continuum of symptomatology and a variable effect on fertility. Patients may present with secondary amenorrhea, hypomenorrhea, or severe dysmenorrhea, but this is variable; among 2151 cases of Asherman's syndrome, Schenker and Margalioth (8) found normal menses in only 6%, while Lancet and Kessler (11) found abnormalities such as hypomenorrhea in 29 of 185 women (16%) and amenorrhea in only 10%. The usual reason that Asherman's syndrome is diagnosed is that these patients have infertility or recurrent fetal wastage with a normal menstrual history, or even a history of premature labor, an-

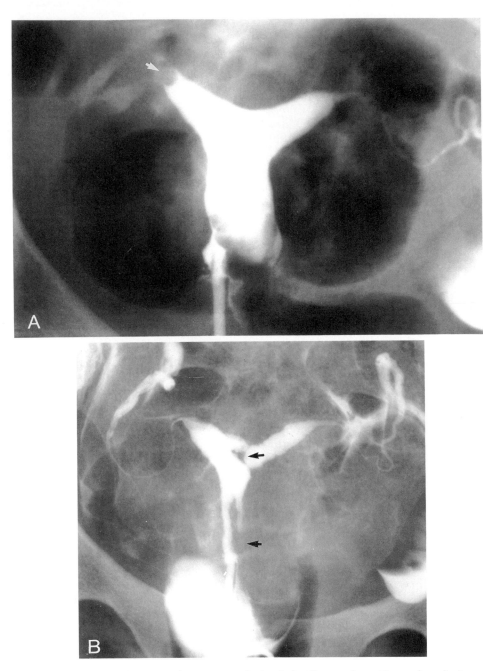

Figure 8.1. **A,** Baseline hysterosalpingogram during infertility workup. Cornual occlusion on the right is noted (*arrow*). **B,** Subsequent hysterosalpingogram on the same patient. In the interim between examinations, a pregnancy was terminated in a first-trimester abortion, which was followed by dilatation and curettage. Note the synechiae (*arrows*) in the midzone of the uterine body and in the lower uterine segment.

tepartum fetal death, and uterine rupture, and the evaluation for these obstetric complications leads to the diagnosis (8, 11). The diagnosis is usually made by hysterosalpingography. This inconstant clinical presentation is the result of the marked variability of both the extent and the location of the synechiae. The lesions of Asherman's syndrome may be found in any portion of the uterus and may involve the entire uterine cavity or only a small area. Synechiae located in the cornua may result in tubal occlusion. Stenosis or atresia of the internal cervical os may cause partial or complete obstruction to menstrual flow and significant dysmenorrhea. Since endometriosis is more likely in these patients, fertility may be severely hampered. If implantation occurs, continued development of the placenta may be impaired and result in first- or second-trimester abortion. Other obstetric complications or mishaps may occur, including premature delivery, malpresentation, premature separation of the placenta, and placenta accreta, a condition in which the placenta becomes markedly adherent to the myometrium, resulting in incomplete postpartum separation (12).

CLASSIFICATION OF INTRAUTERINE ADHESIONS

A grading system to describe the extent of intrauterine synechiae would be useful as an objective means to evaluate improvement after a therapeutic attempt as well as to provide prognostic criteria for the physician and the patient. The grade of severity should have a positive correlation with menstrual dysfunction, infertility, and complications of pregnancy. To date, although several schemes for classification have been proposed, no one has been generally accepted, and an extensive study to analyze the utility of the proposed scheme in terms of outcome has not been done. Toaff (13, 14) proposed a classification, based on the extent of the cavity obliteration, that categorizes the condition into four grades (14).

Grade 1. A single, small filling defect, frequently well inside the uterine cavity, occupying up to about one-tenth of the uterine area (Fig. 8.2).

Grade 2. A single, medium-sized filling defect occupying up to one-fifth of the uterine area, or several smaller defects adding up to the same degree of involvement, located inside the uterine cavity, whose outline may show minor indentations but no gross deformation (Fig. 8.3).

Grade 3. A single large, or several smaller, filling defects involving up to about one-third of the uterine cavity, which is deformed or asymmetrical because of marginal adhesions (Fig. 8.4).

Grade 4. Large filling defects occupying most of a severely deformed uterine cavity (Figs. 8.5 and 8.6).

This classification was published before the widespread use of hysteroscopy, so a hysteroscopic classification has been proposed (11):

Class I (Slight)	Less than ⅓ cavity, both ostia visible.
Class II (Medium)	⅓ to ½ cavity, one ostium visible.
Class III (Severe)	Greater than ½ cavity, no ostium visible.

The American Fertility Society Classification of Intrauterine Adhesions (Fig. 8.7) combines both hysterosalpingographic and hysteroscopic criteria and develops a score from 0 to 12.

DIAGNOSIS OF INTRAUTERINE ADHESIONS

Synechiae are scars that have formed as part of the healing process in the potential space of the uterine cavity

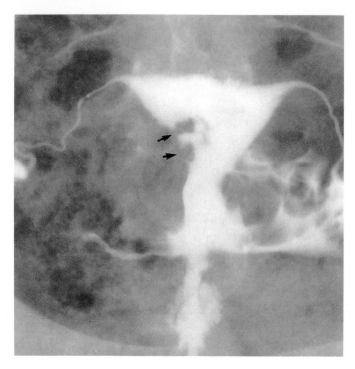

Figure 8.2.   Minimal synechiae formation (*arrows*) along the lateral wall of the uterine body.

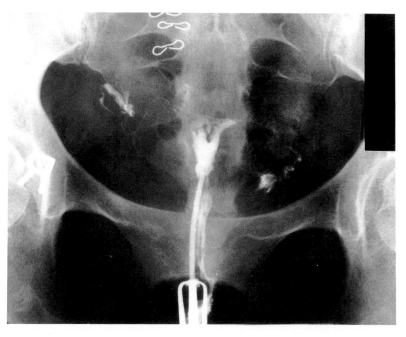

Figure 8.3.   Several irregular synechiae localized to the fundus and upper portion of the uterine body in this patient with a history of abortion and dilatation and curettage.

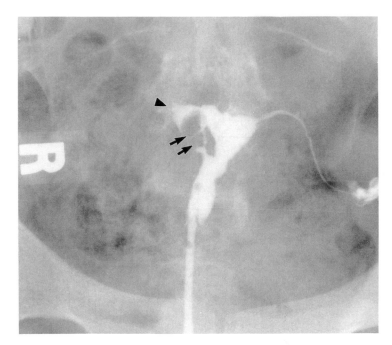

Figure 8.4. Moderately extensive synechiae formation involving the right half of the uterine body (*arrows*). In addition, adhesions have obliterated the ostium of the right fallopian tube (*arrowhead*).

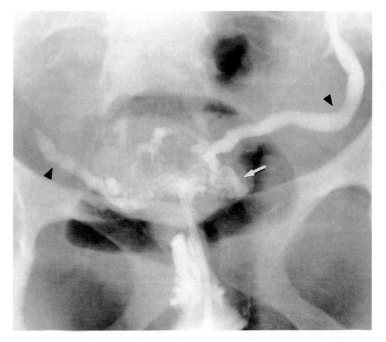

Figure 8.5. Extensive synechiae formation obliterating virtually the entire cavity of the uterine body. Myometrial intravasation (*arrow*) is observed, and there is obvious filling of major uterine and the ovarian veins (*arrowheads*).

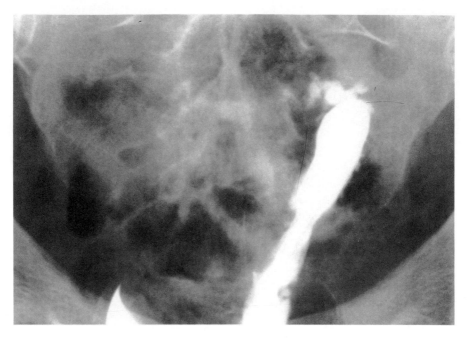

Figure 8.6.   Extensive deformity of the uterine cavity secondary to extensive synechiae formation as demonstrated at hysteroscopy. Adhesive changes have occluded both fallopian tubes at their ostia. The appearance simulates a unicornuate uterus.

when the traumatized uterine walls are held in apposition. The history may suggest the diagnosis, particularly since the otherwise unusual condition hypomenorrhea is common. There is frequently difficulty in sounding the uterine cavity or obtaining tissue for an endometrial biopsy. A "gritty" sensation may be detected when the biopsy is attempted.

More often, however, the diagnosis is unsuspected and is made at hysterosalpingography. Synechiae are frequently listed along with polyps, myomata, and uterine septum as "filling defects" within the uterine cavity as seen at hysterosalpingography. Generally speaking, however, the appearance of the scars is characteristic (Fig. 8.8). Neoplastic filling defects of the uterine cavity and retained products of conception are characteristically round with smooth edges and homogeneous in density. Synechiae, on the other hand, are stellate, irregular, and frequently inhomogeneous if contrast

material enters pockets of no or little adherence. Indeed, the apparent filling defect at hysterosalpingography is not due to a mass lesion within the uterine cavity but rather reflects a constant area of apposition of the anterior and posterior walls of the uterus with failure of distention of the cavity in the area of synechiae formation (Fig. 8.9).

If the diagnosis of intrauterine adhesions is suspected prior to the radiographic examination, a short cannula should be used so as not to disrupt adhesions in the cervical canal or lower uterine segment. It is, of course, important to ensure that the uterine cavity is adequately assessed. This requires sufficient traction to counteract any appreciable anteflexion or retroflexion of the uterus and to permit visualization of the uterine cavity in its entirety (Figs. 8.10 and 8.11). Undue pressure should not be used to introduce the contrast agent. In some cases of severe intrauterine adhesion for-

Patient's Name _____ Date _____ Chart # _____

Age _____ G _____ P _____ Sp Ab _____ VTP _____ Ectopic _____ Infertile Yes _____ No _____

Other Significant History (i.e. surgery, infection, etc.) _____

HSG _____ Sonography _____ Photography _____ Laparoscopy _____ Laparotomy _____

Extent of Cavity Involved	<1/3	1/3 - 2/3	>2/3
	1	2	4
Type of Adhesions	Filmy	Filmy & Dense	Dense
	1	2	4
Menstrual Pattern	Normal	Hypomenorrhea	Amenorrhea
	0	2	4

Prognostic Classification HSG* Score   Hysteroscopy Score

Stage I (Mild) 1-4 _____ _____

Stage II (Moderate) 5-8 _____ _____

Stage III (Severe) 9-12 _____ _____

*All adhesions should be considered dense

Treatment (Surgical Procedures): _____

_____

_____

_____

_____

Prognosis for Conception & Subsequent Viable Infant*

_____ Excellent (> 75%)

_____ Good (50-75%)

_____ Fair (25%-50%)

_____ Poor (< 25%)

*Physician's judgment based upon tubal patency.

Recommended Followup Treatment: _____

_____

_____

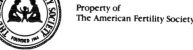

Property of
The American Fertility Society

Additional Findings: _____

_____

_____

_____

_____

DRAWING

HSG Findings

Hysteroscopy Findings

For additional supply write to:
The American Fertility Society
2140 11th Avenue, South
Suite 200
Birmingham, Alabama 35205

Figure 8.7. The American Fertility Society classification of intrauterine adhesions. (From The American Fertility Society classification of adnexal adhesions, distal tubal occlusion, tubal occlusion secondary to tubal ligation, tubal pregnancies, müllerian anomalies and intrauterine adhesions. *Fertil Steril* 49:953, 1988. Reproduced with permission of the publisher, The American Fertility Society.)

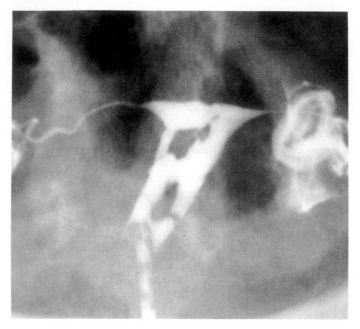

Figure 8.8.   Classic appearance of synechiae presenting as irregular, angular, well-defined filling defects.

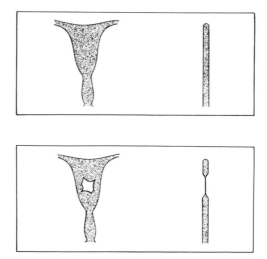

Figure 8.9.   Artistic conception of synechia. *Upper panel* demonstrates normal uterine cavity (distended with contrast medium) in anteroposterior and lateral projections. *Lower panel* reveals that the irregular filling defect seen in the anteroposterior projection is really an area of apposition of the anterior and posterior endometrial surfaces rather than a mass lesion.

mation, contrast material may enter the vascular or lymphatic system (Fig. 8.5). These episodes are usually uncomplicated and present no difficulty to the patient. Because of the frequency of intravasation and vascular embolization,

however, the use of oil-soluble contrast media may be especially ill advised in patients suspected of synechiae (Figs. 8.5 and 8.12).

The intrauterine defects that are characteristic of synechiae are typically

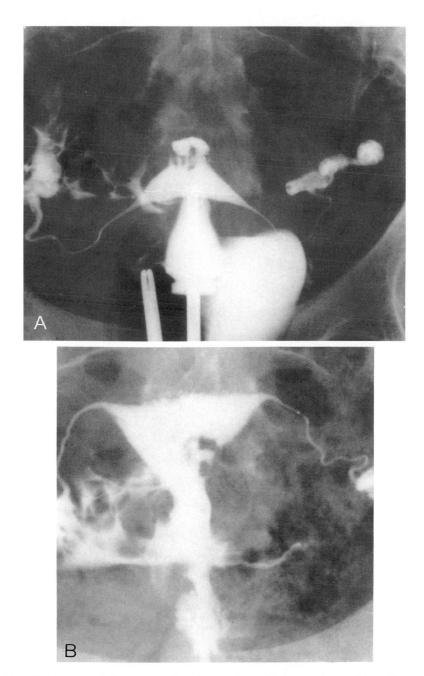

Figure 8.10. **A,** Hysterosalpingogram of patient with multiple small synechiae. One cannot appreciate the presence of the filling defect because of the marked anteflexion of the uterus. **B,** Adequate traction permits better evaluation of the uterine cavity. Multiple small, angular filling defects are noted.

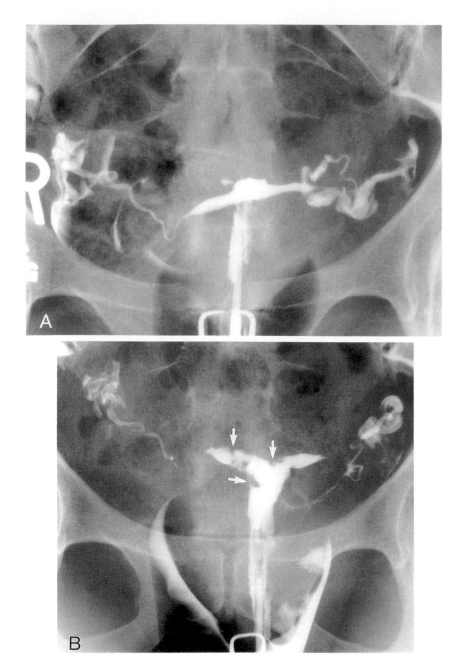

Figure 8.11.   A, Moderately flexed uterus. No abnormality can be identified. **B,** Traction optimizes visualization of the uterine cavity. Numerous small synechiae are demonstrated (*arrows*).

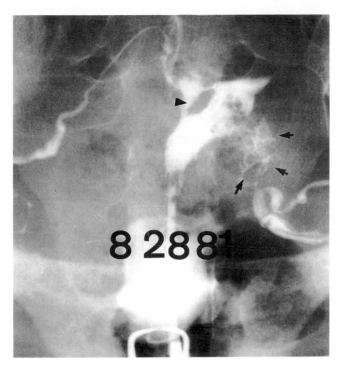

Figure 8.12.   Classic angular appearance of adhesions obliterating a portion of the uterine cavity (*arrowhead*). The cavity is also partially obliterated along the right lateral wall, with resultant extravasation of contrast material into the myometrium (*black arrows*).

irregular, angulated, sharply contoured, and immobile. The position, shape, and number of these adhesions may vary considerably from patient to patient. If localized to the cervical canal, the adhesions may appear quite similar to mesonephric (Gartner) duct remnants (Fig. 8.13). These latter, also described in Chapter 4, present what appear to be linear filling defects in the endocervical canal and may be virtually impossible to distinguish from synechiae; hysteroscopy is needed to make a definitive diagnosis.

Although the diagnosis of intrauterine scarring is usually established at hysterosalpingography, hysteroscopy is necessary for confirmation and further evaluation of the extent of the pathology. The apparent lack of correlation that sometimes occurs when the two procedures are compared is understandable when the differences in the two techniques are considered. The technique of hysteroscopy introduces a viscous medium under pressure, resulting in distention of the uterine cavity and frequently in disruption of some of the adhesions. Synechiae that appear large and well defined at hysterosalpingography may present at hysteroscopy only as filmy, band-like adhesions because of the distention produced during the procedure of hysteroscopy. Perfect correlation between the two procedures is therefore not to be expected. Further, synechiae observed at hysterosalpingography may not be seen at hysteroscopy, which is not meant to imply a false-positive radiographic finding.

TREATMENT AND PROGNOSIS

Although there is some controversy surrounding the proper approach to the

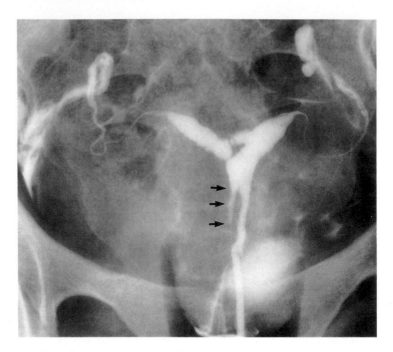

Figure 8.13. Synechiae formation in the uterine body and lower uterine segment. The appearance in the lower uterine segment simulates the radiographic appearance of a mesonephric duct remnant (*arrows*).

patient with intrauterine adhesion formation, nevertheless the essential components of therapy are lysis of adhesions at hysteroscopy or at curettage, placement of some form of device to keep the uterine walls apart, and administration of hormones to induce endometrial proliferation and menstruation (4, 15–22). Most of the controversy revolves around the necessity for antibiotic administration, which is ordinarily employed in the therapy, and corticoid administration, to prevent subsequent formation of adhesions. The recommended devices for intrauterine placement have included intrauterine contraceptive devices (IUDs) of several types, an inflated Foley catheter balloon, and a form made of distensible material molded to fit the uterine cavity. We are now recommending stepwise transcervical lysis, leaving a Foley catheter in place between procedures. We have a patient who required three hyster-

osalpingograms to complete the lysis of adhesions and reclaim the cavity.

With complete cervical stenosis or adhesion formation at the level of the internal os, hysterotomy may be the only approach to the lysis of intrauterine adhesions (9, 23). Using this approach, the uterus is incised in the fundus, and a route of dissection toward the cervix is employed, using either blunt or sharp dissection. Neither technique has been proven superior to the other. Again, a Foley catheter is introduced.

Postoperative hysterosalpingography is essential and is usually performed in the next proliferative phase after discontinuation of the hormonal treatment (Fig. 8.14). It is not unusual to find recurrent adhesion formation, which, it is hoped, will be less than at the initial procedure (Fig. 8.15).

Results of present-day treatment are excellent in terms of symptomatic re-

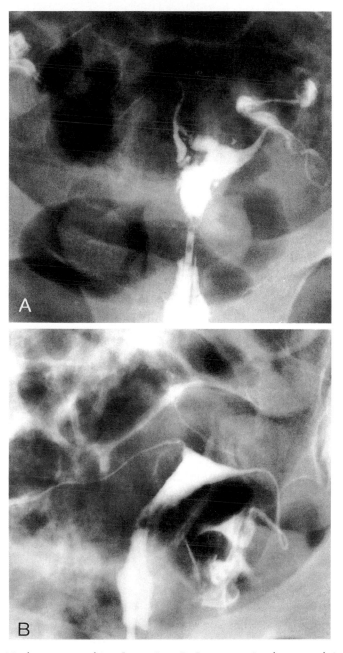

Figure 8.14. **A,** Moderate synechiae formation. **B,** Postoperative hysterosalpingogram demonstrates a normal-appearing uterine cavity.

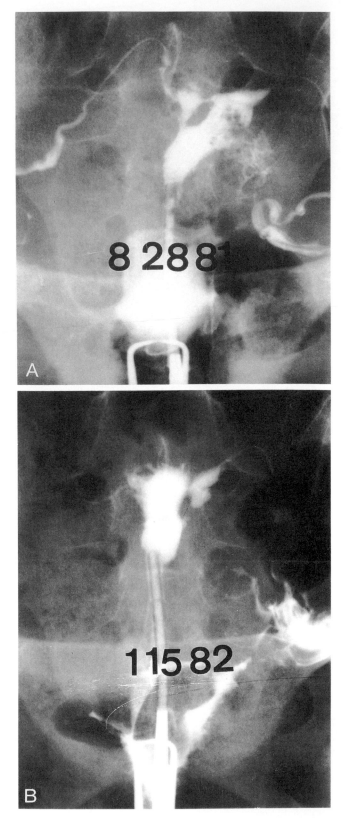

Figure 8.15. Same patient as in Figure 8.12. Intervening surgical therapy for the intrauterine synechiae formation resulted in partial improvement. Considerable uterine cavity deformity due to residual and/or recurrent synechiae is noted.

lief and correction of menstrual disorders, but they remain far from ideal with respect to restoration of fertility (8, 23–29). Most women regain normal menstruation, although about 11% continue to describe hypomenorrhea. The pregnancy rate depends on the severity of the adhesions, the extent of occlusion of the uterine cavity, and the type (filmy or fibromuscular) of adhesion treated; among 187 patients treated, there were term pregnancy rates of 81.3% for those with mild adhesions and 31.9% for those with severe adhesions (22). Overall, about half of women desiring fertility conceive, and among these pregnancies, about 25% abort or have ectopic pregnancies.

Abnormal placentation in patients treated with curettage has been reported in 5 to 31% of cases. With hysteroscopy, the occurrence may be much lower, as only one case of partial placenta accreta was reported among 187 women treated by hysteroscopic lysis of adhesions (22). Freidman et al. (28) reported uterine dehiscence, placenta increta, and uterine sacculation in different cases, with two of the three treated at hysteroscopy, and Deaton et al. (29) reported a case of uterine rupture. Overall, serious obstetric complications are encountered more frequently than is normal. Of particular concern is the high incidence of placenta accreta, most probably caused by an abnormal adherence of placental tissue to sites of the severed adhesions adjacent to the myometrium, where the lack of decidua basalis is most evident. Thus, restoration of menstruation after treatment of intrauterine adhesions does not necessarily imply normal fertility, and the ensuing pregnancy may be subject to a number of complications. Pregnancies in women who have had treatment for intrauterine adhesions are potentially hazardous and should therefore be regarded as having a high risk for complications.

REFERENCES

1. Fritsch J: Einfall von volligen Schwund der Gebermutterhohle nach Auskratzung. *Zentralbl Gynakol* 52:337, 1894.
2. Asherman J: Amenorrhea traumatica (atretica). *J Obstet Gynaecol Br Emp* 55:23, 1948.
3. Asherman J: Traumatic intrauterine adhesions. *J Obstet Gynaecol Br Commonw* 57:892, 1950.
4. Taylor PJ, Cumming DC, Hill PJ: Significance of intrauterine adhesions detected hysteroscopically in eumenorrheic infertile women and role of antecedent curettage in their formation. *Am J Obstet Gynecol* 139:239, 1981.
5. Rabau E, David A: Intrauterine adhesions: Etiology, prevention and treatment. *Obstet Gynecol* 22:626, 1963.
6. March CM, Israel R: Intrauterine adhesions secondary to elective abortion. Hysteroscopic diagnosis and management. *Obstet Gynecol* 48:422, 1976.
7. Polishuk WZ, Anteby SO, Weinstein D: Puerperal endometritis and intrauterine adhesions. *Int Surg* 60:418, 1975.
8. Schenker JG, Margalioth EJ: Intrauterine adhesions: An updated appraisal. *Fertil Steril* 37:593, 1982.
9. Jensen PA, Stromme WB: Amenorrhea secondary to puerperal curettage (Asherman's syndrome). *Am J Obstet Gynecol* 113:150, 1972.
10. Schenker JG, Yaffe H: Induction of intrauterine adhesions in experimental animals and in women. *Isr J Med Sci* 14:261, 1978.
11. Lancet M, Kessler I: A review of Asherman's syndrome, and results of modern treatment. *Int J Fertil* 33:14, 1988.
12. Breen JL, Neubecker R, Gregori CA, Franklin JE Jr: Placenta accreta, increta and percreta. A survey of 40 cases. *Obstet Gynecol* 49:343, 1977.
13. Toaff R: Amenorrea e ipomenorrea traumatics (Sindrome di Asherman). *Atti Soc Ital Ginecol* 49:258, 1962.
14. Toaff R, Ballas S: Traumatic hypomenorrhea-amenorrhea (Asherman's syndrome). *Fertil Steril* 30:379, 1978.
15. Danezis J, Souplis A, Papathanassiou Z: Conservative correction of uterine anomalies in cases of congenital and post-traumatic infertility. *Int J Fertil* 23:118, 1978.
16. Sugimoto O: Diagnostic and therapeutic hysteroscopy for traumatic intrauterine

adhesions. *Am J Obstet Gynecol* 131:539, 1978.

17. Badawy S, Nusbaum M: Intrauterine synechiae—etiological factors and effect of treatment on reproductive function. *Infertility* 2:303, 1979.

18. Ikeda T, Morita A, Imamura A, Mori I: The separation procedure for intrauterine adhesion (synechiae uteri) under roentgenographic view. *Fertil Steril* 36:333, 1981.

19. Siegler AM, Kontopoulos VG: Lysis of intrauterine adhesions under hysteroscopic control. A report of 25 operations. *J Reprod Med* 26:372, 1981.

20. Neuwirth RS, Hussein AR, Schiffman BM, Amin HK: Hysteroscopic resection of intrauterine scars using a new technique. *Obstet Gynecol* 60:111, 1982.

21. Hamou J, Salat-Barous J, Siegler AM: Diagnosis and treatment of intrauterine adhesions by microhysteroscopy. *Fertil Steril* 39:321, 1983.

22. Valle RF, Sciarra JJ: Intrauterine adhesions: Hysteroscopic diagnosis, classification, treatment, and reproductive outcome. *Am J Obstet Gynecol* 158:1459, 1988.

23. Jewelewicz R, Khalaf S, Neuwirth RS, Vande Wiele RL: Obstetric complications after treatment of intrauterine synechiae (Asherman's syndrome). *Obstet Gynecol* 47:701, 1976.

24. Georgkopoulos P: Placenta accreta following lysis of uterine synechiae (Asherman's syndrome). *J Obstet Gynaecol Br Commonw* 81:730, 1974.

25. Oelsner G, David A, Insler V, Serr DM: Outcome of pregnancy after treatment of intrauterine adhesions. *Obstet Gynecol* 44:341, 1974.

26. Caspi E, Perpinial S: Reproductive performances after treatment of intrauterine adhesions. *Int J Fertil* 20:249, 1975.

27. Bergquist CA, Rock JA, Jones HW Jr: Pregnancy outcome following treatment of intrauterine adhesions. *Int J Fertil* 26:107, 1981.

28. Friedman A, DeFazio J, DeCherney A: Severe obstetric complications after aggressive treatment of Asherman's syndrome. *Obstet Gynecol* 67:864, 1986.

29. Deaton JL, Maier D, Andreoli J: Spontaneous uterine rupture during pregnancy after treatment of Asherman's syndrome. *Am J Obstet Gynecol* 160:1053, 1989.

9

Hysterosalpingography of the Fallopian Tube

Tubal factors are thought to be responsible for some 30 to 50% of all infertility problems and require prompt and accurate assessment. Hysterosalpingography is usually the initial diagnostic tool employed in assessing tubal disease because of its ease, accuracy, and cost effectiveness. Diagnostic laparoscopy, however, frequently plays a significant role in tubal assessment. It is practical to view these two diagnostic procedures as complementary rather than competitive tools in the search for fallopian tube abnormalities (1–6).

Radionuclide hysterosalpingography to evaluate tubal patency has been described as an innocuous technique with a 94% efficiency (7). Technetium-labeled human serum albumin microspheres placed in the posterior vaginal fornix migrate spontaneously to the peritoneal cavity, and their progress can be followed by using a gamma camera. Free pelvic activity can be demonstrated at 40 to 180 minutes and documented by activity found in peritoneal fluid aspirated by culdocentesis (8). The radiation dose to the ovaries may be excessive, however, and the method yields only limited information.

Conventional hysterosalpingography can be done easily on an outpatient basis without anesthesia or significant premedication. In addition to visualizing tubal patency and configuration, it permits evaluation of the uterine cavity. Disadvantages include occasional inability to differentiate cornual spasm from occlusion, as well as the inability to diagnose peritubal or adnexal disease, although

Karasick and Goldfarb (9) conclude that hysterosalpingography is the diagnostic procedure of choice in the initial investigation of infertility.

Diagnostic laparoscopy permits accurate assessment of tubal patency by the retrograde injection of a colored dye, such as dilute methylene blue or indigo carmine, which can be seen to emerge from the fimbriated ends of the tube. Cornual occlusion due to spasm is less likely with laparoscopy because of the general anesthesia needed for the procedure. However, both laparoscopy and hysterosalpingography may result in faulty assessment of tubal occlusion. If results from the two procedures contradict one another, any data signifying tubal patency should be accepted. The ability of laparoscopy to find evidence of peritubal and adnexal disease is a distinct advantage of this procedure.

Some data suggest that pregnancy rates may be increased for the 3 to 4 months following hysterosalpingography (10–12). This seems to hold true whether oil- or water-soluble contrast material is used, although advocates of oil-soluble media report that the incidence of pregnancy is doubled, from 13% with aqueous to 29% with oil-soluble agents (11). In either event, the procedure may possibly have therapeutic as well as diagnostic value.

Tubal dysfunction and disease can take several forms: tubal occlusion, which may be proximal, midposition, distal, or combined; hydrosalpinx, which can be patent or obstructed; and intratubal lesions, which can include destruction of ciliated and nonciliated cells of the tubal epithelium, intratubal polyps, and salpingitis isthmica nodosa. Large series have been reported tabulating the abnormalities diagnosed (13–15); these are of limited use because of population and technique differences.

ABNORMALITIES OF THE UTEROTUBAL JUNCTION

The normal uterotubal junction at hysterosalpingography has a diamond or wedge shape in the intramural segment of the fallopian tube (see Chapter 3) and has been described as an "endometrial funnel" (16). The length of the intramural tube as measured on extirpated specimens varies from 5 to 14 mm. A true anatomic sphincter is absent; however, the intramural tube has an inner longitudinal muscle layer, which functions with the middle circular layer of muscle to induce a constricting action in this area of the oviduct. Cornual spasm occurring during hysterosalpingography can give the appearance of tubal occlusion; this may or may not be reversed by the intravenous administration of antispasmodics. In our practice, glucagon has been valuable (17) (Fig. 9.1). Cornual occlusion can also occur during the secretory phase of the cycle if protruding secretory endometrium is pushed into the ostium and blocks the opening of the uterotubal junction. Polyps or papillations of the mucosa of the intramural portion of the tube are occasionally observed (Fig. 9.2) and, according to some reports, can contribute to the diagnosis of occlusion (18, 19). We have not experienced any instances of tubal occlusion secondary to such polyps. Furthermore, although polyps were diagnosed in 31 of 174 (18%) of hysterosalpingograms (19), there was no difference in conception rates in women with or without tubo-cornual polyps, probably related to their failure to occlude the tubes. It is likely that most of

these findings are merely the result of redundancy of the endosalpinx rather than true polyp formation. However, synechia formation at the tubal ostium may cause obstruction. During hysterosalpingography, it is important to move the uterus in relation to the tube, straightening the convoluted intramural portions so that contrast medium is more likely to pass; pulling down on the tenaculum, then pushing up while injecting contrast material will often accomplish this.

Few studies have systematically investigated uterotubal junction pathology causing obstruction. Excised tubal segments from women with uterotubal junction obstruction indicate that the most frequent lesion is obliterative fibrosis (in 38%) (Fig. 9.3), followed by salpingitis isthmica nodosa (24%), intramucosal endometriosis (14%), and chronic tubal inflammation (21%) (20) (Fig. 9.4). In marked contrast, Sulak et al. (21) found no specific reason for tubal occlusions in 11 of 18 cases diagnosed at both hysterosalpingography and laparoscopy, and amorphous material "plugs" in 6 cases. That tubal debris, mucoid plugs, and light adhesions cause cornual occlusion may account for the success of nonsurgical fallopian tube recanalization in restoring tubal patency (22–24) (See Chapter 10).

ABNORMALITIES OF THE ISTHMUS AND AMPULLARY PORTION

Obstruction at the isthmic and ampullary portions of the fallopian tubes can be due to infection, sterilization procedures, and congenital anomalies. Tubal occlusion secondary to infectious processes may occur at any portion of the tube (25). Siegler (26) evaluated 1000 consecutive salpingograms and found unilateral tubal occlusion in 27.7% and bilateral blockage in 11.1%. Cornual occlusion was most common, followed

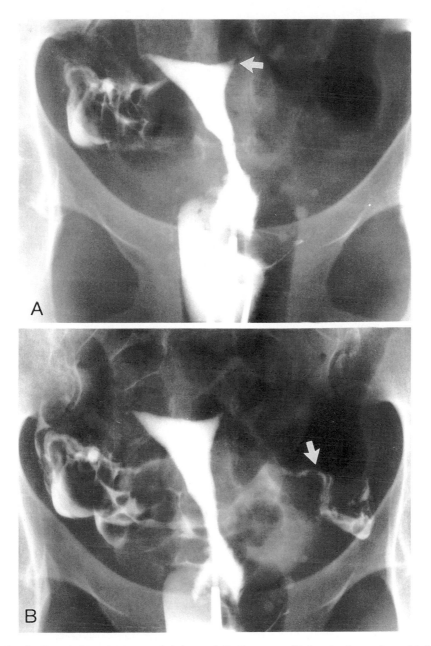

Figure 9.1. **A,** Cornual occlusion on left (*arrow*). **B,** Patency of left tube (*arrow*) established after intravenous administration of 1 ml glucagon.

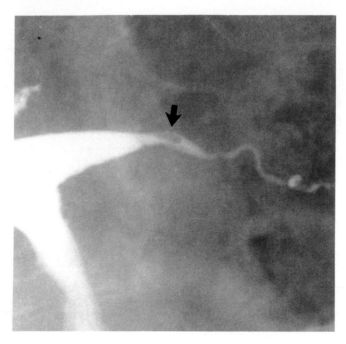

Figure 9.2.   Small polyp in the intramural or interstitial segment of the left fallopian tube (*arrow*).

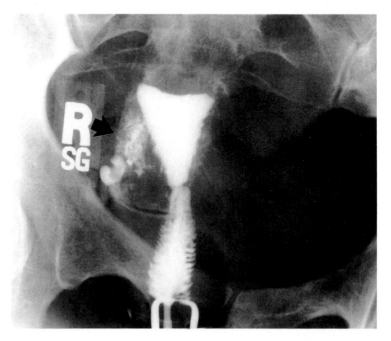

Figure 9.3.   Obstructive changes at the uterotubal junction bilaterally secondary to obstructive inflammatory fibrosis. Note the extravasated contrast medium filling the abundant venous channels within the myometrium (*arrow*).

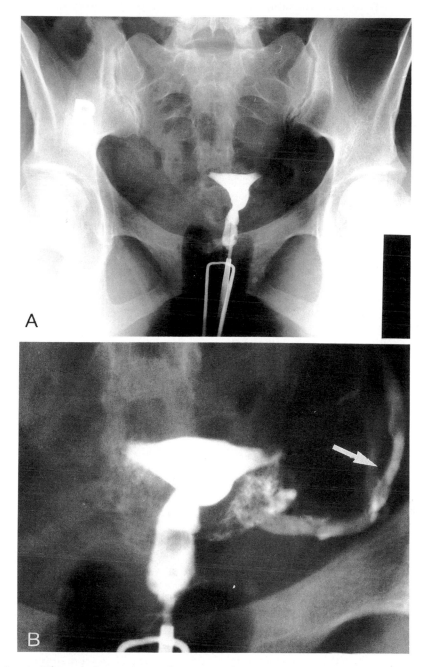

Figure 9.4. **A,** Bilateral obstruction at the cornua due to previous infection. **B,** Continued introduction of contrast medium results in intravasation of contrast medium into the myometrium and vascular structures. The ovarian vein (*arrow*) is well filled.

closely by obstruction in the ampullary segment of the tube (Fig. 9.5). Postinflammatory obstruction in the isthmic segment was found in only 5% of his series. Since the myometrial width cannot be distinguished by hysterosalpingography, it is sometimes difficult to differentiate between intramural and isthmic obstruction. Peritubal adhesion formation and tubal tuberculosis involving the isthmic-ampullary segment can cause midportion obstruction. The normal rugal patterns may or may not be seen, and occasionally rugae are observed in markedly dilated, diseased tubes. Crohn's disease, or regional enteritis, and ulcerative colitis may induce a significant inflammatory process and can be associated with tubal occlusion as well as adhesive disease. *Chlamydia*, which is frequently associated with subclinical infection, is likely to cause fimbrial disease. The use of an intrauterine device (IUD) for contraception has also been associated with adnexal adhesions and fimbrial occlusion. In general, the etiologic agent associated with tuboovarian infection and adhesion formation cannot be distinguished by radiographic or pathologic findings. Pelvic tuberculosis may be an exception.

Poststerilization tubal obstruction is predictable from history, and the purpose of hysterosalpingography is usually to confirm the occlusion or to determine the length of the proximal portion of the tube if reanastomosis is being considered. However, Groff et al. (27) concluded that routine preoperative hysterosalpingography is not warranted, as the site of tubal occlusion was not predictive of a repairable tube, cornual occlusion was overdiagnosed, and estimated proximal tubal length was unreliable.

The investigative technique of hysterosalpingography performed in the poststerilization patient to determine successful tubal occlusion may increase the incidence of fistula formation and recanalization, particularly if done early in the postoperative period; this is discussed further in Chapter 11.

Congenital anomalies of the fallopian tube are rare but may include accessory ostia, multiple lumina, diverticula, and total tubal duplication; complete absence of the fallopian tube; and segmental absence of a portion of the fallopian tube (Fig. 9.6). Accessory tubes are thought to contribute to infertility by capturing oocytes that otherwise would have entered the normal tube, and perhaps by increasing the incidence of ectopic pregnancy; they are found in about 0.6% of women (28). Accessory tubes are visualized at hysterosalpingography only if communication with the tubal lumen or fimbrial pickup of contrast medium occurs. Segmental absence may be caused by tubal torsion or twisting with interruption of the blood supply; it supposedly cannot be congenital in origin, so an acquired etiology should be sought (29, 30). Complete torsion of ovary and tube on the pedicle may result in necrosis and sloughing of the tissue; this has been identified later at open surgical procedures as calcified tissue in the cul-de-sac, but the hysterosalpingographic appearance has not been reported.

Other abnormalities of the fallopian tube include polyps in the intramural portion (Fig. 9.2) or, less commonly, in the proximal isthmic portion. Polyps may be diagnosed in 1.2 to 2.7% of hysterosalpingograms (31–33), although a tissue diagnosis is usually lacking. In tubes examined for pathology after salpingectomy, 11% reportedly contained polyps (16). Infertility has been reported in 27 to 53% of patients diagnosed at hysterosalpingography to have polyps (32), but it is likely that these are simply incidental findings. Surgical management has been uniformly poor: removal of the affected segment of tube, with subsequent uterine implantation of the distal portion (31), and microsurgical resection (33) have not led to pregnancy. This suggests that the

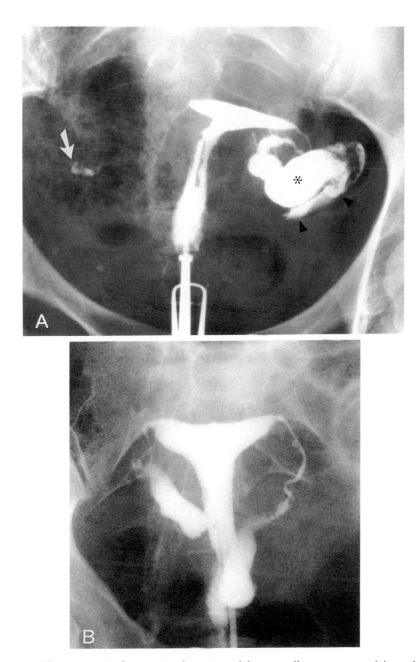

Figure 9.5. **A,** Obstruction in the proximal portion of the ampullary segment of the right fallopian tube (*arrow*). Note the peritubal collection of contrast material on the left (*arrowheads*), reflecting inflammatory changes around the left hydrosalpinx (*asterisk*). **B,** Bilateral tubal occlusions occurring in distal portions of the ampullae. Tubes are displaced and fixed deep in the pelvis.

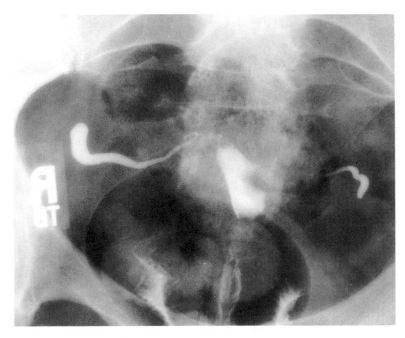

Figure 9.6.   Atresia of the ampullary portion of the fallopian tube. The etiology is uncertain but may reflect intrauterine interruption of vascular supply.

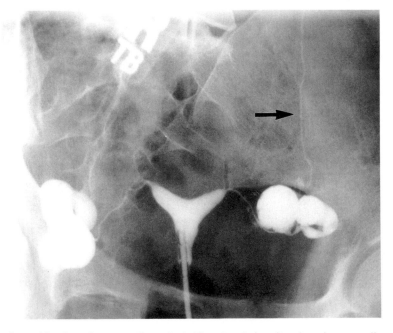

Figure 9.7.   Bilateral hydrosalpinges. The tubal dilatation is localized to the ampullary portion of the tubes. Note the filling of a lymphatic channel from the left peritubal region (*arrow*).

infertility might better be explained by another etiology, because tubal implantation and reanastomosis procedures ordinarily have a higher reported pregnancy rate when performed for frankly obstructing tubal disease.

DISTAL FIMBRIAL OBSTRUCTION

The finding of a distal hydrosalpinx suggests acute or chronic infectious disease as the etiology of the occlusion, and a history of pelvic inflammatory disease or an IUD for contraception is often obtained. On the other hand, pelvic inflammatory disease may be totally "silent" with no recollection of acute infection; most patients found to have hydrosalpinges at laparoscopy will not recall an episode of pelvic infection (34). Chronic obstruction at the fimbriated end, whatever the etiologic process, leads to dilatation, mucosal damage, and destruction of the ciliated cells normally lining the tube (Fig. 9.7), although on occasion a normal rugal pattern may be preserved (Figs. 9.8 and 9.9). The appearance of hysterosalpingography is characteristic if sufficient contrast material is introduced to fill the dilated tube. Partial filling may give the appearance of a normal, nondilated tube, so it is very important to be sure that the salpinx is completely filled (Figs. 9.10, 9.11). Contrast media must be dispersed freely in the peritoneal cavity to demonstrate patency, and a delayed film may be helpful to clarify peritoneal spilling (Fig. 9.12). If uncertainty exists, continued introduction of more contrast agent or carbon dioxide is warranted (Fig. 9.13). On occasion, this may result in the introduction of contrast medium into the lymphatics or the venous vasculature (Fig. 9.7).

Occasionally, a collection of contrast medium surrounding the ampullary portion of the tube is seen associated with a patent or nonobstructed hydrosalpinx. This appearance may persist on the delayed film. Such pooling of contrast medium, often outlined with a "halo" appearance around the dilated ampulla

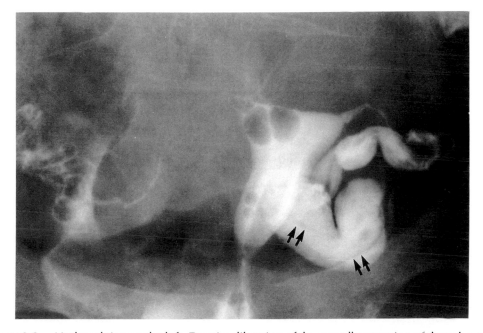

Figure 9.8.   Hydrosalpinx on the left. Despite dilatation of the ampullary portion of the tube, rugal folds are intact (*arrows*).

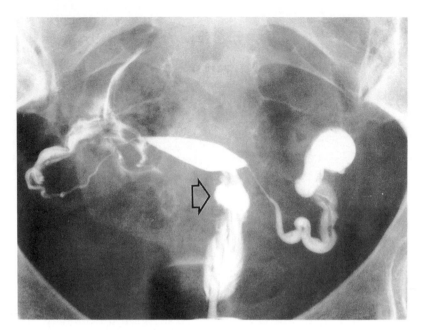

Figure 9.9. Hydrosalpinx on the left with a normal and patent tube on the right. Both normal and abnormal fallopian tubes demonstrate the presence of rugal folds. Incidental note is made of the diverticula-like collection of contrast in the lower uterine segment, the result of a previous cesarean section (*open arrow*).

(Figs. 9.5, 9.14), reflects associated peritubal adhesions and is usually the result of the same process responsible for the formation of the hydrosalpinx.

Recent advances in endoscopy have permitted the development of a technique of translaparoscopic salpingoscopy to evaluate the ampullary segment of the tube and to take microbiopsies of tubal epithelium (35). The mucosal fold pattern could be visualized more accurately than at hysterosalpingography. Salpingoscopy only occasionally failed to confirm a hydrosalpinx diagnosed at hysterosalpingography.

SALPINGITIS ISTHMICA NODOSA

Salpingitis isthmica nodosa (SIN) is the descriptive term for nodular thickenings of the isthmic and occasionally ampullary portion of one or both fallopian tubes (36–38). Radiologically, this con-

dition is characterized by a honeycombed accumulation of radiocontrast material in the wall of the fallopian tube, giving the appearance of multiple small diverticuli (36) (Figs. 9.15 to 9.17). These punctate accumulations of contrast medium are distributed in the isthmic, isthmic-cornual, or isthmic ampullary segments. The area sometimes resembles the branches of a tree or a bush, with a complex maze of opaque channels; more commonly, the image is that of a cluster of diverticula or outpouchings, with persistence of contrast material in these pouches on delayed films.

Pathologically, these nodular areas are characterized by inpouchings and invaginations of normal endosalpinx surrounded by a hypertrophied myosalpinx. There are alveolar-like, slit-like, or cystic irregular spaces in the myosalpinx. These cavities or pockets may be empty or may contain a homogenous coagulum, desquamated epithelial cells, macrophages

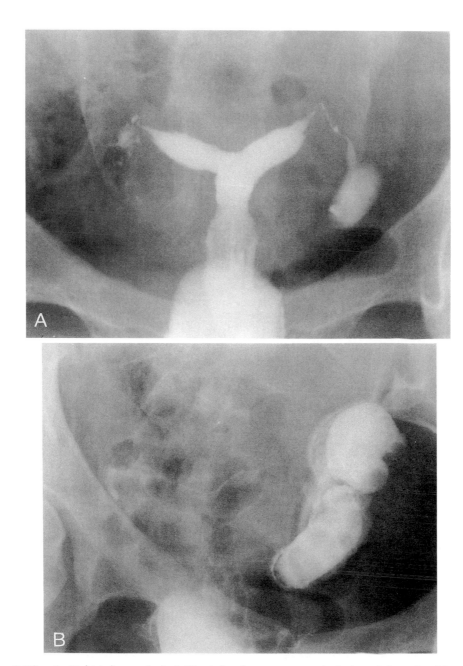

Figure 9.10. **A,** Right tube occluded. The left tube appears occluded, and there is a bicornuate uterus. **B,** Further filling demonstrates the extent of a very large hydrosalpinx on the left.

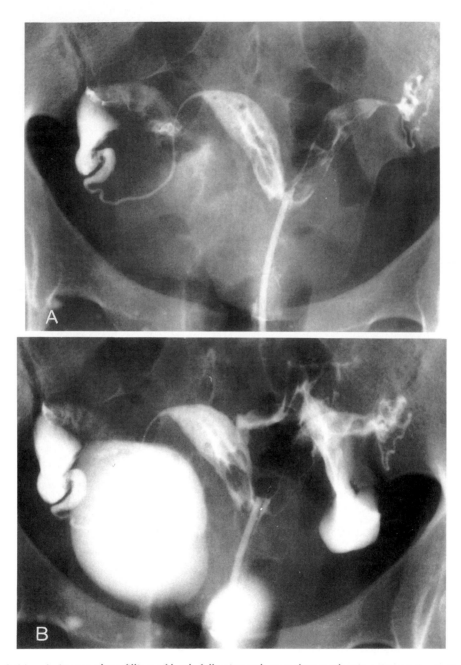

Figure 9.11.   A, Incomplete filling of both fallopian tubes makes evaluation uncertain. **B,** Further introduction of contrast medium demonstrates a huge obstructed hydrosalpinx on the right. The left fallopian tube is patent.

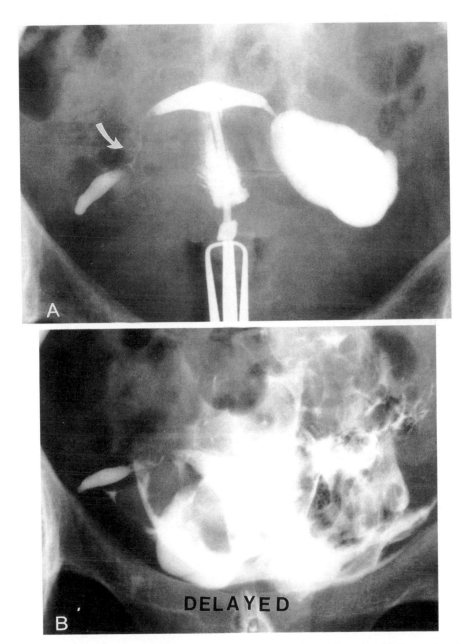

Figure 9.12. **A,** Right tube is occluded in the ampulla. Note the salpingitis isthmica nodosa (*arrow*). The left tube is markedly dilated and appears occluded. **B,** Delayed film demonstrates that the left tube is patent, as the contrast material spills into the peritoneal cavity.

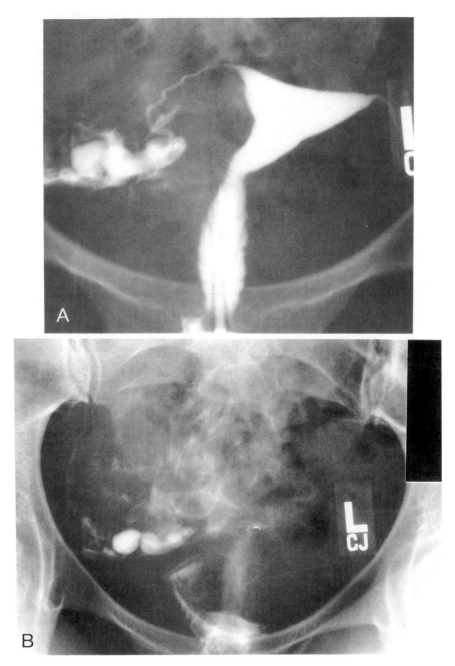

Figure 9.13.   A, Ampullary portion of the right fallopian tube is minimally dilated and clearly patent. **B,** Delayed film demonstrates retained contrast material within the slightly dilated right fallopian tube. This retention, associated with the dilatation, supports the diagnosis of postinflammatory change.

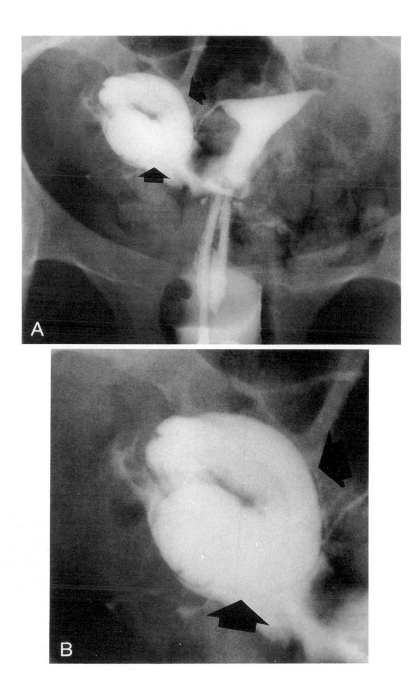

Figure 9.14. **A,** Right fallopian tube demonstrates a patent hydrosalpinx, with contrast material entering a discrete peritubal collection. A "halo sign" is seen separating the fallopian tube from the peritubal contrast (*arrows*). **B,** Magnification view of **A.**

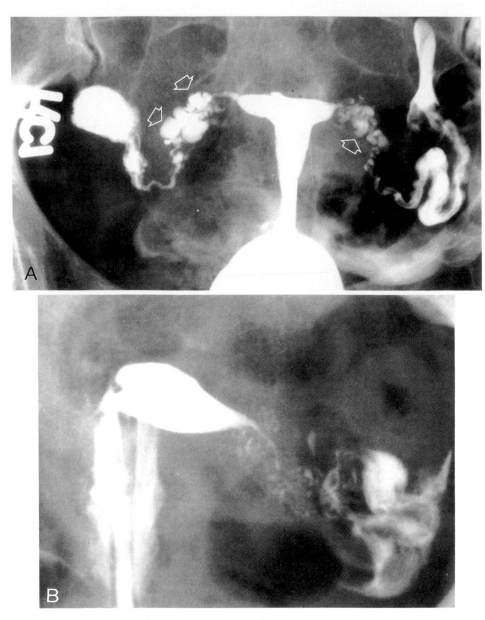

Figure 9.15.   A, Salpingitis isthmica nodosa. Note the numerous large, diverticula-like collections of contrast in the isthmic segment of the left fallopian tube. (Courtesy of T. A. Baramki, Baltimore, MD.) **B,** Another example of salpingitis isthmica nodosa. Collections are smaller but quite numerous and equally characteristic.

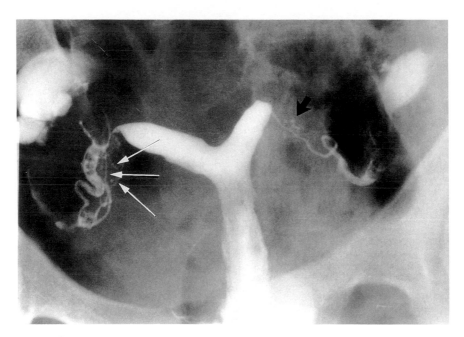

Figure 9.16. Salpingitis isthmica nodosa, bilateral. Both tubes demonstrate ampullary hydrosalpinges. The right fallopian tube shows several diverticula as well as lacy linear tracts of contrast medium (*arrows*). The left fallopian tube shows the more characteristic appearance of small diverticula-like collections in the isthmic segment of the tube (*black arrow*).

with or without phagocytized brown pigment, and occasionally a purulent exudate (39).

Salpingitis isthmica nodosa appears almost exclusively to involve the isthmic segment of the tube, which has a powerful muscle coat and a very dense adrenergic motor innervation. The etiology of SIN could be a postinfectious process, the result of endosalpingeal metaplasia, or, unlikely, a congenital or development defect. Salpingitis isthmica nodosa could also be a late morphologic expression of chronic tubal spasm. Some patients with SIN have external endometriosis in other parts of the pelvis, but other studies (37) have excluded endometriosis, suggesting that the two conditions are not identical but may exist independently. Both acute and chronic infection have been identified in resected nodules, and even the name salpingitis isthmica nodosa, as coined by Chiari (40), denotes the inflammatory origin of the lesion, its predomi-

nant location, and its nodular gross appearance. Evidence of previous inflammatory disease, including gonococcal infection, has been reported in the majority of cases diagnosed (38).

Von Recklinghausen (41) in 1896 proposed that the findings of SIN were due to wolffian rests, since embryologically the tubal isthmus is the region where the müllerian and wolffian ducts cross. However, examination of tubal tissue from embryos, term female infants, and older prepubertal girls has failed to demonstrate the lesion (39). Although various etiologies have been recorded for SIN, it seems likely that the process is postinflammatory in origin, with proliferation of normal epithelium in the tubal isthmus, slow penetration into the tubal wall forming a labyrinth of pathways and cysts, and finally secondary muscular hypertrophy. It is clearly a progressive lesion, with change demonstrable in only 12 months (42).

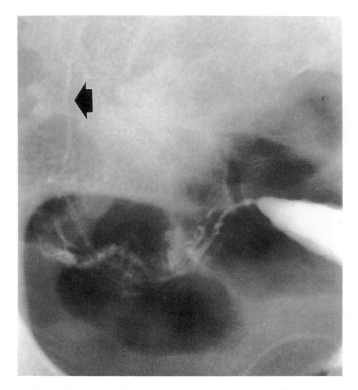

Figure 9.17.   Salpingitis isthmica nodosa. Numerous rounded and linear collections of contrast material associated with the isthmic segment of the right fallopian tube. In addition to these small diverticula-like collections, some of the linear pattern is believed to reflect lymphatic drainage with a prominent lymphatic channel directed cephalad (*arrow*).

Salpingitis isthmica nodosa appears to be associated with either subfertility or infertility. Tubal occlusion is not characteristic, and most cases of SIN have tubal patency, with a honeycombed appearance in the isthmic area of the tube, with or without associated hydrosalpinx. As expected, there is an increased incidence of ectopic pregnancy, 75% of which are found in the isthmus or ampulla (38, 43, 44). In many specimens no communication can be demonstrated between the main tubal lumen and the trophoblastic tissue, suggesting implantation in a diverticulum (45). Interestingly, tubal pregnancies are more common in the right than in the left tube; 49% of women with ectopic pregnancies have SIN nodules, with 30% having nodules in the right tube compared to 19% with nodules in the left (43).

Salpingitis isthmica nodosa cannot be detected by pelvic examination but may be observed at diagnostic laparoscopy, and is determined by palpation during open surgical procedures. From a hysterosalpingographic standpoint, the diagnosis of SIN is easily established, is not uncommon, and can be expected in at least 4% of hysterosalpingographies (38). The remainder of the tube may appear normal and patent, but hydrosalpinx is common. Approximately 50% of patients with SIN have tubal occlusion distal to the SIN, with frequent evidence of tubal damage on the contralateral side.

OTHER FINDINGS

The fallopian tube may appear to be coiled on itself in a corkscrew type of pattern or have poor mobility suggestive of adhesive disease. The convoluted tube with a corkscrew appearance on radiographic examination has been described as being associated with the finding of endometriosis at laparoscopy (46). Peritubal adhesions are associated with ampullary dilatation, a peritubal halo effect due to a double-contour appearance of the tubal wall, vertically positioned tubes, loculation of spillage of contrast medium in the peritoneal cavity, and convoluted tubes, with the last two criteria correlating best with the presence of adhesions (9). Significant peritubal and periovarian adhesions and a laterally shortened and scarred broad ligament are found that contribute to the convoluted pattern (Fig. 9.18). This abnormality may be associated with retrograde menstruation, which in turn could be responsible for the induction of endometriosis and peritubal adhesion formation.

This corkscrew configuration of the tube is not the only way that peritubal disease can present. A beaded appearance suggesting minimal tubal dilatation with a series of short constrictions has similar significance (Fig. 9.19). With peritubal inflammatory disease, the tube may appear crowded and folded on itself. This configuration is persistent even when viewed in varying degrees of obliquity. Generally, peritubal adhesive disease is not associated with tubal occlusion, although exceptions occur.

The classic etiologic factors for peritubal adhesive disease are endometriosis and gonococcal pelvic inflammatory disease (PID). Other processes include nongonococcal PID, IUD with associated subclinical pelvic infection, *Chlamydia*, tuberculosis, and Crohn's disease (Figs. 9.20 to 9.22).

HYSTEROGRAPHIC DIAGNOSIS OF TUBERCULOSIS

Genital tuberculosis is now rare, but characteristic abnormalities found at hysterosalpingography suggest that further

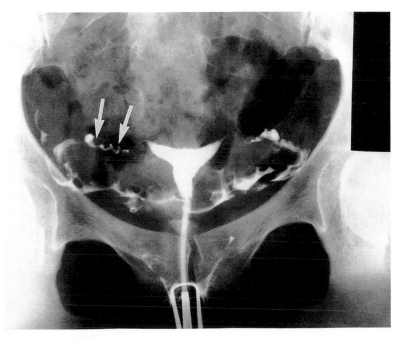

Figure 9.18. Endometriosis proven at laparoscopy. Note the corkscrew-like configuration of the isthmic and proximal ampullary portions of the fallopian tubes (*arrows*), an observation often seen with peritubal inflammatory diseases.

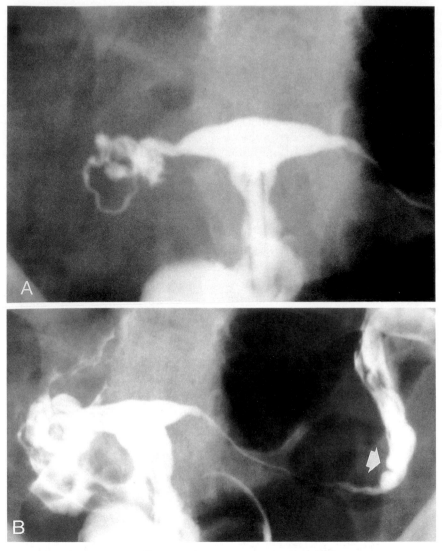

Figure 9.19.   A, Endometriosis. Fallopian tubes are patent but are distorted and crowded together. **B,** Endometriosis. The ampullary segment of the left tube is characterized by segmental dilatations not unlike links of sausage (*arrow*).

studies should be done in some women to identify the disease. Genital tuberculosis affects the tube more than the uterus, resulting in destruction of normal tissue, occlusion of the tubes, and partial or complete sclerosis of the uterine cavity, or an ulcerated appearance (47). The tubal ampulla and isthmus become constricted and rigid, resulting in a sewer pipe appearance with a rounded blunt end, complete obstruction, and the absence of rugae (Fig. 9.23). Alternating dilatation and constriction result in a "rosary bead" pattern. Calcified pelvic lymph nodes and smaller areas of calcified material in the region of the tubes may also be observed. Fistulous extension from the tubes, appearing like diverticula, and vascular or lymphatic intravasation of contrast material are occasionally noted.

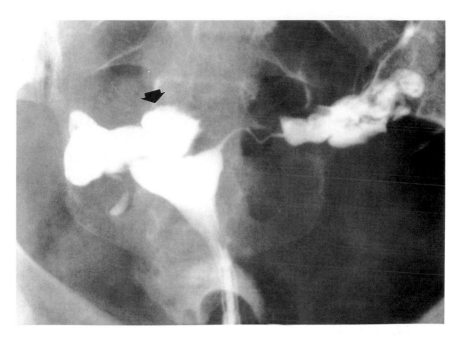

Figure 9.20. Crohn's disease. Essentially normal left adnexa. The right fallopian tube is distorted with a rather crowded, clustered appearance and some dilatation of the distal end of the tube. A peritubal collection of contrast material (*arrow*) further reflects the inflammatory process surrounding the adnexa.

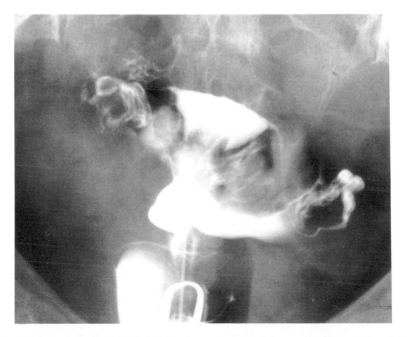

Figure 9.21. Crohn's disease. The left fallopian tube is within normal limits. The right fallopian tube again shows a crowded, distorted configuration. The tube is patent and no significant dilatation is evident. Exploration confirmed extensive peritubal inflammatory change with no obstruction.

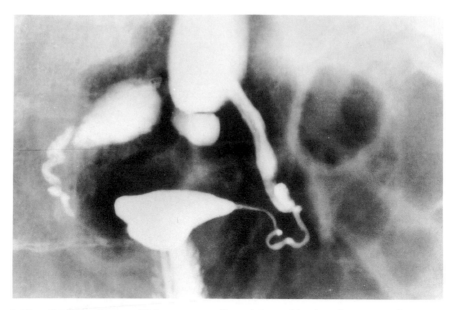

Figure 9.22.   Crohn's disease. This pattern reflects bilateral hydrosalpinges and is not typical for peritubal inflammatory change. One must speculate whether this patient had both Crohn's disease and pelvic inflammatory disease.

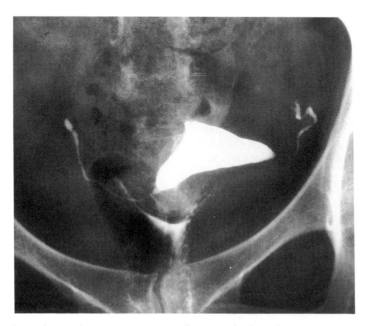

Figure 9.23.   Tuberculosis. The cavity is essentially normal. The tubes appear narrowed, irregular, and uneven. There is no significant dilatation despite the bilateral obstruction.

Hysterosalpingography performed in the patient with active genital tuberculosis or acute salpingitis of any origin can spread infection to the peritoneal cavity or the extragenital organs. When the condition is suspected at hysterosalpingography, culture of the tubercle bacillus or histologic examination of endometrial tissue is mandatory.

Klein and coworkers (48) established criteria for the diagnosis of pelvic tuberculosis:

1. Calcified lymph nodes or smaller, irregular calcifications in the adnexal area.
2. Obstruction of the fallopian tube in the zone of transition between the isthmus and the ampulla.
3. Multiple constrictions along the course of the fallopian tube.
4. Endometrial adhesions and/or deformity or obliteration of the endometrial cavity, in the absence of a history of curettage or abortion.

Although the disease is rare, its radiographic appearance is characteristic and, if observed, mandates further diagnostic evaluation.

PREVENTION OF ACUTE PELVIC INFLAMMATORY DISEASE AFTER HYSTEROSALPINGOGRAPHY

Hysterosalpingography provides useful information about the uterine cavity and fallopian tubes in the evaluation of the infertile patient, and not infrequently may uncover significant pathology; however, it has the potential of activating an infectious process. The examination is therefore not without some risk of complication. The development of acute pelvic inflammatory disease (PID) following hysterosalpingography and the possibility of resultant diminished fertility are of serious concern. The incidence of severe PID after hysterosalpingography has

been reported to be as low as 0.3% and as high as 3.4% (49–53). This obviously depends on many factors, not the least of which is a reflection of the patient population studied. Risk factors for infection after hysterosalpingography have been examined, but a proposed scoring system of these risks successfully predicted only 8 of the 14 identified infections (50). Prophylactic ampicillin and tetracycline were reportedly ineffective in preventing serious infections in women having hysterosalpingography. On the other hand, Pittaway and coworkers (49) studied 278 women undergoing hysterosalpingography for infertility, and identified four (1.4%) who developed acute pelvic inflammatory disease. All cases of PID following hysterosalpingography occurred in women with dilated tubes; among those women with dilated tubes, 11.4% developed PID. Patent hydrosalpinx signified a greater risk than tubal obstruction, because three or four patients afflicted had dilated but nonobstructed tubes despite the fact that 75% of all hydrosalpinges in this series were occluded.

Administration of antibiotics may be indicated before performance of hysterosalpingography if the possibility of activating infection is suspected. If such an abnormality is identified at hysterosalpingography, antibiotics should be instituted at the time of the procedure. All patients with tubal dilatation should therefore receive antibiotics. We have advocated the use of doxycycline 100 mg, two tablets on diagnosis, and one twice daily for a total of 5 days. To our knowledge, this regimen has successfully prevented the development of such an acute inflammatory process.

REFERENCES

1. Hutchins CJ: Laparoscopy and hysterosalpingography in the assessment of tubal patency. *Obstet Gynecol* 49:325, 1977.
2. Taylor PJ: Correlation in infertility: Symptomatology, hysterosalpingogra-

phy, laparoscopy and hysteroscopy. *J Reprod Med* 18:339, 1977.

3. Philipsen T, Hansen BB: Comparative study of hysterosalpingography and laparoscopy in infertile patients. *Acta Obstet Gynecol Scand* 60:149, 1981.

4. Duff DE, Fried AM, Wilson EA, Haack DG: Hysterosalpingography and laparoscopy: A comparative study. *AJR* 141:761, 1983.

5. Snowden EU, Jarrett JC II, Dawood MY: Comparison of diagnostic accuracy of laparoscopy, hysteroscopy, and hysterosalpingography in evaluation of female infertility. *Fertil Steril* 41:709, 1983.

6. Randolph JR, Ying YK, Maier DB, Schmidt CL, Riddick DH: Comparison of real-time ultrasonography and hysterosalpingography in the evaluation of uterine abnormalities and tubal patency. *Fertil Steril* 46:828, 1986.

7. McCalley MG, Braunstein P, Stone S, Henderson P, Egbert R: Radionuclide hysterosalpingography for evaluation of fallopian tube patency. *J Nucl Med* 26:874, 1985.

8. Becker W, Steck T, Albert P, Borner W: Hysterosalpingoscintigraphy: A simple and accurate method of evaluating fallopian tube patency. *Nucl Med* 27:252, 1988.

9. Karasick S, Goldfarb AF: Peritubal adhesions in infertile women: Diagnosis with hysterosalpingography. *AJR* 152:777, 1989.

10. Mackey RA, Glass RH, Olson LE, Vaidya R: Pregnancy following hysterosalpingography with oil and water soluble dye. *Fertil Steril* 22:504, 1971.

11. DeCherney AH, Kort H, Barney JB, DeVore GR: Increased pregnancy rate with oil-soluble hysterosalpingography dye. *Fertil Steril* 33:407, 1980.

12. Soules MR, Spandoni LR: Oil versus aqueous media for hysterosalpingography: A continuing debate based on many opinions and few facts. *Fertil Steril* 38:1, 1982.

13. Pontifex G, Trichopoulos D, Karpathios S: Hysterosalpingography in the diagnosis of infertility (statistical analysis of 3437 cases). *Fertil Steril* 23:1972.

14. Lapido OA: An evaluation of 576 hysterosalpingograms on infertile women. *Infertility* 2:63, 1979.

15. Acton CM, Devit JM, Ryan EA: Hysterosalpingography in infertility: An experience of 3,631 examinations. *Aust NZ J Obstet Gynecol* 28:127, 1988.

16. Lisa JR, Gioia JD, Rubin IC: Observation on the interstitial portion of the fallopian tube. *Surg Gynecol Obstet* 99:159, 1954.

17. Winfield AC, Pittaway DE, Maxson W, Daniell J, Wentz AC: Apparent cornual occlusion in hysterosalpingography: Reversal by glucagon. *AJR* 139:525, 1982.

18. Merchant RN, Prabhu SR, Chougale A: Uterotubal junction—morphology and clinical aspects. *Int J Fertil* 28:199, 1983.

19. Glazener CMA, Loveden LM, Richardson SJ, Jeans WD, Hull MGR: Tubo-cornual polyps: Their relevance in subfertility. *Hum Reprod* 2:59, 1987.

20. Fortier KJ, Haney AF: The pathologic spectrum of uterotubal junction obstruction. *Obstet Gynecol* 65:93, 1985.

21. Sulak PJ, Letterie GS, Coddington CC, Hayslip CC, Woodward JE, Klein TA: Histology of proximal tubal occlusion. *Fertil Steril* 48:437, 1987.

22. Thurmond AS: Nonsurgical fallopian tube recanalization for treatment of infertility. *Radiology* 174:371, 1990.

23. Thurmond AS, Rosch J: Fallopian tubes: Improved technique for catheterization. *Radiology* 174:572, 1990.

24. Lang EK, Dunaway HE Jr, Roniger WE: Selective osteal salpingography and transvaginal catheter dilatation in the diagnosis and treatment of fallopian tube obstruction. *AJR* 154:735, 1990.

25. Nordenskjold F, Ahlgren M: Laparoscopy in female infertility. *Acta Obstet Gynecol Scand* 62:609, 1983.

26. Siegler AM: *Hysterosalpingography*, ed. 2. New York: Medcom Press, 1974.

27. Groff TR, Edelstein JA, Schenken RS: Hysterosalpingography in the preoperative evaluation of tubal anastomosis candidates. *Fertil Steril* 53:417, 1990.

28. Beyth Y, Kopolovic J: Accessory tubes: A possible contributing factor in infertility. *Fertil Steril* 38:382, 1982.

29. Richardson DA, Evans MI, Talerman A, Maroulis GB: Segmental absence of the mid-portion of the fallopian tube. *Fertil Steril* 37:577, 1982.

30. Silverman AY, Greenberg EI: Absence of a segment of the proximal portion of a fallopian tube. *Obstet Gynecol* 62:90S, 1983.

31. Gordts S, Boechx W, Vasquez G, Brosens I: Microsurgical resection of intramural tubal polyps. *Fertil Steril* 40:258, 1983.

32. David MP, Ben-Zwi D, Langer L: Tubal intramural polyps and their relationship to infertility. *Fertil Steril* 35:526, 1981.

33. Stangell JJ, Chervenak FA, Mouradian-

Davidian M: Microsurgical resection of bilateral fallopian tube polyps. *Fertil Steril* 35:580, 1981.

34. Rosenfeld DL, Seidman SM, Bronson RA, Scholl GM: Unsuspected chronic pelvic inflammatory disease in the infertile female. *Fertil Steril* 39:44, 1983.

35. Puttemans P, Brosens I, Delattin P, Vasquez G, Boechx W: Salpingoscopy versus hysterosalpingography in hydrosalpinges. *Hum Reprod* 2:535:1987.

36. Honore LH: Salpingitis isthmica nodosa in female infertility and ectopic tubal pregnancy. *Fertil Steril* 29:164, 1978.

37. Tulandi T, Wilson RE, Arroent GH, McInnes RA: Fertility aspect of women with tubal diverticulosis: A 5-year follow-up. *Fertil Steril* 40:260, 1983.

38. Creasy JL, Clark RL, Cuttino JT, Groff TR: Salpingitis isthmica nodosa: Radiologic and clinical correlates. *Radiology* 154:597, 1985.

39. Kontopoulos VG, Wang CF, Siegler AM: The impact of salpingitis isthmica nodosa on infertility. *Infertility* 1:137, 1978.

40. Chiari H: Zur pathologischen anatomie des eileitercatarrhas. *Zeittschr Heilkl* 8:457, 1887.

41. Von Recklinghausen F: *Die Anenomyome und Cystadenome der Uterus and Tubenwandung.* Berlin: A. Hirschwald, 1896, p 247.

42. McComb PF, Rowe T: Salpingitis isthmica nodosa: Evidence it is a progressive disease. *Fertil Steril* 51:542, 1989.

43. Persaud V: Etiology of tubal ectopic pregnancy: Radiologic and pathologic studies. *Obstet Gynecol* 36:257, 1970.

44. Homm RJ, Holtz G, Garvin AJ: Isthmic ectopic pregnancy and salpingitis isthmica nodosa. *Fertil Steril* 48:756, 1987.

45. Stewart DB, Skinner SM: Tubal ectopic pregnancy. *Manitoba Med Rev* 47:552, 1967.

46. Cohen BM, Katz M: The significance of the convoluted oviduct in the infertile woman. *J Reprod Med* 21:31, 1978.

47. Nogales-Ortiz F, Tarancon I, Nogales FF: The pathology of female genital tuberculosis. *Obstet Gynecol* 53:422, 1979.

48. Klein TA, Richmond JA, Mischell DR: Pelvic tuberculosis. *Obstet Gynecol* 48:99, 1976.

49. Pittaway DE, Winfield AC, Maxson W, Daniell J, Herbert C, Wentz AC: Prevention of acute pelvic inflammatory disease after hysterosalpingography: Effect of doxycycline prophylaxis. *Am J Obstet Gynecol* 147:623, 1983.

50. Stumpf PG, March CM: Febrile morbidity following hysterosalpingography: Identification of risk factors and recommendations for prophylaxis. *Fertil Steril* 33:487, 1980.

51. Moller BR, Allen J, Toft B, Hansen KB, Taylor-Robinson D: Pelvic inflammatory disease after hysterosalpingography associated with *Chlamydia trachomatis* and *Mycoplasma hominis*. *Br J Obstet Gynaecol* 91:1181, 1984.

52. Marshak RH, Roole CS, Goldberg MA: Hysterography and hysterosalpingography. *Surg Gynecol Obstet* 91:182, 1950.

53. Measday B: An analysis of the complications of hysterosalpingography. *J Obstet Gynaecol Br Emp* 67:663, 1960.

10

Transcervical Fallopian Tube Catheterization for Management of Proximal Tube Obstruction

Amy S. Thurmond
Miles J. Novy

Fallopian tube disease is a major cause of infertility and is estimated to affect more than 300,000 women in the United States (1). Proximal obstruction of the tube, either unilateral or bilateral, is observed in 10 to 20% of hysterosalpingograms performed to evaluate infertility (2). As a consequence, visualization of the distal tubes is prevented, and there is question whether the proximal tubal obstruction is contributing to the patient's infertility. Proximal tubal obstruction (PTO) has been a frustrating problem, since underfilling of the tube, muscular "spasm," and mechanical occlusion from a variety of causes are not easily differentiated from one another by conventional hysterosalpingography or even at laparoscopy. Particularly frustrating for the infertility surgeon has been the resection of an obstructed cornual or proximal isthmic segment of oviduct that is subsequently shown to be normal or to have minimal histopathologic findings. Indeed, in the authors' earlier experiences, antegrade tubal cannulation with flexible wireguides at the time of an isthmic salpingotomy was successful in establishing tubal patency in the majority of women who were taken to laparotomy for persistent PTO without need for resection of the obstructed segment. Such observations, together with a background experience in angiography by one of the au-

thors, led to the development of coaxial catheterization techniques for transcervical fallopian tube catheterization and selective salpingography (3, 4).

In this chapter, we describe the techniques for fluoroscopic and hysteroscopic catheterization of the proximal oviduct. The methods, the issues of patient selection, and the results of fallopian tube catheterization are discussed in the context of the pathophysiology of PTO. New developments in diagnostic and therapeutic applications of transcervical catheterization methods are briefly considered.

PATHOPHYSIOLOGY OF PROXIMAL TUBAL OBSTRUCTION

The uterine cavity, in its cornual portion, tapers to form an endometrial funnel. The ostium of the intramural portion of the fallopian tube appears as a circular opening (0.5 to 1.5 mm in diameter) at the end of the endometrial funnel. At hysteroscopy, using carbon dioxide as a distending medium, the ostium can be seen to open and close several times per minute. The circular mucosal fold, which demarcates the edge of the ostium, often appears on hysterosalpingograms as an indentation between the endometrial funnel and the tubal antrum (Fig. 10.1).

192

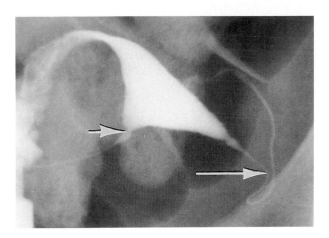

Figure 10.1. A normal hysterosalpingogram. The circular mucosal fold that demarcates the edge of the tubal ostium is well demonstrated (*short arrow*). The interstitial-isthmic junction can usually only be estimated from the hysterosalpingogram; however, it often occurs at a bend in the tube (*long arrow*).

It has been mistaken for a sphincter, although a true sphincter is absent in this location. The periodic closure of the tubal ostium is due to contractions of the surrounding myometrium.

The length of the intramural tube varies between 8 and 14 mm. Its course is straight or curved in 60% and convoluted in 40% of patients (5). The bulge-like dilatation of the inner tubal antrum tapers in the middle and outer thirds of the intramural tube to a diameter of 0.5 to 1.0 mm. Estimates of the lumen size vary, in part, due to the presence of mucosal folds, luminal secretions, and muscular contractions. Three muscle layers can be identified at the uterotubal junction and in the proximal isthmus: the innermost longitudinal, the intermediate circular, and the outer longitudinal or spiral layer. The circular layer is the most prominent, and changes in tone are likely to affect the lumen diameter or resistance to contrast media. As the tube enters the uterus, both outer spiral and circular muscle layers disappear, leaving only the inner longitudinal layer intact in the interstitial segment.

Temporary obstruction of the proximal tube does occur and is presumably due to tubal spasm (Fig. 10.2). The smooth muscle, vasculature, and epithelium (endosalpinx) of the fallopian tube are exquisitely sensitive to the actions of estrogens and progesterone (6). The oviduct is supplied with both parasympathetic and sympathetic nerves. It is the circular muscle layer that is most heavily innervated. Neurons containing vasoactive intestinal peptide (VIP) have also been demonstrated in the fallopian tube, with particularly high concentrations at the uterotubal junction. Smooth muscle from the isthmus responds to VIP with a reduction in motor activity. Substance P and oxytocin increase isthmic contractile activity (6). Norepinephrine is the main catecholamine detected in the human fallopian tube, particularly in the isthmus. During the menstrual cycle, there are cyclic variations in the quantity and distribution of catecholamines, in the numbers of adrenergic receptors and steroid hormone receptors, and in epithelial morphology. The concentration of norepinephrine in the proximal oviduct is highest during the immediate preovulatory period, when estradiol concentration is maximal; isthmic motor activity is increased at this stage (7). α-Adrenergic

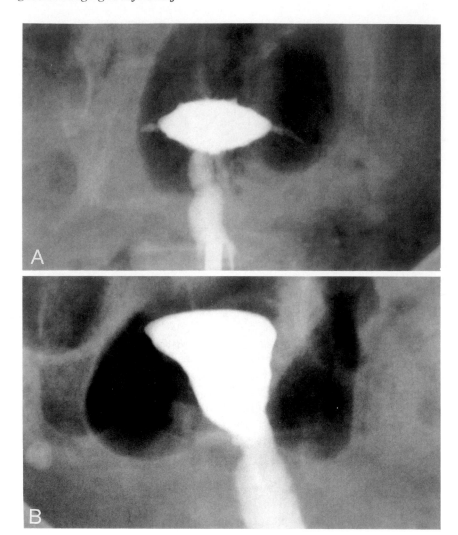

Figure 10.2.   This woman, who had a history of bilateral distal tuboplasty, was evaluated prior to fallopian tube catheterization. Three postoperative hysterosalpingograms showed bilateral proximal tubal obstruction. The fourth hysterosalpingogram showed left tubal patency and persistent right PTO. Presumably, the cause of persistent PTO, in this case, was spasm. The patient subsequently conceived without any other intervention. **A,** Initial postoperative hysterosalpingogram showed bilateral PTO. **B,** Subsequent hysterosalpingogram 1 month later showed bilateral PTO. **C,** Hysterosalpingogram 6 months later confirmed bilateral PTO. **D,** The fourth postoperative hysterosalpingogram showed a patent left tube and persistent right PTO.

receptors of both subtypes in the fallopian tube are generally stimulatory, whereas β receptors (primarily β_2) inhibit contractility. Throughout the cycle, β receptor activity generally predominates in isthmic circular muscle, except around the time of ovulation, when α receptor activity is increased. After ovulation, as plasma progesterone levels rise above 2 ng/ml, the response to norepinephrine is reversed and isthmic relaxation coincides with dominance of β receptor activity once again. Cyclic nucleotides and prostaglandins also modulate smooth muscle tone in the oviduct. Prostaglandin $F_{2\alpha}$ causes an increase in contractility of isth-

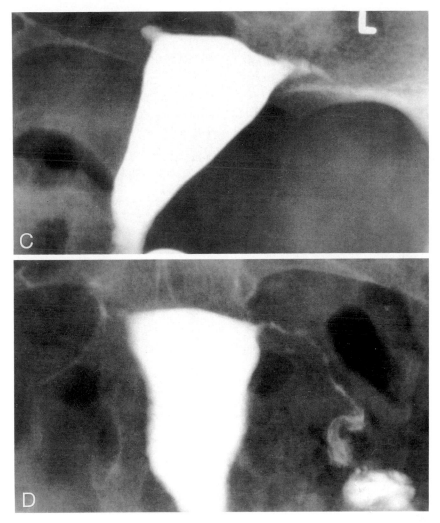

Figure 10.2.   **C** and **D.**

mic circular muscle, while prostaglandin E_2 is generally inhibitory. Although many agents—including dibutyl cyclic **AMP**, indomethacin, β_2 agonists, and α-adrenergic antagonists—have been demonstrated to relax the circular muscle layer in vitro, their in vivo effects are variable or uncertain (6).

It is possible that tubal secretions may occlude the proximal tube. Ciliogenesis and secretory activity of the tubal epithelium are estrogen-dependent processes that are antagonized by progesterone. Deciliation, atrophy of the epithe-

lium, a decrease in tissue water, and a reduction in secretory activity accompany the postovulatory rise in plasma progesterone. Studies in monkeys show evidence of considerable apocrine secretory activity in the isthmus but not in the ampulla during the preovulatory period (6). Not infrequently, granular and membranous products of apocrine secretion pack the isthmic lumen to the point where it is completely occupied by these secretions. Scanning electron micrography of the human isthmus strongly suggests that there is a decrease in the lumen diameter before ovulation in comparison with the postovulatory phase (6). It is reasonable, therefore, that ovum transport may be impeded by decreased compliance of the tubal wall or viscosity of the luminal contents, both of which are hormonally dependent. In this regard, it is noteworthy that spermatozoa can negotiate the isthmic lumen at a time in the cycle when fluid flow between the uterine cavity and ampulla is blocked (8).

Diagnostic hysterosalpingography is traditionally performed before ovulation to prevent the accidental exposure of an embryo to radiation during a fertile cycle. One can see from the above discussion that this may be the time when the tubes are most prone to obstruction from spasm or secretions. On the other hand, examination performed in the postovulatory phase may be limited by the thickened secretory endometrium, which can block the tubal ostium.

The previous approach to managing patients with cornual obstruction was to repeat the hysterosalpingogram with an adjunctive spasmolytic agent prior to performing a laparoscopy or reconstructive surgery. Several smooth muscle relaxants were investigated, including glucagon, diazepam, isoxsuprine, and general anesthesia, but success was limited (2). For this reason, we abandoned pharmacologic methods and now use transcervical catheterization techniques to evaluate proximal tubal obstruction.

PATHOLOGY OF PROXIMAL TUBAL OBSTRUCTION

The etiology of PTO is frequently unclear, but infection and subsequent inflammation or fibrosis are leading causes in all series reported (9). Cornual or isthmic occlusion can occur after chlamydia or gonococcal salpingitis or as a consequence of postabortal or postpartum endometritis. Histopathologic findings in resected proximal tubal segments include

Table 10.1.   Conditions Associated with Proximal Tubal Obstruction or Occlusion

Muscular spasm
Stromal edema
Mucosal agglutination
Amorphous material
Viscous secretions
Salpingitis isthmica nodosa
Adenomyosis
Tuberculosis
Chronic salpingitis
Fibrosis
Leiomyomata
Cornual polyps
Endosalpingiosis
Congenital atresia

obliterative fibrosis, salpingitis isthmica nodosa (SIN), and chronic inflammation (10–12). Together, these lesions account for 70 to 85% of anatomical occlusions at the uterotubal junction (Table 10.1). Granulomatous or "giant cell" salpingitis is relatively uncommon but is seen with tuberculosis, foreign bodies, and some parasitic infestations. Other causes of PTO include cornual polyps, fibroids, and endometriosis. Intraluminal endometriosis occurs in approximately 10% of tubes resected for proximal occlusion and may exist without relation to visible lesions elsewhere in the pelvis (10, 11). Müllerian anomalies of the fallopian tube are rare, but cornual occlusion is seen with variants of unicornuate uterus, and atresia of tubal segments (including the proximal isthmus) is known to occur (13). Fibrosis of the tubal lumen or poststerilization isthmic occlusion is often marked by a pre-stenotic bulge or dilatation that is distinguished from a tapered lumen usually seen with other causes of tubal obstruction (Fig. 10.3). However, the appearance of the tube at the site of occlusion does not accurately predict the cause, and a pre-stenotic bulge may also occur in a tube that is apparently occluded only by debris (Fig. 10.4).

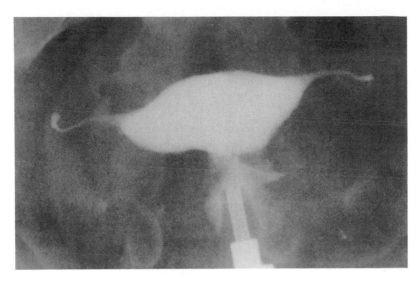

Figure 10.3. This woman had cautery sterilization. Both tubes are occluded in the mid-isthmic portion, and there is mild focal dilation of the tube just proximal to the obstruction.

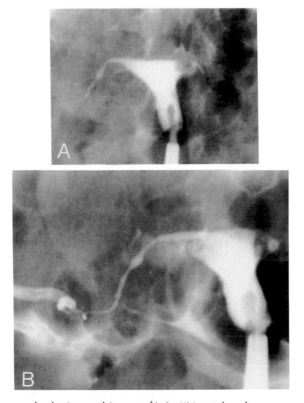

Figure 10.4. This woman had a 3-year history of infertility and underwent successful fluoroscopic recanalization on both sides for bilateral proximal tubal obstruction. The patient conceived within a week of the procedure. **A,** The tubes are occluded in the isthmic portion, and there is a mild focal dilation of the tubes just proximal to the obstruction. **B,** Intratubal salpingogram following successful recanalization on the right side.

Several authors have noted a lack of major histologic findings in about 10 to 20% of patients despite a persistent cornual block (9, 11, 12, 14). According to Sulak and coworkers (14), amorphous material was present in the tubal lumen, possibly forming a cast in six of 18 (33%) patients with PTO. In three patients (17%), the tubes were completely normal without occlusion. In only seven of the 18 patients (39%) was tubal occlusion with either fibrous obliteration or SIN documented histologically. Thus, in at least 50% of the patients examined histologically, PTO was caused by a temporary entity such as spasm or loose mechanical obstruction.

PATIENT SELECTION AND MANAGEMENT

The algorithm shown in Figure 10.5 summarizes our current strategy for eval-uating the patient with cornual obstruction found on conventional hysterosalpingography or laparoscopy. If the hysterosalpingography is done to confirm postoperative patency, or if the patient is otherwise not a candidate for laparoscopy (e.g., previous laparoscopy with normal pelvic findings or low suspicion for pelvic disease), fallopian tube catheterization is performed fluoroscopically. If cornual patency is not demonstrated by selective salpingography or fallopian tube recanalization, hysteroscopic catheterization with laparoscopy or laparotomy is a logical follow-up study. Conversely, if abnormal pelvic findings are known or suspected to coexist or if there is a large uterine mass, PTO is initially investigated by hysteroscopic fallopian tube catheterization in conjunction with laparoscopy or laparotomy. Thus, pelvic or uterine disease can be treated under the same anaesthetic. If hysteroscopic catheteriza-

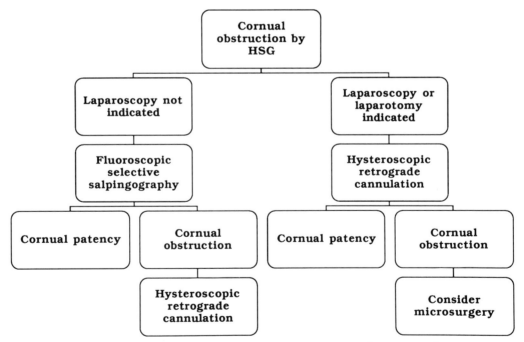

Figure 10.5.   Algorithm showing the recommended management of patients with proximal tubal obstruction. (From Novy MJ, Thurmond AS, Patton P, Uchida BT, Rosch J: Diagnosis of cornual obstruction by transcervical fallopian tube cannulation. *Fertil Steril* 50:434, 1988. Reprinted by permission of the publisher, The American Fertility Society.

gross SIN or fibrosis, fluoroscopic catheterization may be subsequently tried. Proximal tubal obstruction that is not correctable by fluoroscopic or hysteroscopic catheterization methods may require surgical resection and reanastomosis. Fortunately, the deep transmural segment of the tube is spared in more than 80% of cases with PTO, and microsurgical anastomosis (with its higher success rate and lower morbidity compared to tubouterine implantation) is nearly always possible when the proximal oviduct is occluded, despite attempts at catheterization.

FLUOROSCOPIC CATHETERIZATION

Patient Preparation

The procedure is performed during the follicular phase of the patient's menstrual cycle at least 2 days after bleeding has stopped (to prevent the flushing of blood into the fallopian tubes or peritoneal cavity), and before the patient has ovulated. The patient receives doxycycline 100 mg p.o. b.i.d. for 5 days starting 2 days before the procedure, or 200 mg p.o. just before the procedure followed by 100 mg p.o. b.i.d. for 5 days (15). Aseptic technique is used. Small doses of midazolam and fentanyl citrate may be given intravenously before and during the procedure as needed.

Technique

A vacuum cup type hysterosalpingography device is applied to the external cervix[a]. This provides a sterile conduit through which catheters can be advanced (Figure 10.6) and allows the application

---

[a]Thurmond-Rosch Hysterocath, Cook Inc., Bloomington, IN, or Cook OB/Gyn, Spencer, IN.

of traction on the uterus without a tenaculum (16). A conventional hysterosalpingogram is performed initially, which allows localization of the uterine cornua. Diluted water-soluble contrast medium is used so as not to obscure visualization of the catheters. A coaxial catheter system is used to engage the tubal ostium and then to catheterize the proximal fallopian tube (17). A 9 F Teflon sheath and 5.5 F polyethylene catheter are advanced over a 0.035-inch-diameter (0.089 cm) J guidewire. The 9 F sheath is placed in the lower third of the uterus to stabilize the system, and the 5.5 F catheter is advanced to the uterine cornu. For final positioning of the 5.5 F catheter in the tubal ostium, a 0.035-inch straight wire is helpful. The guidewire is removed, and full-strength contrast agent is injected to confirm positioning and to attempt visualization of the tube. If proximal tubal obstruction persists, a 0.015-inch-diameter (0.038 cm) guidewire with platinum tip and 3 F Teflon catheter are advanced together into the fallopian tube, and an attempt is made to recanalize the obstruction with to-and-fro probing movements of the guidewire. If there is undue resistance to probing with the guidewire, or if it is evident that there is an acute angulation in the fallopian tube, the small guidewire and catheter are exchanged for a softer, tapered system (18). When the guidewire passes the obstruction, the catheter is advanced coaxially over the guidewire, the guidewire is removed, and contrast agent is injected through the small catheter. If injection indicates satisfactory recanalization, the small catheter is withdrawn, and contrast agent is injected through the 5.5 F catheter (which has remained in place in the tubal ostium) to better visualize the entire tube, particularly the site of recanalization.

If the contralateral side is also blocked, the procedure is repeated by reinserting the 0.035 J guide and directing the 5.5 F catheter to the contralateral

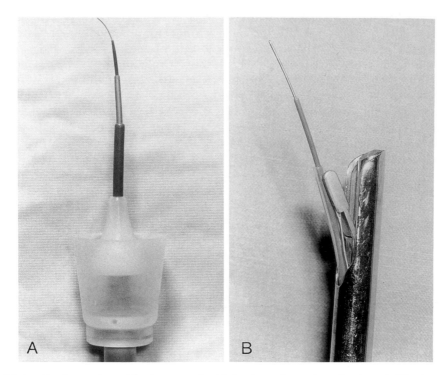

Figure 10.6.   Equipment used for transcervical fallopian tube catheterization. **A,** The Hysterocath used for fluoroscopic catheterization, with the 9 F sheath, the 5.5 F catheter, 3 F catheter, and 0.015-in.-diameter platinum tip guidewire protruding from its acorn tip. The only other equipment is a 0.035-in.-diameter J-tipped guidewire, which is used to help place the 5.5 F catheter in the uterine cornu. **B,** The tip of the Hysteroscope, with the 5.5 F clear outer cannula, the 3 F catheter, and 0.018-in.-diameter guidewire protruding.

cornu. At the conclusion of the procedure, the 5.5 F catheter is drawn back into the uterus, and contrast agent is injected for a postcatheterization hysterosalpingogram.

Postcatheterization Follow-up

Patients usually have a few days of mild vaginal bleeding and occasionally mild cramping and bloating after the procedure. They can return to normal activities, including intercourse, the following day. Patients should see their gynecologist for consideration of treatment of any other infertility problems such as ovulatory dysfunction or semen abnormalities, and should be promptly evaluated for symptoms of pregnancy so that ectopic gestation can be excluded.

Patency Rates

Using the equipment and technique described above, reported success rates for catheterization of the fallopian tubes and visualization of distal tubal anatomy range from 75 to 92% (19). Perforation of a tube occurs in about 5% of cases. Adverse consequences of perforation have not been reported, and additional monitoring or treatment has not been necessary (19).

Tubal Findings

Approximately one-third of patients who undergo fallopian tube catheterization for proximal tubal obstruction (unilateral or bilateral) have normal-appearing tubes following the procedure (Fig.

10.7). Another one-third also have normal tubes; however, the appearance of the peritoneal spill suggests peritubal adhesions. Of the remaining patients, approximately 8% will have a small dilation at the site of the recanalization (Fig. 10.4), and an unequal number will demonstrate frank salpingitis isthmica nodosa. Approximately 8% will have a distal occlusion or hydrosalpinx demonstrated, and about 10% will have unsuccessful attempts at recanalization.

Pregnancy Rates

Evaluation of any treatment for infertility is difficult because of the many clinical variables involved. We evaluated the therapeutic effect of fallopian tube catheterization in 20 carefully selected patients in whom PTO was thought to be the primary or sole cause of infertility (17). All had bilateral proximal tubal obstruction identified by at least two hysterosalpingographies and by laparoscopy, with no distal tubal disease identified by laparoscopy. The average duration of infertility was 4 years. Seven of the 20 women had additional infertility factors. All 20 patients had been recommended for tubal microsurgery or in vitro fertilization but underwent catheter recanalization instead. Recanalization of one or both tubes was successful in 19 women (95%). Fifty-eight percent of the women conceived by 1 year, without receiving any other therapy, and all pregnancies were intrauterine. Evaluation of a similar group of patients at another institution revealed comparable pregnancy results (19).

In a clinically more heterogeneous group of 100 women with unilateral or bilateral proximal tubal obstruction, many without prior laparoscopy, we found catheterization was successful in visualizing the tubes in 86 (Table 10.2) (17). A variety of tubal findings were identified as described above. Short-term follow-up in the women with patent tubes following the procedure revealed a 33% intrauterine pregnancy rate and a 6% ectopic pregnancy rate (average follow-up 7 months). All of the patients with ectopic pregnancies had either laparoscopically proven peritubal adhesions or a history of tubal surgery. All ectopic pregnancies were located in the ampulla of the tube, several centimeters distal to the site of catheterization. We attribute the lower intrauterine pregnancy rate and the higher number of ectopic pregnancies in this group to a different spectrum of underlying pathologic conditions, including more diffuse tubal disease.

Reocclusion Rate

The tubal reocclusion rate is difficult to determine because, in part, it is time dependent. In patients who do not conceive, it appears that approximately 50% of tubes reocclude by six months (19). If we assume that the tubes are patent in the patients who conceive, this gives an approximate reocclusion rate of 25% (Table 10.2). Repeat catheter recanalization is technically possible, and pregnancies have resulted after the second procedure (unpublished data).

HYSTEROSCOPIC CATHETERIZATION

Technique

Retrograde fallopian tube catheterization by hysteroscopy is performed under general anesthesia at the time of concurrent laparoscopy or laparotomy (4). A hysteroscope with an operating channel is required (Fig. 10.6). Carbon dioxide is the preferred distention medium, but liquid distention media are also suitable.

Hysteroscopic tubal catheterization for proximal obstruction is not recommended in an office setting, because it is

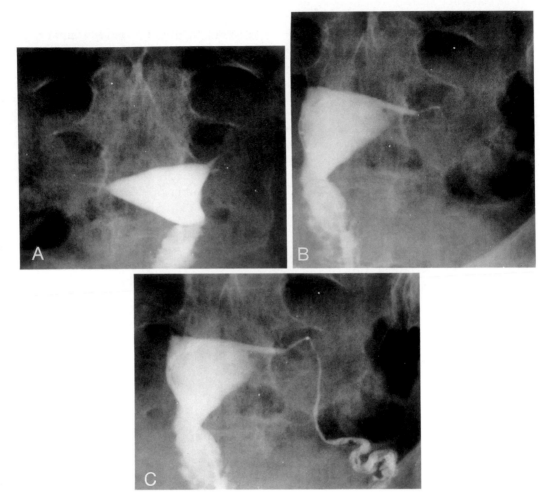

Figure 10.7. A 35-year-old woman with infertility and bilateral proximal tubal obstruction. She had bilateral PTO confirmed by laparoscopy followed by laparotomy with resection of the right salpingitis isthmica nodosa and tubal reanastomosis. On the left side, the surgeon described cob-web-like adhesions filling the endosalpinx, and he did not operate on this tube. Postoperatively, both tubes showed persistent PTO. Fluoroscopic recanalization was successful on the left side but not on the right side. **A,** Preoperative hysterosalpingogram showed bilateral PTO. **B,** Postoperative hysterosalpingography showed bilateral PTO, similar to the preoperative examination. A left selective salpingogram confirmed an obstruction approximately 1.5 cm from the tubal ostium. **C,** The obstruction was successfully passed by probing with the guidewire, and an intratubal salpingogram confirmed a successful recanalization. (Catheter tip marked by radiopaque bead.) **D,** The obstruction on the right, which was at the site of the surgical anastomosis, was initially probed with a 0.015-in. platinum-tipped guidewire. **E,** When undue resistance was encountered, a softer, tapered guidewire was used; however, it also did not pass the site of obstruction. **F,** Subsequent intratubal injection of contrast agent showed a small area of extravasation from a perforation at the surgical anastomosis.

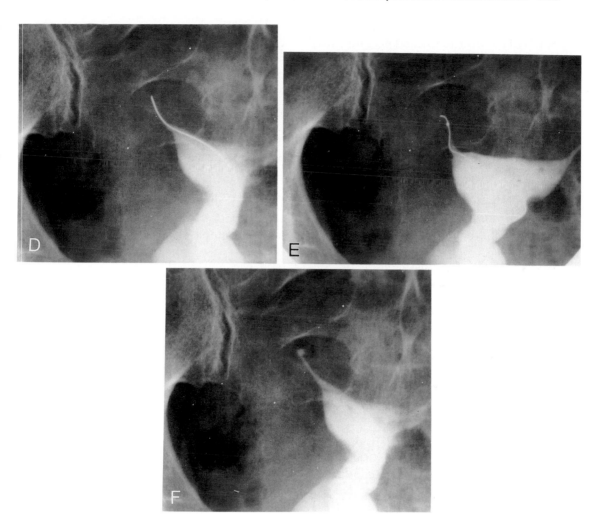

Figure 10.7.   D, E, and **F.**

Table 10.2.   Results of Fluoroscopic Transcervical Fallopian Tube Recanalization for Proximal Tubal Obstruction

Author	Number of Patients	Successful Visualization (at Least One Tube)	Early Pregnancy Rate	Ectopic Pregnancy Rate	Estimated 6-Month Patency
		%	%	%	%
Thurmond (17)	100	86	39	6	75
Platia (20)	21	76	38	13	75
Confino (21)	77	92	35	1	82

difficult to distinguish between successful relief of an obstruction and perforation of the tube without the benefit of laparoscopic visualization or documentation by fluoroscopy.

The tubal catheterization set consists of a 30 or 35 cm 5.5 F clear Teflon outer cannula with metal obturator that is introduced through the perforated rubber nipple of the hysteroscope operating channel.[b] The 5.5 F Teflon cannula is fitted with a plastic Y-adapter that ends in Luer-lok hubs. The straight arm of the adapter is sealed with a screw cap when not in use. This portal is available for irrigation, suction, and injection of contrast media or dye into the uterine cavity when desired. The outer arm of the Y-adapter is fitted with a "stop-leak" Luer-lok fitting with an adjustable O ring that provides a gas-tight seal around the 3 F Teflon inner catheter (tapered to 2.5 F in its distal 3 cm). A Teflon-coated, Cope-type stainless steel guidewire 0.018 inch (0.043 cm) in diameter with flexible blunt tip completes the catheterization set. Guidewires of smaller diameter (0.015 inch) with platinum tip and greater flexibility are recommended as useful accessories. Modifications of the catheter assembly are available for flexible hysteroscopes.

After the tubal ostium is visualized, the 5.5 F outer catheter is directed toward the tubal ostium and wedged in the endometrial funnel or tubal antrum. The 3 F Teflon catheter and guidewire are then introduced coaxially, as described in the fluoroscopic approach. The flexibility of the guidewire is increased as it protrudes farther from the end of the catheter. Advancement of the guidewire through the uterotubal junction is observed under laparoscopy with video display of the guidewire movement in the proximal oviduct. Laparoscopic assis-

tance with a blunt probe or atraumatic grasping instrument may be necessary to straighten the cornual isthmic junction to prevent perforation. Upon entering the isthmus, the guidewire is withdrawn, and indigo carmine dye or contrast medium is injected through the 3 F catheter to evaluate the patency of the distal oviduct.

Results

Hysteroscopic fallopian tube catheterization for PTO with direct visualization by laparoscopy or laparotomy has been successful in demonstrating patency in 72 to 92% of tubes attempted (4, 22). When smaller, more flexible guidewires are used, the perforation rate is similar to that with fluoroscopic cannulation, about 5%. A postcannulation patency rate of 73% has been reported on follow-up hysterosalpingography (22). We have observed an intrauterine pregnancy rate of 47%, with an ectopic pregnancy rate of 8% in 50 patients after a median follow-up period of 12 months (unpublished data). Due to the patient selection process (Fig. 10.5), patients who undergo hysteroscopic tubal catheterization usually have other pathologic findings in addition to PTO, including pelvic adhesions, distal tubal occlusion, endometriosis, or Asherman's syndrome (4, 22).

ULTRASOUND-GUIDED FALLOPIAN TUBE CATHETERIZATION

Ultrasound has been used to guide transvaginal catheterization of normal fallopian tubes. Unfortunately, visualization of small catheters in the fallopian tube has been difficult. The small catheters are not echogenic enough, and because of the tortuosity of the fallopian tube and the inherent limitations of ultra-

---

[b]Cook OB/Gyn, Spencer, IN.

sound, more work is needed in this area (unpublished data). This is, nonetheless, an area of active interest since it is postulated that transvaginal placement of gametes or developing embryos in the fallopian tube may result in higher pregnancy rates compared to uterine placement (23).

CURRENT CONTROVERSIES

The years from 1987 to 1990 were marked by debate in the literature regarding the concept of transcervical fallopian tube catheterization. Over this short period of time, former skeptics became ardent proponents of this new technique (21, 24). There is little disagreement about which patients should have hysteroscopic-laparoscopic catheterization for PTO and which patients should have fluoroscopic catheterization. There may be variation in patient selection between institutions, depending on the level of cooperation between radiologists and gynecologists. There has been disagreement, however, about the technical aspects and catheter systems used for fluoroscopic catheterization. The generic equipment required is a hysterosalpingography device for gaining access to the uterus, and catheters and guidewires for use in the fallopian tube. We have described a vacuum-cup device that is used to opacify the uterine cavity and to allow introduction of fallopian tube catheters (16). An acorn-tip cannula with a tenaculum (25) and a double balloon device (21) have been described as well and have their merits. Regarding the actual fallopian tube catheterization, all methods currently described share a common coaxial methodology, which consists of advancing a small catheter over a flexible guidewire. Some authors advocate using a balloon catheter over the guidewire (21). It is hypothesized that inflation of the balloon in the cornual region or in the tube may result in improved long-term

patency of the fallopian tube when compared to flushing with a simple coaxial catheter (21). So far, however, recanalization rates, post-procedure pregnancy rates, and reocclusion rates are similar for the balloon techniques and the non-balloon techniques (Table 10.2). Thus, while balloon catheterization is particularly suited for vascular stenoses, simple coaxial catheterization is tailored to the conditions found in the proximal fallopian tube (Table 10.1). This method achieves the goals of tubal patency and tubal visualization without the increased cost of balloon catheters.

FUTURE DIRECTIONS

The demonstrated feasibility and success of transcervical catheterization in the diagnosis of PTO have paved the way for other diagnostic and therapeutic applications of this technique. Access to the fallopian tube, as provided by transcervical catheterization, has the potential to increase our understanding of tubal physiology and to improve other treatments that are currently performed surgically. Fluoroscopic transcervical catheterization and selective salpingography have been used to diagnose ectopic pregnancy. Following diagnosis, nonsurgical treatment of tubal gestation has been performed by injecting small doses of methotrexate through the catheter (26). Hysteroscopic catheterization has been used in conjunction with fiberoptics to allow falloposcopy (27). If visual observation of the tubal lumen can be perfected in the proximal fallopian tube as well as in its distal segment, it will permit improved diagnosis and confirmation of a variety of defects. Another exciting future application of transcervical fallopian tube catheterization may be tubal sterilization, both permanent and reversible (unpublished data). This would allow sterilization to be performed in an outpatient setting without anesthesia.

CONCLUSION

Patients benefit from the improved diagnosis that fallopian tube catheterization affords. Hysteroscopic catheterization or fluoroscopic catheterization with selective salpingography results in tubal visualization in at least 85% of patients with proximal tubal obstruction. Successful hysteroscopic or fluoroscopic catheterization may spare the patient tubal resection and reanastomosis for minimal or absent disease, or may help to direct subsequent surgical or medical treatment. The therapeutic benefit of fallopian tube catheterization with recanalization is more difficult to prove. It may not be possible to directly compare the pregnancy rates following these newer techniques with the pregnancy rates following the established surgical procedures in which the pathologic cause is usually known. Nonetheless, it is quite clear that establishing tubal patency via fallopian tube catheterization does allow some women with proximal tubal obstruction to conceive.

REFERENCES

1. Serafini P, Batzofin J: Diagnosis of female infertility: a comprehensive approach. *J Reprod Med* 34:29, 1989.
2. Thurmond AS, Novy M, Rosch J: Terbutaline in diagnosis of interstitial fallopian tube obstruction. *Invest Radiol* 23:209, 1988.
3. Thurmond AS, Novy MJ, Uchida BT, Rosch J: Fallopian tube obstruction: Selective salpingography and recanalization. *Radiology* 163:511, 1987.
4. Novy MJ, Thurmond AS, Patton P, Uchida BT, Rosch J: Diagnosis of cornual obstruction by transcervical fallopian tube cannulation. *Fertil Steril* 50:434, 1988.
5. Merchant RN, Prabhu SR, Schougale A: Uterotubal junction—Morphology and clinical aspects. *Int J Fertil* 28:199, 1983.
6. Jansen RPS: Endocrine response in the fallopian tube. *Endocr Rev* 5:525, 1984.
7. Helm G, Owman C, Rosengren E, Sjoberg NO: Regional and cyclic variations in catecholamine concentration of the human fallopian tube. *Biol Reprod* 26:553, 1982.
8. Edgar DG, Asdell SA: Spermatozoa in the female genital tract. *J Endocrinol* 21:321, 1960.
9. Musich JR, Behrman SJ: Surgical management of tubal obstruction at the uterotubal junction. *Fertil Steril* 40:423, 1983.
10. Fortier KJ, Haney AF: The pathologic spectrum of uterotubal junction obstruction. *Obstet Gynecol* 65:93, 1985.
11. Donnez J, Casanas-Roux R: Prognostic factors influencing the pregnancy rate after microsurgical cornual anastomosis. *Fertil Steril* 46:1089, 1986.
12. Gillett WR, Herbison GP: Tubocornual anastomosis: Surgical considerations and coexistent infertility factors in determining the prognosis. *Fertil Steril* 51:241, 1989.
13. Silverman AY, Greenberg EI: Absence of a segment of the proximal portion of a fallopian tube. *Obstet Gynecol* 62:90S–91S, 1983.
14. Sulak PJ, Letterie GS, Coddington CC, Hayslip CC, Woodward JE, Klein TA: Histology of proximal tubal occlusion. *Fertil Steril* 48:437, 1987.
15. Pittaway DE, Winfield AC, Maxson W, Daniell J, Herbert C, Wentz AC: Prevention of acute pelvic inflammatory disease after hysterosalpingography: Efficacy of doxycycline prophylaxis. *Am J Obstet Gynecol* 147:623, 1983.
16. Thurmond AS, Uchida BT, Rosch J: Device for hysterosalpingography and fallopian tube catheterization. *Radiology* 174:571, 1990.
17. Thurmond AS, Rosch J: Nonsurgical fallopian tube recanalization for treatment of infertility. *Radiology* 174:371, 1990.
18. Thurmond AS, Rosch J: Fallopian tubes: Improved technique for catheterization. *Radiology* 174:572, 1990.
19. Thurmond AS: Selective salpingography and fallopian tube recanalization. *AJR* 156:33, 1991.
20. Platia M, Chang R, Loriaux DL, Doppman JL: Therapeutic potential of transvaginal recanalization for proximal fallopian tube obstruction. American Fertility Society Program and Abstracts: 45th Annual Meeting, San Francisco, CA, November 14, 1989:S24 (abstract 0-056).
21. Confino E, Tur-Kaspa I, DeCherney AH, et al: Transcervical balloon tuboplasty—A multicenter study. *JAMA* 264:2079, 1990.

22. Deaton JL, Gibson M, Riddick DH, Brumsted JR: Diagnosis and treatment of cornual obstruction using a flexible tip guidewire. *Fertil Steril* 53:232, 1990.
23. Jansen RPS, Anderson JC, Sutherland PD: Nonoperative embryo transfer to the fallopian tube. *N Engl J Med* 319:288, 1988.
24. DeCherney AH: Anything you can do I can do better . . . or differently! *Fertil Steril* 48:374, 1987.
25. LaBerge JM, Ponec DJ, Gordon RL: Fallopian tube catheterization: Modified fluoroscopic technique. *Radiology* 176:283, 1990.
26. Risquez F, Mathieson J, Pariente D, Foulot H, Dubuisson JB, Bonnin A, Cedard L, Zorn JR: Diagnosis and treatment of ectopic pregnancy by retrograde selective salpingography and intraluminal methotrexate injection: Work in progress. *Hum Reprod* 5:759, 1990.
27. Kerin J, Daykhovsky L, Grundfest W, Surrey E: Falloposcopy. *J Reprod Med* 35:606, 1990.

11

Postoperative Findings at Hysterosalpingography

in collaboration with Carl M. Herbert III

Operative procedures performed on the cervix, uterus, or fallopian tubes may leave characteristic findings on postoperative hysterosalpingography. Depending on the potential for an operation to recreate normal anatomic relationships, these findings can be subtle or quite obvious. The postoperative HSG provides a simple and rapid evaluation for both the patient and surgeon, and generates information that may be helpful in establishing a realistic prognosis and directing future care.

SURGICAL PROCEDURES ON THE UTERUS

Correction of Congenital Anomalies

Only perhaps 25% of women with a "double uterus" have reproductive problems, and present with recurrent pregnancy wastage or premature delivery. Experience suggests that each successive pregnancy is likely to be carried for a longer duration until finally a viable pregnancy results. In women who have aborted early, progesterone supplementation may permit the pregnancy to be carried. Therefore, an operative procedure to correct either a septate or a bicornuate uterus may be unnecessary in most women. However, if a corrective procedure is performed, a postoperative hysterogram is necessary, primarily to diagnose the formation of intrauterine adhesions.

Unification procedures performed on bicornuate or septate uteri do result in characteristic findings at hysterosalpingography. The Jones procedure (1), used for the septate uterus, is a wedge metroplasty and removes the septum entirely (Fig. 11.1). The postoperative hysterosalpingogram shows a narrow fundus with a small wedge-like septum or arcuate pattern, a smaller uterine cavity, and two small lateral "dog ears" (Figs. 11.2 to 11.4). The Tompkins procedure splits the septum by bivalving the uterus in an anteroposterior direction, dissects the septum away from the fundus, and closes the defect, leaving a wider fundus and larger uterine cavity (Figs. 11.5 and 11.6). The Strassman procedure, which splits the septum across the fundus, also results in a wider cavity but with a different line of incision, and is used only with a bicornuate and not with a septate uterus. Fullterm delivery rates of about 80% are to be expected after surgical unification, and are essentially the same for all the procedures described. On occasion, a septum may be resected by hysteroscopic technique. No dysfunction or specific radiographic findings characterize such a metroplasty. Such procedures are, as a matter of fact, gaining in popularity, and the results often show little stigma of surgery (Fig. 11.7). Synechiae may form after any of these surgical procedures (Fig. 11.8).

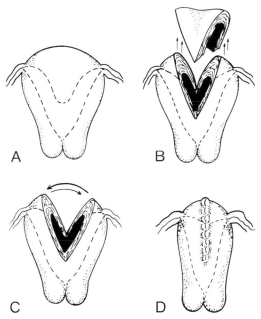

Figure 11.1. Jones procedure. The septum is removed in its entirety (**B**) and the cavity is closed (**C**). The cornua are brought closer together and the fundus is narrowed (**D**).

The uterus didelphys, which is duplicated throughout, does not lend itself to surgical correction, nor is this indicated. However, excision of a rudimentary or noncommunicating uterine horn, especially one that contains a pregnancy, is sometimes necessary. Occasionally, in the past, surgical establishment of communication between the two chambers was carried out (Fig. 11.9). A vaginal septum may be removed for patient comfort or obstetric convenience. The reproductive performance of the didelphic uterus is usually good, and a primary surgical approach may result in damage to a functional organ.

Tumor Resection

The leiomyoma (fibromyoma) is the most common uterine tumor. These tumors are characterized by location as subserosal, intramural, and submucosal. Removal of a subserosal fibromyoma usu-

ally leaves no characteristic hysterosalpingographic finding. Myomata in intramural or submucous locations may cause considerable distortion of the uterine cavity preoperatively and leave defects after their removal.

Following myomectomy, with removal of single or multiple myomata, the uterine cavity may remain as misshapen as it was before the operation was performed (Fig. 11.10); however, the cavity usually reverts to a normal appearance (Fig. 11.11). Submucosal fibromyomas of various sizes are often removed transcervically under hysteroscopic guidance. Such fibromyomas are often surprisingly bulky, but their removal no longer requires a laparotomy with a transfundal uterine incision (Fig. 11.12). Removal of larger myomata, especially transmural myomata with encroachment into the uterine cavity, may create a new abnormality, intrauterine synechiae, which can be diagnosed at follow-up hysterosalpingography (Fig. 11.13). Resection of myomata may also cause tubal obstruction or induce mechanical problems and blockage in the cornual areas (Fig. 11.14).

After resection of endometrial polyps, deformity is rare and the cavity usually is normal in appearance (Fig. 11.15). Similarly, resection of synechiae may restore a normal appearance to the cavity (Fig. 11.16) or could result in scar reformation.

Other Procedures

The most common of all postoperative findings is the scar left by a lower-segment cesarean section. This is ordinarily a jagged, wedge-like, sharp-contoured defect in the area of the lower segment (Fig. 11.17), and is characteristic of this operative procedure during an antecedent pregnancy. Some scars are large saccular defects and others have a wide base suggestive of poor healing of the uterine

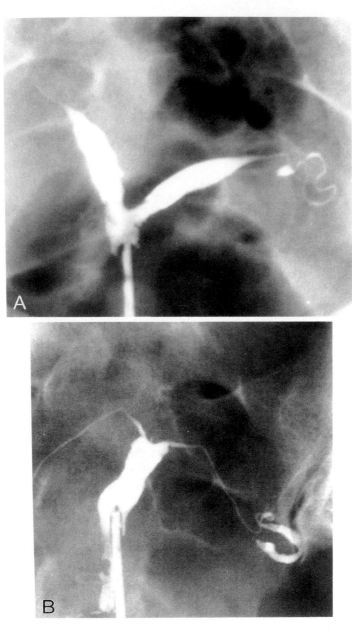

Figure 11.2.   Characteristic hysterosalpingographic pattern of a Jones wedge procedure for correction of a septate uterus. Note the narrow fundus and approximated cornua. **A,** Preoperative. **B,** Postoperative. (Courtesy of Howard W. Jones, Jr., Norfolk, VA.)

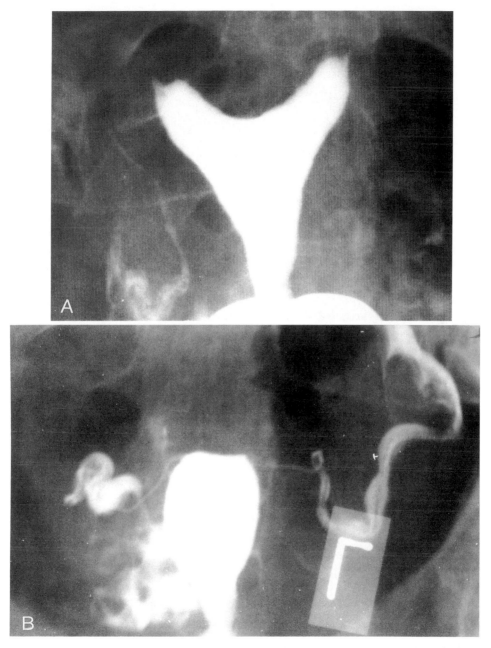

Figure 11.3. Jones procedure for correction of septate uterus. **A,** Preoperative. **B,** Postoperative. (Courtesy of Howard W. Jones, Jr., Norfolk, VA.)

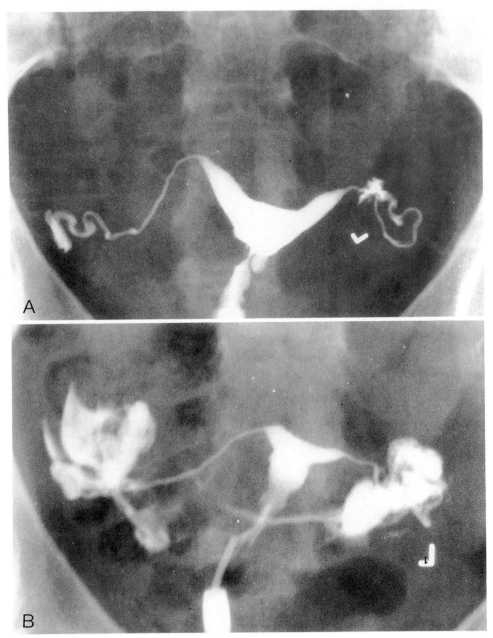

Figure 11.4.   Jones procedure for correction of septate uterus. **A,** Preoperative. **B,** Postoperative. (Courtesy of Howard W. Jones, Jr., Norfolk, VA.)

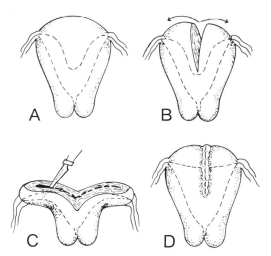

Figure 11.5. Tompkins procedure. The septum is dissected from the fundus (**C**). Closure results in a relatively wide fundal configuration (**D**).

incision (Fig. 11.18). Dog ear-like diverticula may also be observed (Fig. 11.19).

There should be no hysterosalpingographic changes induced by dilatation and curettage, although a widened internal os is thought by some to be the result of overdistention during dilatation and evacuation. Removal of a nonviable second-trimester fetus or a large submucous fibromyoma may require dilatation of the internal os to 5 cm or more. Nevertheless, there is no definitive evidence that this leaves permanent excessive dilatation of the cervix postoperatively.

Uterine perforation by a rigid injection cannula or a probe is occasionally diagnosed. More often, the instrument is buried in the myometrial wall (Fig. 11.20). The procedure should be immediately terminated, and no contrast material should be injected. When there is a strong suspicion of perforation, the patient should be admitted for observation, with close attention to the development of symptoms of blood loss, fever, and abdominal pain; antibiotic administration may be required.

SURGICAL PROCEDURES ON THE FALLOPIAN TUBES

Hysterographic Follow-up of Sterilization Procedures

Sterilization procedures and techniques have changed over the years for the purpose of simplifying the procedure and improving success rates (Fig. 11.21). There has been modification and improvement of older methods of tubal occlusion such as ligation and fulguration. Recent successful developments include the application of clips or bands to the tubes, whereas the placement of various chemicals or plugs introduced transcervically into the tubes has proved disappointing.

Tubal ligation to prevent the passage of sperm and ova is one of the oldest forms of tubal occlusion. Various combinations of simple ligation, crushing, division and burial of the stump, and simple resection are commonly used (2). The Pomeroy technique is the most frequently performed of all simple ligation techniques, with a low failure rate worldwide. With this technique, suture is tied around a "knuckle" of the isthmic-ampullary segment of tube. This portion of tube is surgically removed.

In the Uchida technique, the proximal ligated stump is buried between the peritoneal surfaces of the mesosalpinx. With fimbriectomy, the fimbria and a portion of the ampulla of each tube are removed. Both the Pomeroy and Uchida techniques result in virtually identical hysterosalpingographic pictures (Figs. 11.22 and 11.23). The film may show a blunted end, fistula formation, or distal patency, and most abnormalities are seen beginning at the midisthmic area (3). With a proximal isthmic resection, the intramural portion of the tube may not fill with contrast medium.

In the Irving technique, the tubes are divided between two absorbable lig-

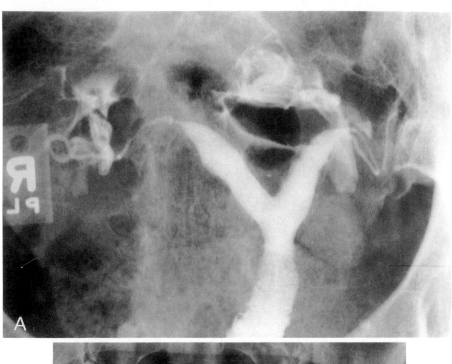

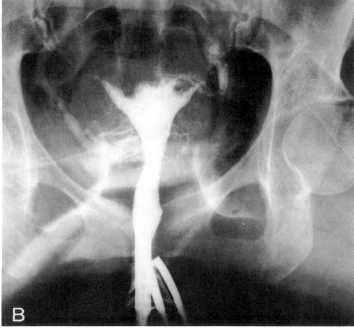

Figure 11.6.   A, Septate uterus in a woman with a history of multiple spontaneous abortions. **B,** Postoperative appearance after septum resection via the Tompkins procedure. The irregular appearance at the fundus is not unusual.

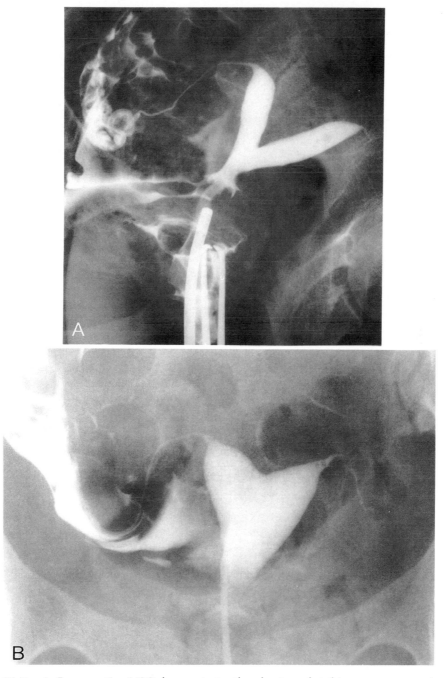

Figure 11.7. **A,** Preoperative HSG demonstrates the classic and striking appearance of a septate uterus in a patient with a history of mid- and late-term fetal loss. **B,** Following laser resection of the septum as a hysteroscopic procedure; minimal distortion persists.

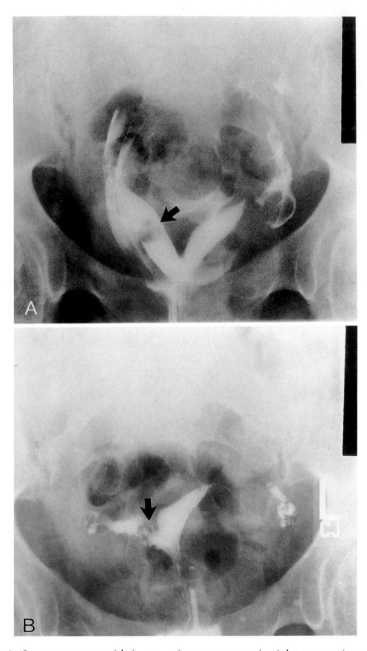

Figure 11.8.   A, Septate uterus with intrauterine pregnancy in right cornua (*arrow*). Subsequent pregnancy was lost. **B,** Postoperative hysterosalpingogram following reunification procedure. There is localized synechia formation in the right cornua (*arrow*).

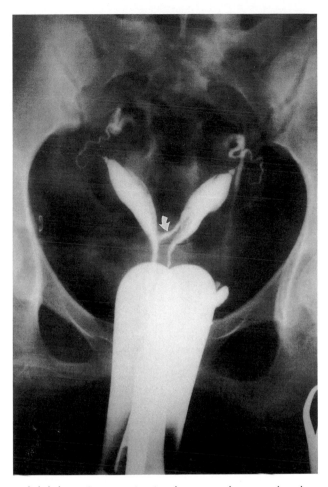

Figure 11.9. Uterus didelphys. Communication between the two chambers was created surgically (*arrow*). This operation is no longer performed.

atures, and the proximal stump is buried in the uterine myometrium, usually posteriorly. At follow-up hysterosalpingography, the proximal part of the tube will be bent upon itself. The radiographic picture is unique and striking, as contrast is distributed in varying amounts in the uterine myometrium, depending on the patency of the buried tubal segment (Fig. 11.24). The contrast clears rapidly after the injection.

Most ligation techniques were originally devised to be done postpartum through a small abdominal incision. In the past 20 years, interval sterilization pro-

cedures have been adapted to the laparoscope. Laparoscopic fulguration uses a combination of coagulation and cutting current and attempts to destroy one or more portions of the tube.

When laparoscopic fulguration techniques were first developed and their efficacy was under investigation, several groups designed studies to test patency using hysterosalpingography in the postoperative period. This was revealed to be a mistake. Jordan et al. (4) initially performed salpingography at 6 weeks, but when 22 of 60 women had spillage of contrast, it was deduced that the "depress-

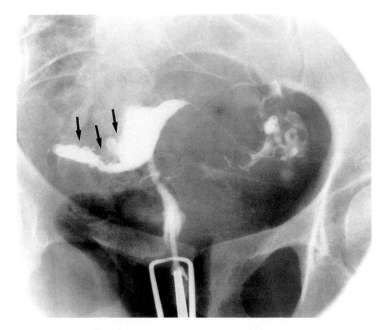

Figure 11.10.   Appearance following resection of a fundal fibromyoma. Note the marked irregularity of the fundus (*arrows*), the result of cavity distortion and scarring.

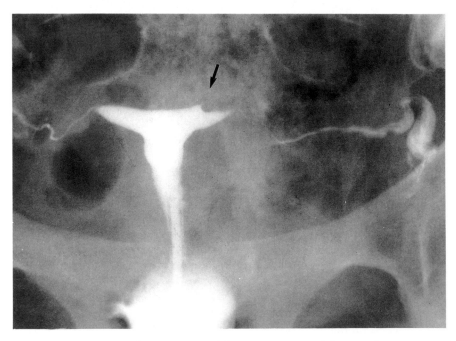

Figure 11.11.   Virtually normal appearance of the uterine cavity following the resection of a large fundal fibromyoma. Note the small deformity near the left cornua (*arrow*).

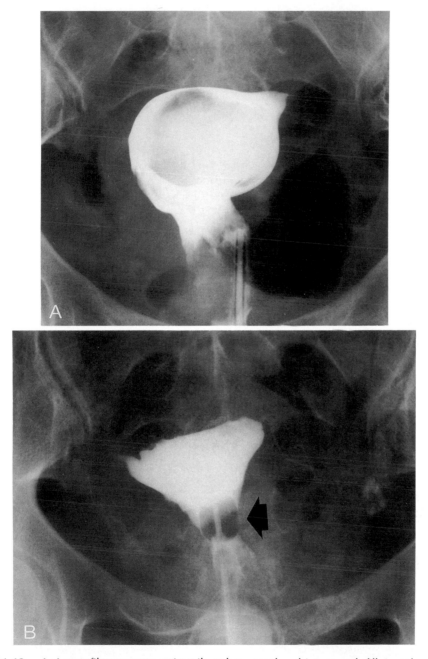

Figure 11.12. **A,** Large fibromyoma, primarily submucosal and intramural, fills much of the endometrial cavity. **B,** Following transcervical hysteroscopic resection. The cavity is virtually normal in appearance.

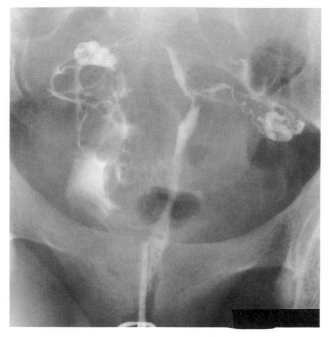

Figure 11.13. Significant deformity of the endometrial cavity following myomectomy at laparotomy.

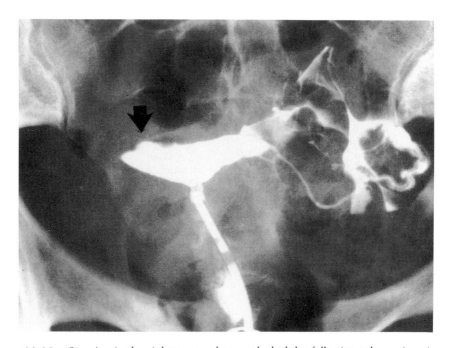

Figure 11.14. Scarring in the right cornua has occluded the fallopian tube ostium (*arrow*).

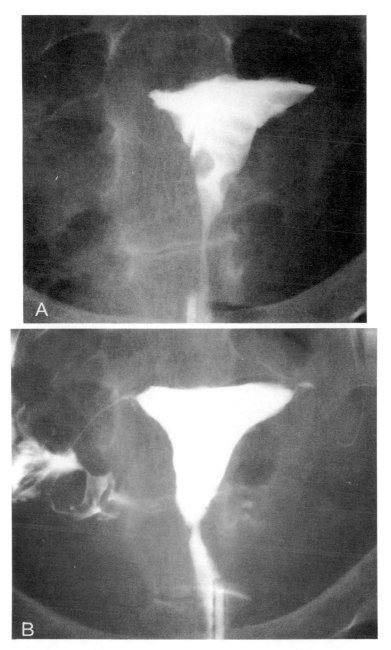

Figure 11.15. **A,** Multiple endometrial polyps throughout the uterine cavity. **B,** Hysterosalpingogram following hysteroscopic resection and curettage. The cavity now has a normal appearance.

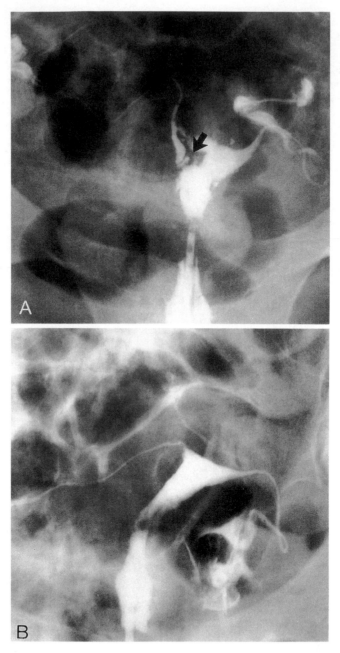

Figure 11.16.   A, Synechia formation (*arrow*). **B,** Hysterosalpingogram following hysteroscopic resection and uterine cavity distention with Foley catheter for 2 weeks. Normal-appearing cavity results.

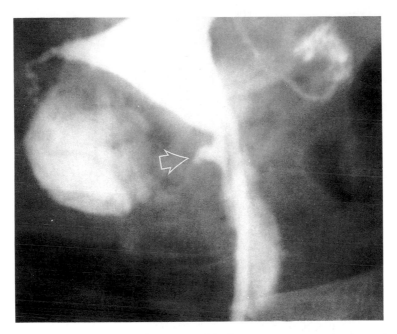

Figure 11.17. Typical appearance of deformity of the lower uterine segment (*arrow*) secondary to previous cesarean section.

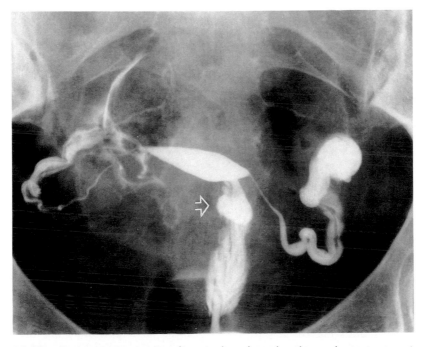

Figure 11.18. Postcesarean section diverticulum, broad and saccular in contour (*arrow*).

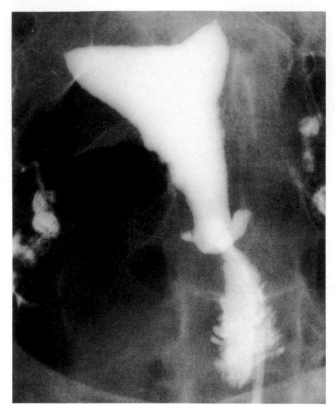

Figure 11.19.   Bilateral diverticular outpouching resulting from cesarean section in the past.

ingly high rate of spill" was because the hysterosalpingography was being performed before the tube had fully fibrosed, thus forcing a fistula (Fig. 11.25). When the salpingogram was performed at or beyond 12 weeks, only eight of 383 patients were diagnosed to show spillage. Others (5–7) confirmed these findings. Although Sheikh (5) recommended follow-up with hysterosalpingography in teaching institutions and when inexperienced operators were learning the technique of sterilization procedures, routine hysterosalpingography cannot be recommended if fulguration is the method of tubal occlusion.

Tantalum clips for sterilization are applied to the tube via specially designed pliers, and failures may result if a clip opens slightly, renewing tubal patency, or cuts through the tube leading to recanalization. Spring-loaded clips have been judged more effective than the tantalum clip (Fig. 11.26); the hysterosalpingographic pictures may not allow differentiation between the two types of clips.

Bands, including the Falope ring, may be applied by any approach except transcervically. Electrocautery is not required, and the ring is slipped over a loop of tube that has been drawn into a special applicator; the blood supply is interrupted and eventually the tube undergoes fibrosis. The characteristic hysterosalpingographic picture is that of tubal obstruction adjacent to a radiopaque band, which is the Falope ring (Fig. 11.27). Some physicians have been uncomfortable about the placement of a single clip or Falope ring, and, not infrequently, more than a single ring can be found on a patient who has undergone this form of sterilization (Fig. 11.28).

Tissue adhesives have been used to

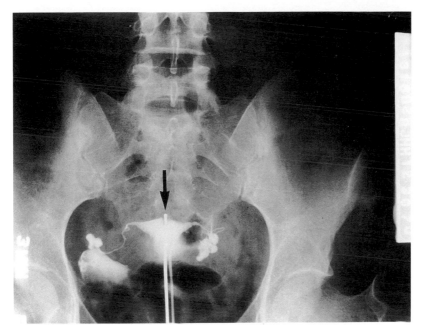

Figure 11.20. Probe inadvertently embedded in the myometrium (*arrow*). Occasionally such instrumentation may traverse the muscular wall and enter the peritoneal cavity.

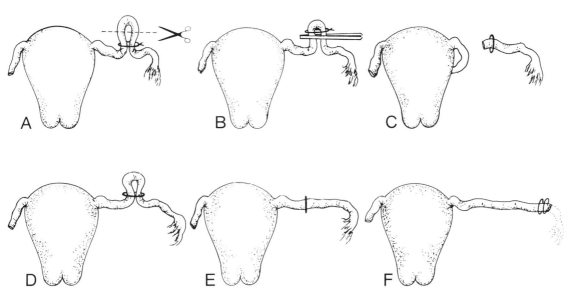

Figure 11.21. Various techniques of tubal ligation and interruption currently encountered. **A,** Pomeroy. **B,** Madlener. **C,** Irving. **D,** Falope ring.[a] **E,** Hulka clip.[b] **F,** Fimbriectomy.

form a plug, and sclerosing chemicals, including quinacrine and silver nitrate,

have been employed in the past attempting to destroy the inner lining of the tube with subsequent fibrosis. More recently, solid Silastic intratubal devices, polyethylene and Teflon plugs, and silver-impregnated silicone plugs (8) have been in-

[a]Cabot Medical Corp., Langhorn, PA.
[b]Richard Wolf Medical Instruments, Rosemont, IL.

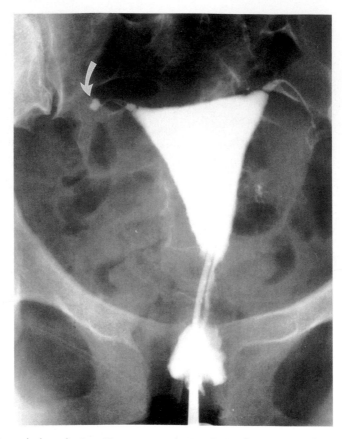

Figure 11.22. Posttubal occlusion (Pomeroy technique). Occlusions are characteristically in the isthmic segment and often show slight bulbous dilatation at the point of obstruction (*arrow*).

stilled transcervically to accomplish tubal occlusion (Fig. 11.29). The major advantage of these techniques is their potential reversibility and the ability to apply them transcervically without general anesthesia. The major disadvantages include the specially designed instrumentation, the above-average operator skill required for insertion, and a higher than acceptable failure rate secondary to dislodgment.

Tubal Anastomosis and Implantation

A major reason for hysterosalpingography in the sterilized patient is when reanastomosis is being contemplated. Requests for reversal of tubal sterilization

are not uncommon. The proximal tubal segment may not remain normal after ligation procedures, especially following fulguration, so preoperative evaluation may be helpful before anastomosis is undertaken (Figs. 11.23 and 11.30). The length of the proximal segment is important, as the prospect for a normal pregnancy is influenced by the length of the repaired tube (9). About 75% of patients with more than 4 cm of tube on the longest side successfully conceive, but few become pregnant after surgical anastomosis that results in tubes of less than 3.0 cm. For pregnancy, the presence of both the fimbria and the ampullary segment is important. At least 1 cm of ampulla must remain intact, but this cannot be evaluated radiographically in the occluded

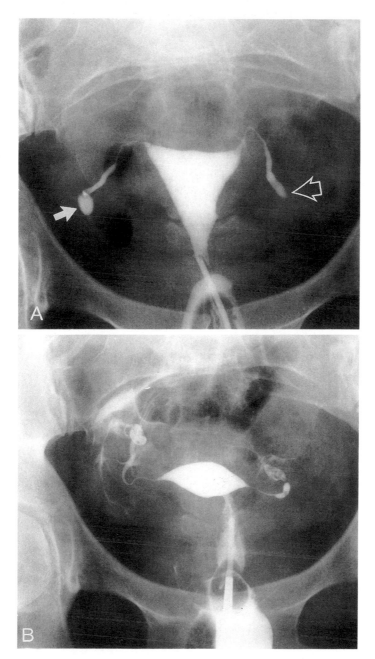

Figure 11.23. A, Bilateral tubal occlusions with prominent dilatation at the terminal end of the right tube (*arrow*), and a club-like termination of the left tube (*open arrow*). **B,** Same patient following successful reanastomosis. Both tubes are patent.

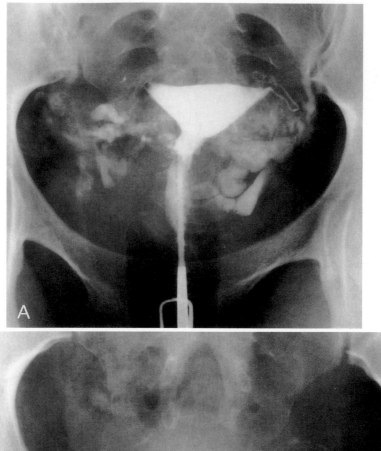

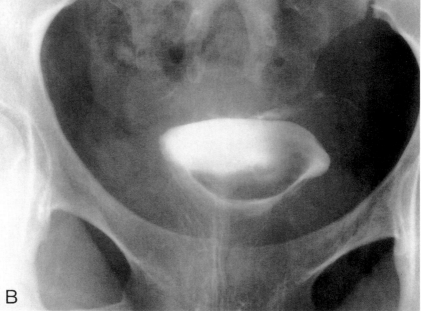

Figure 11.24.   A, Irving procedure for tubal occlusion. The severed end of the proximal segment of the tube is embedded in the myometrium. The contrast material thus fills the venous channels draining the uterus. **B,** Delayed film (same study), within a few minutes, shows emptying of the vascular channels seen in **A.**

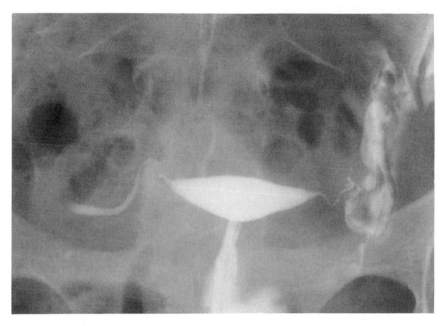

Figure 11.25. Recanalization has resulted in a patent left fallopian tube following bilateral Pomeroy ligations.

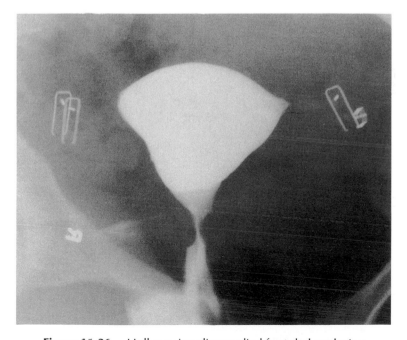

Figure 11.26. Hulka spring clips applied for tubal occlusion.

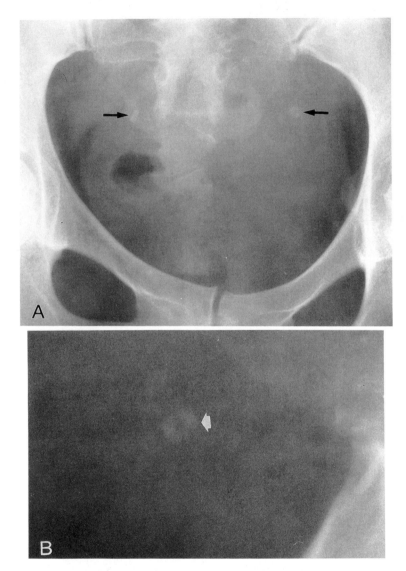

Figure 11.27.   **A,** Falope rings (*arrows*) applied for tubal occlusion. This appearance may, on occasion, be confused with ureteral calculi in some symptomatic patients. **B,** Note the characteristic ring-like appearance (*arrow*).

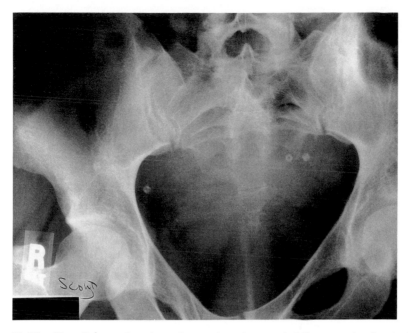

Figure 11.28. Two Falope rings have been placed on each fallopian tube for occlusion.

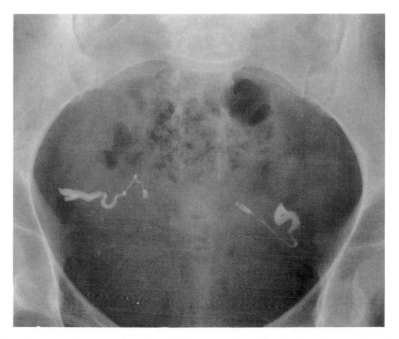

Figure 11.29. Characteristic appearance of fallopian tubes filled with silicone plugs for occlusion. Radiopaque appearance results from silver salts impregnating the silicone.

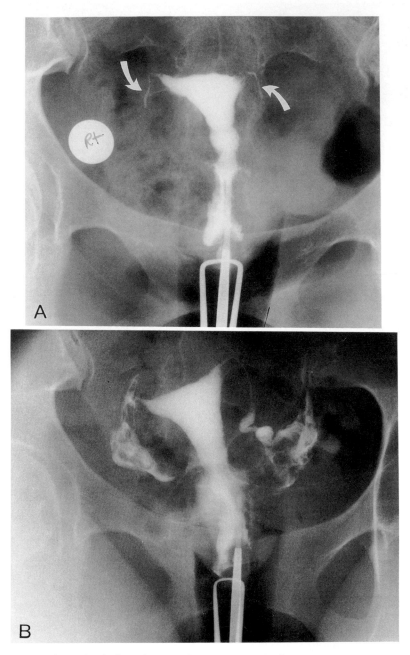

Figure 11.30.   A, Bilateral tubal occlusions. Prior to a surgical attempt to reanastomose the occluded tube segments, the position of the separation must be assessed. Note that the isthmic segment of the tube is ample for plastic repair (*arrows*) and suggests that an adequate portion of the distal tube remains. **B,** Successful tubal reanastomoses. Both tubes are patent.

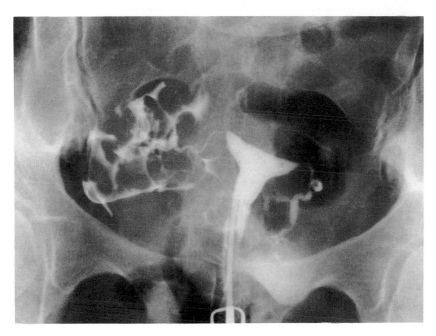

Figure 11.31.   Successful tubal reanastomoses. Both tubes are patent. The location of repair is difficult to identify.

tube. The hysterosalpingogram can demonstrate the length of the proximal segment to aid in planning the reversal procedure, but failure to fill intramural segments may be secondary to resistance caused by the more distal occlusion and may not represent true cornual occlusion. In a recent study, only 12% of tubes with hysterosalpingographic evidence of cornual occlusion after tubal ligation were found to be occluded at the time of the anastomosis procedure (10). These authors concluded that a preoperative hysterosalpingogram did not provide adequate reliable information to justify performing this procedure. However, visualization of the uterine cavity is an added benefit to the diagnosis of unsuspected intrauterine pathology such as polyps or submucous myomata. Alternatively, this portion of the investigation can be performed as an office hysteroscopy procedure.

Postoperative findings characteristic of fallopian tube operations are many and variable (11) (Fig. 11.31). In the case of an ampullary-isthmic tubal anastomosis, the tubal lumen will vary in size on either side of the anastomosis, with the degree of difference depending on where the anastomosis was done (Figs. 11.32, 11.33, and 11.34). As a further example, the cornual area may have lost its characteristic wedge-like appearance if a "cork borer" technique is used for implanting the tube into the uterine cavity in the cornual region (Fig. 11.35).

Tubal repair may also be accomplished for cornual occlusion by a technique in which the myometrium is "shaved" down until a patent interstitial lumen is found. Anastomosis is then carried out, which likely leaves the cornual area with its usual anatomic configuration, or at least less distortion than when the area is opened with a uterine reamer (Fig. 11.36).

A technique occasionally encountered but now rarely performed implants the proximal portion of the tube into the

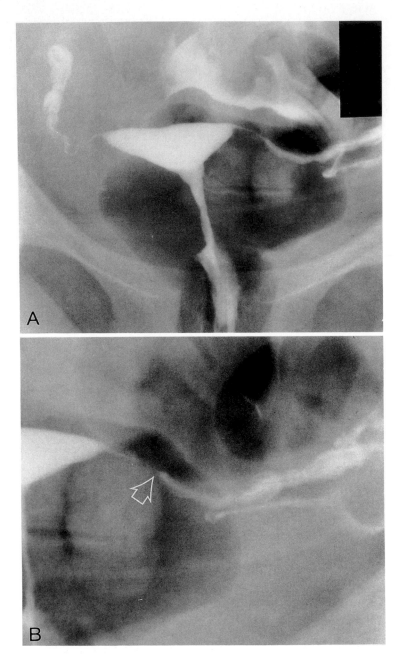

Figure 11.32.   **A,** Location of tubal anastomosis can be identified by the sudden change in caliber of the fallopian tube, as seen in the enlarged view (**B**) (*arrow*).

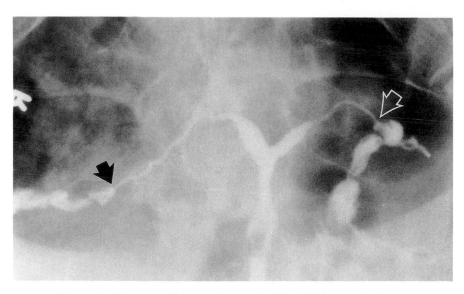

Figure 11.33.   Dramatic change in diameter (*arrows*) of the fallopian tube lumen following successful reanastomosis.

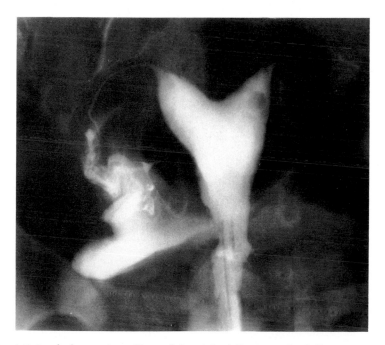

Figure 11.34.   Minimal change in caliber of the right fallopian tube following anastomosis. The exact location of the surgical site is difficult to identify with certainty.

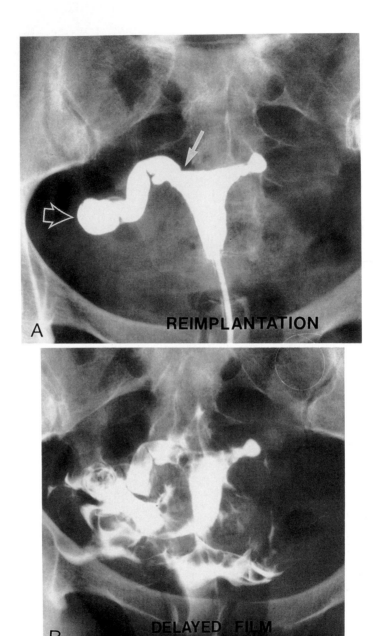

Figure 11.35.   A, Reimplantation of the right fallopian tube into the cornua following a "cork borer" technique to establish an adequate lumen (*arrow*). The dilated ampullary portion of the tube was opened at the same time (*open arrow*). The left fallopian tube is obstructed. **B,** Delayed film demonstrates that the right fallopian tube is patent, although deformity persists.

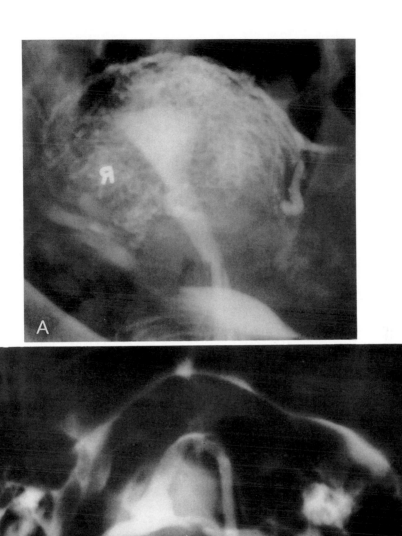

Figure 11.36. **A,** Bilateral cornual occlusion. Extravasation of contrast material in the myometrium and vascular channels is related to the obstruction and increased pressure in the endometrial cavity. **B,** Reimplantation with very little deformity at the uterolateral junction (*arrow*).

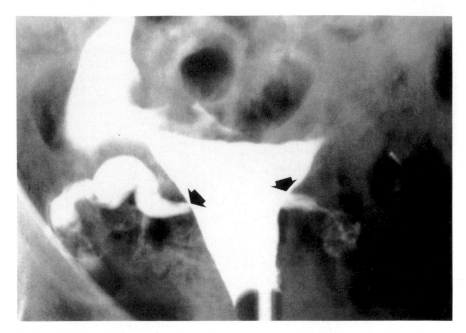

Figure 11.37. Hysterosalpingogram following a uterotubal implantation of the Peterson type. Note the low position of the tubal insertion (*arrows*) in reference to the fundus. (Courtesy of T. A. Baramki and F. Bottiglieri, Baltimore, MD.)

uterine cavity at a site adjacent to the cornua, usually in the posterior fundus or below the fundal level (Fig. 11.37) (12). Although initial results were encouraging, this procedure has proved less efficacious than anastomosis procedures and is therefore used infrequently. With the advent of tubal recanalization techniques, the need for many of these surgical operations has been obviated (see Chapter 10).

Distal Neosalpingostomy

One of the most dramatic radiographic changes is the postoperative appearance of a repaired hydrosalpinx. Surgical incision and repair now can be performed either by laparoscopy or using the conventional microsurgical techniques during an open laparotomy. The postoperative hysterosalpingogram may reveal complete decompression of the hydrosalpinx with or without evidence of damage to the endothelial surface. How-

ever, more frequently some degree of tubal dilatation persists (Fig. 11.38). Frequently, the normal rugae may be obliterated, which suggests that the thin-walled hydrosalpinx may have few ciliated or nonciliated endothelial cells left. Rugae may sometimes be seen in hydrosalpinges, although these may have a thickened appearance suggesting intratubal edema or the presence of postinflammatory folds. The presence or absence of rugae, however, has no predictive value for pregnancy success.

SALPINGOSTOMY FOR REMOVAL OF AN ECTOPIC PREGNANCY

Linear incisions over an ectopic pregnancy with evacuation of the tubal products of conception can be accomplished by laparoscopy or by more conventional methods at laparotomy. The postoperative hysterosalpingographic picture will vary with the degree of damage and may demonstrate complete oc-

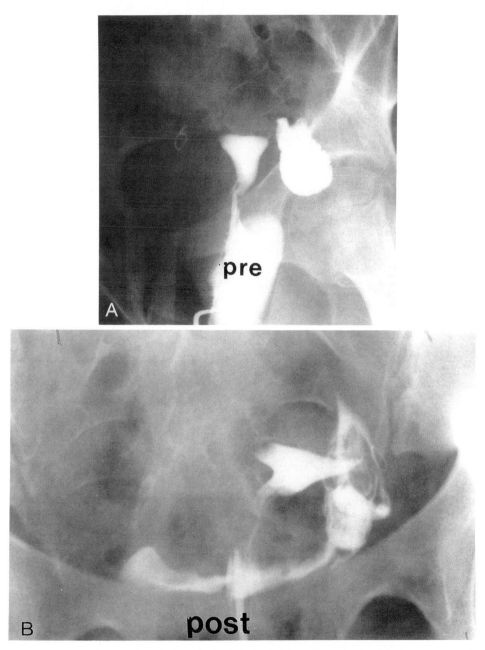

Figure 11.38.   A, Marked hydrosalpinx on the left. The right fallopian tube has been surgically re-moved. **B,** Following laser laparoscopic surgery, the dilatation persists but there is obvious tubal patency.

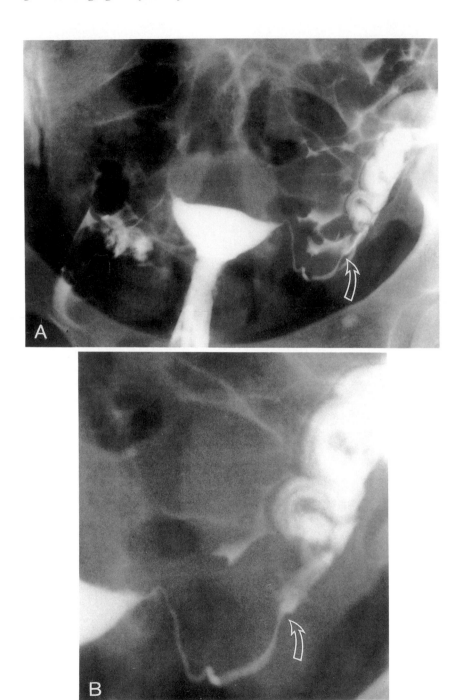

Figure 11.39.   **A,** Bilateral laser salpingostomies. Ectopic pregnancies have necessitated surgery to both fallopian tubes. The site of surgery is identifiable (*arrow*), but only minimal deformity is recognized. **B,** Enlarged view of **A.**

clusion, fistula formation, or even a tubal lumen indistinguishable from normal (Fig. 11.39).

Information obtained from a hysterosalpingogram postoperatively following the removal of an ectopic pregnancy in a single tube is mandatory to ensure that tubal patency is maintained. This information may also be helpful in directing a patient's future care even if two fallopian tubes are present.

REFERENCES

1. Rock JA, Jones WH Jr: The clinical management of the double uterus. *Fertil Steril* 28:798, 1977.
2. Wortman J: Tubal sterilization—review of methods. *Popul Rep C*, May 1976.
3. Ayers JWT, Johnson RS, Ansbacher R, Menon M, LaFerla JJ, Roberts JA: Sterilization failures with bipolar tubal cautery. *Fertil Steril* 42:526, 1984.
4. Jordan JA, Edwards RL, Pearson J, Maskery PJK: Laparoscopic sterilization and follow-up hysterosalpingogram. *Br J Obstet Gynaecol* 78:460, 1971.
5. Sheikh HH: Hysterosalpingographic follow-up of laparoscopic sterilization. *Am J Obstet Gynecol* 126:181, 1976.
6. Sheikh HH: Hysterosalpingographic follow-up of the partial salpingectomy type of sterilization. *Am J Obstet Gynecol* 128:858, 1977.
7. Grunert GM: Late tubal patency following tubal ligation. *Fertil Steril* 35:406, 1981.
8. Dan SJ, Goldstein MS: Fallopian tube occlusion with silicone: Radiographic appearance. *Radiology* 151:603, 1984.
9. Silber SJ, Cohen R: Microsurgical reversal of female sterilization: The role of tubal length. *Fertil Steril* 33:598, 1980.
10. Groff TR, Edelstein JA, Schenken RS: Hysterosalpingography in the preoperative evaluation of tubal anastomosis candidates. *Fertil Steril* 53:417, 1990.
11. Schwimmer M, Heiken JP, McClennan BL: Postoperative hysterosalpingogram: Radiographic surgical correlation. *Radiology* 157:313, 1985.
12. Peterson EP, Musich JR, Behrman SJ: Uterotubal implantation and obstetrical outcome after previous sterilization. *Am J Obstet Gynecol* 128:662, 1977.

12

Transvaginal Sonography in Gynecologic Infertility

Arthur C. Fleischer
Donna M. Kepple
Carl M. Herbert III
George A. Hill

The increased utilization and availability of transvaginal (TV) transducer probes have had a major impact on the management and treatment of patients with gynecologic infertility. Specifically, transvaginal sonography (TVS) has its greatest clinical impact in precise monitoring of follicular development, guided follicular or cyst aspiration, and guided transcervical cannulization of the fallopian tube (1). Another application of TVS includes evaluation of the adequacy of endometrial development. Color Doppler sonography obtained with a transvaginal probe provides a means of evaluating the vascular perfusion of the ovary and uterus—additional parameters that may be important in optimizing treatment.

INSTRUMENTATION

There are several types of transvaginal transducer probes available (Figs. 12.1 and 12.2). The most common types use either a single mechanically sectored element, a curvilinear array, or a phased linear array. Each produces a sector field of view usually encompassing 80 to 95° with a 10-cm depth. They also vary as to their transducer contact surface or "footprint" size. For more superficial structures (within 5 cm), a larger footprint al-

lows greater line density and resolution. Some probes contain multiple transducers and can be changed according to the depth of the area of interest. For example, a 5.0-MHz transducer is used to image structures in the far field (beyond 5 cm), whereas a 7.5-MHz transducer can be used in the near field. This transducer probe also allows the operator to angle the beam by turning a thumbwheel on the probe's shaft. This allows visualization of side wall structures, for example, without angulation of the probe itself.

Needle guides are needed for accurate aspiration/biopsy using a TV probe. These attachments maintain the needle path within the beam. Ones that are flush to the shaft of the probe are preferred over those that are outrigged, since the chance for irritation of the anterior urethral area is less.

The probe should be disinfected between uses. We recommend the use between studies of a spray that has bacteriocidal and virucidal effects (e.g., Sporocidin[a]). Before insertion into the vagina, a condom is placed over the shaft of the probe. Usually, there are sufficient vaginal secretions for adequate contact;

---

[a]Sporocidin International, Rockville, MD.

242

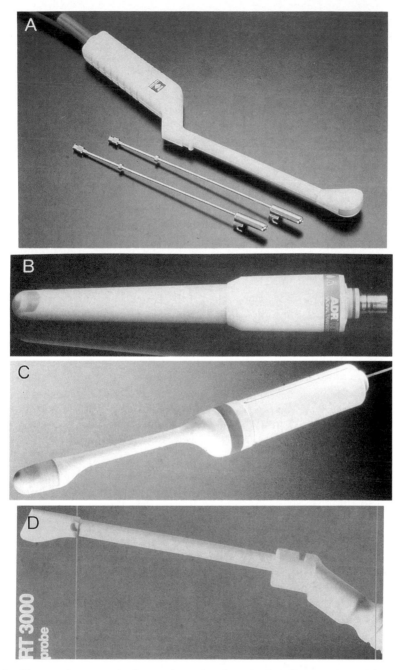

Figure. 12.1. Types of transvaginal transducer/probes. **A,** Curvilinear array with attachable 16- and 18-gauge needle guides. **B,** Single-element mechanical sector. **C,** Multiple-element mechanical sector. The probe rotates a 5.0-MHz and a 7.5-MHz transducer within its housing. **D,** Phased linear array.

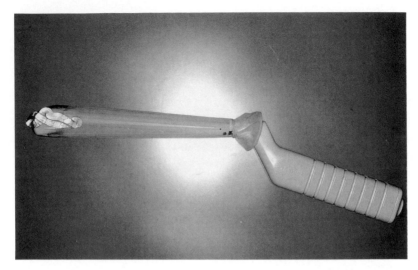

Figure. 12.2. Prepared probe with condom covering secured to shaft with rubber bands and gel placed on the outer surface of the condom.

occasionally, a small amount of gel is needed on the condom to afford adequate transmission.

FOLLICULAR MONITORING

As stated previously, TVS has a vital role in depicting follicular development in patients treated for infertility that can be traced to disorders of ovulation (2). Although the maturity of the oocyte is only indirectly inferred by the size of the follicle, the sonographic information can be coupled with serum estradiol values to provide an accurate assessment of the presence or absence and number of mature follicles (3, 4). The anatomic information obtained with TVS concerning the size and development of maturing follicles and corpora lutea can be used to distinguish physiologic from "insufficient" cycles with abnormal folliculogenesis or possible luteal phase inadequacy (LPI) (5, 6). For example, the maximal follicle size in insufficient cycles has been reported to be significantly less than in normal ones, and the absence of a corpus luteum was found more often in insufficient cycles (6). In addition, the undesirable development of multiple immature follicles rather than development of a single dominant follicle can be recognized in patients with polycystic ovaries (7).

Although its actual contribution to infertility is controversial, some authors describe an abnormality in ovulation termed luteinized unruptured follicle (LUF) syndrome as a cause of unexplained infertility (8). In this disorder, there is failure of extrusion of the oocyte, which remains trapped within the follicle. The presence of this abnormality can be confirmed only by observation at laparoscopy of the absence of a stigma (a healed rent where ovulation occurred) in the ovarian capsule. Since this may not be present as little as 2 hours postovulation, the presence of this syndrome is difficult to confirm. With TVS, one can observe failure of the follicle to deflate and the absence of intraperitoneal fluid associated with ovulation. This syndrome may be more common in women with endometriosis and may not be present on consecutive cycles (6, 8).

Some have also reported on the "empty follicle syndrome," in which a cumulus cannot be identified within the follicle (9). Although it is tempting to use TVS to assess whether or not an oocyte is present, it is felt that sonographic absence of the cumulus does not have sufficient reliability at present to confidently diagnose this entity.

Spontaneous Ovulation

At the time of birth, the female neonate has approximately 2 million primary oocytes within each ovary. At menarche, approximately 200,000 remain per ovary. During the childbearing years, approximately 200 oocytes will be ovulated. This indicates that approximately 99.9% of primary oocytes become atretic or do not develop at all.

Maturation of the oocyte and follicle is responsive primarily to changes in follicle-stimulating hormone (FSH) and luteinizing hormone (LH) and may be monitored by circulating levels of estradiol (E_2). With the elaboration and release of FSH in the late secretory phase, there is development of one and sometimes two follicles in a subsequent cycle. Actually, the follicle begins its maturation process several months prior to the actual ovulation of the oocyte. It is not uncommon to observe more than one follicle developing to approximately 10 mm in size, with one becoming dominant and growing and the other regressing. LH reinitiates meiosis of the oocyte, and ovulation typically occurs within 24 to 36 hours of its "surge" in circulating levels. E_2 is synthesized by the granulosa cells and provides important feedback to the pituitary in the production of FSH and LH.

Beginning with menarche, during spontaneous cycles, there is usually development of one or sometimes two dominant follicles. TVS can depict the developing follicles starting when they measure between 3 and 5 mm. In the spontaneous cycle, there is usually one or at the most two follicles that develop to measure approximately 10 mm in size. As the follicle matures, more fluid is elabo-

rated into its center, and the number of granulosa cells lining the inner wall of the follicle increases. The oocyte itself, which is less than a tenth of a millimeter, is surrounded by a cluster of granulosa cells. This complex is termed the cumulus oophorus. It measures approximately 1 mm and can be depicted occasionally along the wall of some mature follicles with TVS. Immediately prior to ovulation the cumulus separates from the wall and floats freely within the center of the follicle. Even with the enhanced resolution afforded by TVS, the attached or floating cumulus is only rarely visualized.

Mature follicles (ones that contain a mature oocyte) typically measure from 17 to 25 mm in average inner dimension (Fig. 12.3) (10). However, within the same individual, the size of a mature follicle is relatively constant from cycle to cycle. Intrafollicular echoes may be observed with mature follicles, probably arising from clusters of granulosa cells that shear off the wall near the time of ovulation. After ovulation, the follicular wall becomes irregular as the follicle becomes "deflated" (Fig. 12.4). The fresh corpus luteum usually appears as a hypoechoic structure with an irregular wall and may contain internal echoes corresponding to hemorrhage. As the corpus luteum develops some 4 to 8 days after ovulation, it appears as an echogenic structure of approximately 15 mm in size. Its wall is thickened due to the process of luteinization (Fig. 12.4).

In addition to delineating changes in follicle size and morphology, TVS can depict the presence of intraperitoneal fluid (Fig. 12.4). It is normal to have approximately 1 to 3 ml in the cul-de-sac throughout the cycle. When ovulation occurs, there is typically between 4 and 5 ml within the cul-de-sac. The intraperitoneal fluid resulting from ovulation may be loculated outside the posterior cul-de-sac, surrounding bowel loops in the lower abdomen and upper pelvis, or in the an-

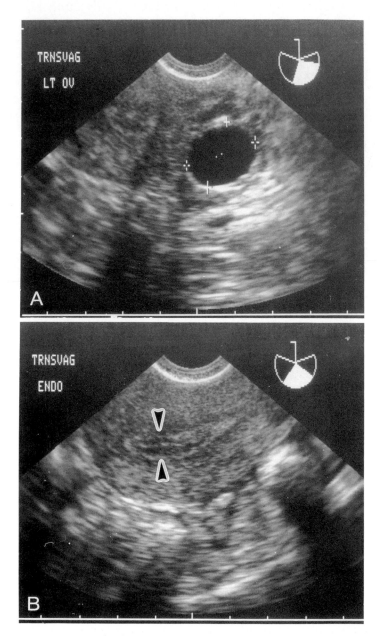

Figure 12.3.   Spontaneous cycle showing normal folliculogenesis. **A,** TVS showing a mature follicle (between *cursors*) within the left ovary. **B,** Typical multilayered endometrium (between *arrowheads*) typically seen in the periovulatory period. **C,** Gray-scale image of transvaginal color Doppler sonogram showing significant diastolic flow in the wall of the corpus luteum.

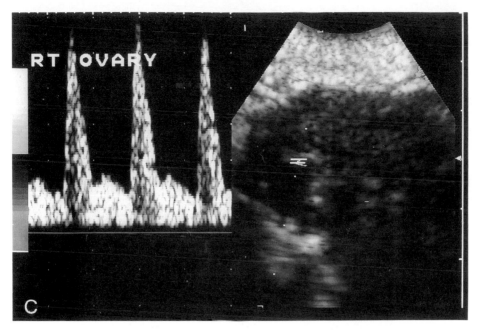

Figure 12.3. C.

terior cul-de-sac superior to the uterine fundus.

Induced Ovulation

In patients whose infertility can be attributed to an ovulation abnormality, ovulation induction is indicated. Ovulation induction is also used in in vitro fertilization-embryo transfer (IVF-ET) to increase the number of oocytes aspirated, which in turn increases the number of fertilized concepti that may be transferred, thereby increasing the chance of pregnancy.

The two medications that are most commonly used for ovulation induction include clomiphene citrate (CC) and human menopausal gonadotropin (hMG). Although both medications result in the development of multiple follicles, they act by different mechanisms. TVS has a vital role in monitoring follicular development in women receiving medication for ovulation induction (3, 4).

Patients undergoing ovulation induction are usually examined every other day beginning between cycle days 7 and 9. For patients undergoing IVF-ET, patients begin to be examined by TVS earlier in their cycles and usually daily in an attempt to carefully monitor follicular development.

CC is considered an estrogen antagonist and exerts its effect by binding estrogen receptor sites in the pituitary and hypothalamus. This leads to increased FSH secretion by the pituitary, thereby recruiting more follicles. Since the process of selection and dominance may be overridden, multiple, relatively synchronous follicles usually develop (Figs. 12.5 and 12.6). Although the preovulatory E_2-LH feedback may be intact in CC-treated patients with an intact hypothalamus, most patients are given human chorionic gonadotropin (hCG) to induce final follicular and oocyte maturation.

Follicular development with CC can be quite different than that observed in spontaneous cycles. Specifically, each follicle seems to develop at an individual rate and at times may be accelerated or slowed down. Therefore, the largest fol-

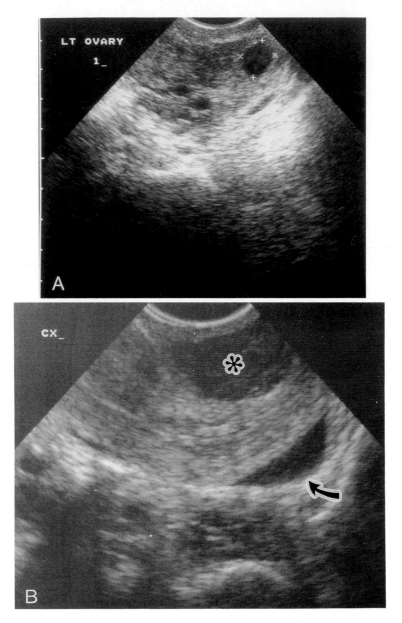

Figure 12.4.   Postovulatory changes. **A,** Thickened, serrated wall of postovulatory follicle (between *cursors*). **B,** "New" intraperitoneal fluid posterior to cervix (*curved arrow*). *Asterisk* shows completely collapsed bladder.

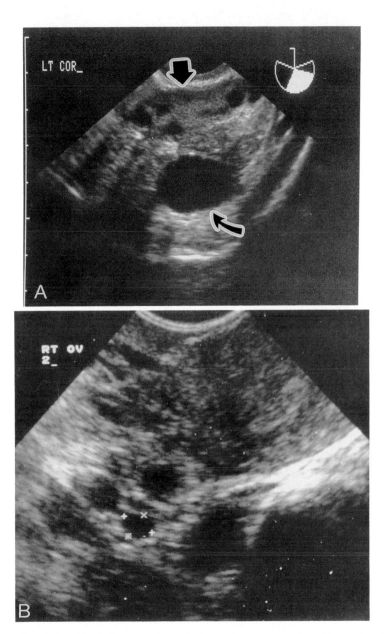

Figure 12.5. TVS mimics of a follicle. **A,** Rounded cystic structure (*curved arrow*) adjacent to but not within the left ovary representing a paraovarian cyst (*arrow*). **B,** Iliac artery (between *cursors*) seen in the short axis.

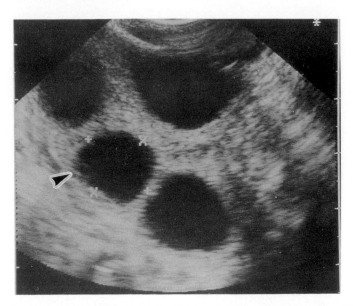

Figure 12.6.   Multiple mature follicles resulting from ovulation induction using Clomid.[b] A cumulus is seen (*arrowhead*) within the one that is measured.

licle on a given date may not be the same 2 days later and may not even be the same one that is most mature. Furthermore, correlation of E_2 and follicle sizes is poor, and the maximum preovulatory diameter can range from 19 to 24 mm.

As opposed to CC, treatment with hMG does not require an intact hypothalamus or pituitary. In hMG-treated patients, there seem to be two distinct patterns of follicular development (3). In amenorrheic women with no exogenous estrogen, estrogenic activity, and dormant ovaries, the response to endogenous gonadotropins is to develop a small number of large follicles (Fig. 12.6). The growth rate and E_2 secretion are linear, correlate well, and are of equal predictive value. A high pregnancy rate is achieved in this group. In contrast, patients with estrogenic activity who harbor antral follicles at different stages of development react very differently (Fig. 12.7). Stimulation of these patients requires less hMG and usually results in the rapid recruit-

ment of many follicles with different growth rates in varying degrees of E_2 secretory capacity. Also, the rate at which E_2 increases is exponential, increasing the risk of hyperstimulation. Thus, there is a dissociation between follicle size and E_2 levels, suggesting that growth rate and functional maturity are asynchronous. This group of women particularly benefits from combined E_2 and follicular monitoring with TVS. Because hMG contains both FSH and LH and a spontaneous LH surge is less frequent when inducing follicular development with hMG, hCG may be required to induce final follicular maturation. TVS delineation of follicle size is crucial, since hCG is best administered once follicles reach 15 to 18 mm in size.

For IVF, follicles are typically aspirated when they reach 15 to 18 mm in average dimension and when there is evidence by estradiol values of a mature follicle (approximately 400 pg/ml/mature follicle) (11). Another sonographic sign of a mature follicle is the presence of low-level, intrafollicular echoes. These echoes probably arise from clumps of granulosa cells that have separated from

[b]Merrell Dow U.S.A.

the follicular wall. In one study involving patients who underwent ovulation induction and were scanned transabdominally, a higher pregnancy rate was achieved in patients whose follicles demonstrated these intrafollicular echoes than those that did not (12).

TVS has an important role in decreasing the likelihood of ovarian hyperstimulation. Ovarian hyperstimulation disorder occurs in various degrees of severity in most patients who undergo ovulation induction, ranging from mild abdominal discomfort (probably due to the distention of the ovarian capsule) to severe circulatory compromise and electrolyte imbalance (probably secondary to ascites or pleural effusions that may develop). The more severe form, ovarian hyperstimulation syndrome (OHSS), is usually associated with massive stromal edema of the ovary. The enlarged ovaries may be prone to torsion. The symptoms associated with OHSS usually begin 5 to 8 days after hCG is given and can be most severe in patients who actually achieve pregnancy. Recent studies have shown that hyperstimulation is unlikely in women whose ovaries contain several large (over 15 mm) follicles and tends to occur when there are multiple small or intermediate-sized follicles (13).

While sonographic findings of bilaterally enlarged ovaries with multiple immature follicles with the presence of intraperitoneal fluid may suggest the possibility of hyperstimulation, this syndrome can be more accurately predicted by extremely high levels of E_2 (over 3,000 pg/ml). Despite the superovulation required for IVF, hyperstimulation is only rarely encountered. This is probably a reflection of the close monitoring that these patients receive but also may be secondary to drainage and collapse of the aspirated follicles. The transabdominal sonographic (TAS) approach is recommended in the initial evaluation of these patients, since transvaginal scanning might involve exerting pressure on very enlarged and tense ovaries.

On TAS, patients with OHSS usually have bilaterally enlarged ovaries (over 10 cm) that may contain several hypoechoic

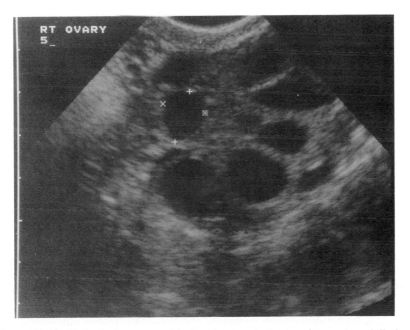

Figure 12.7. Polycystic ovary with development of several immature follicles.

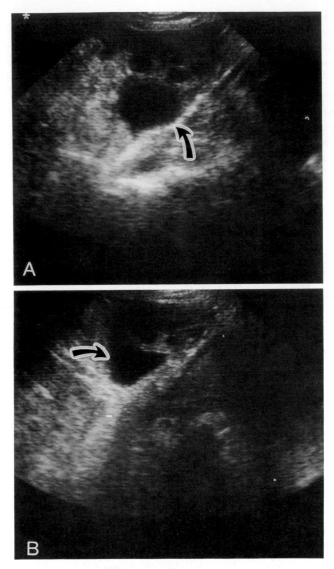

Figure 12.8.   Ovarian hyperstimulation syndrome (OHSS). **A,** TAS of enlarged right ovary with numerous immature follicles and one mature follicle (*curved arrow*). **B,** TAS of enlarged left ovary with numerous follicles surrounded by ascites (*curved arrow*). **C,** Transabdominal duplex Doppler sonogram of enlarged right ovary containing several large follicular cysts. Arterial flow is present. **D,** Same as **C** of left ovary. **E,** Gray-scale image of transabdominal color Doppler sonogram showing flow within an enlarged ovary, thereby excluding the possibility of torsion. The Doppler sample volume is placed on an artery. The accompanying waveform demonstrates typical arterial flow with significant diastolic flow.

areas (Fig. 12.8). The hypoechoic areas may correspond to atretic follicles or regions of hemorrhage within the ovary. By demonstrating the lack of arterial flow, color Doppler sonography may be useful in the detection of ovarian torsion. However, one should realize that the ovary has a dual blood supply: one arising from the adnexal branch of the uterine artery and the other coursing through the infundibulopelvic ligament. Torsion may affect one arterial blood supply more

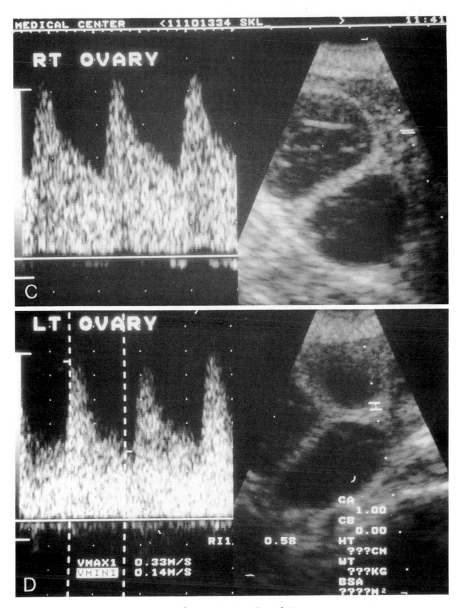

Figure 12.8. C and D.

than the other, resulting in the presence of arterial flow on color Doppler.

OHSS may be associated with very early pregnancy (less than 4 weeks), and no definitive sonographic findings may be found. Intraperitoneal fluid is usually present, a consequence of the serum osmotic imbalance. With supportive medical therapy, this syndrome usually spontaneously regresses.

After induced ovulation, the stimulated follicles usually undergo regression but may persist and enlarge over the remainder of the cycle. The presence of physiologic ovarian cysts (over 3 cm) may preclude attempts at ovulation induction during that cycle, since the previously induced follicles may not have totally regressed and the remaining ovarian tissue may not be as responsive to ovulation in-

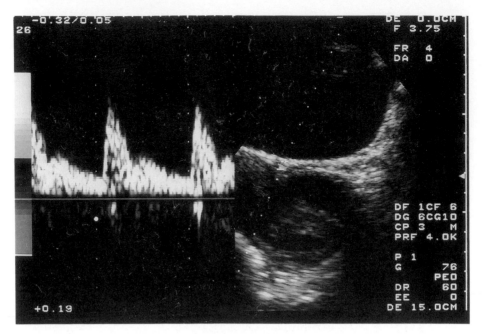

Figure 12.8.   E.

duction medication. Theoretically, the risk of torsion or rupture may also be increased in these women.

TVS can also detect other adnexal masses such as a hydrosalpinx, endometriomas, paraovarian cysts, or peritoneal cysts, which may mimic physiologic cysts or follicles that are either totally anechoic or contain low-level homogeneous echoes (Fig. 12.9). These masses can be differentiated from ovarian cysts since they are extraovarian.

Sonographic monitoring of follicular development is also helpful in decreasing the likelihood of multiple gestations that may occur with fertilization of multiple ova. However, it is difficult to predict which pregnancies will result in multiple births. Clearly, however, when there are more than four mature follicles, the chance for multiple gestation beyond twinning is more probable than if only two or three mature follicles are induced.

GUIDED PROCEDURES

Recently, needle guides have been developed that can be attached to trans-

vaginal probes and greatly facilitate guided follicular aspiration. After the probe is draped with a condom, these needle guides can be placed directly on the transducer probe, allowing for a direct and continuous visualization of the aspirating needle as it is advanced into the ovary (Fig. 12.10). The "line of sight" is generated on the monitor and closely approximates the needle path that will be traversed.

Follicular Aspiration

TVS-guided follicular aspiration is preferable for oocyte retrieval to the previously used laparoscopic techniques. The major advantages to this technique include the use of local and sedation anesthesia rather than general anesthesia, lower chance for operative complications, and quicker recovery time. TVS-guided aspiration can also be performed in an outpatient setting. The success rate, as determined by the number of fertilizable oocytes retrieved and pregnancies produced, is comparable to the laparoscopic technique (Table 12.1) (14). The

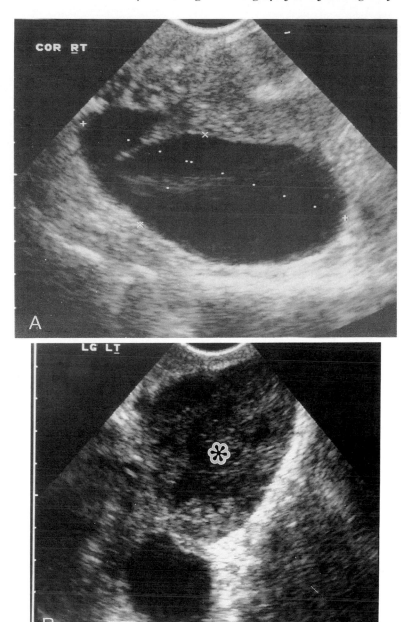

Figure 12.9. Associated adnexal lesions. **A,** Hydrosalpinx of the left tube (between *cursors*). **B,** Torsed endometrioma (*asterisk*) with adjacent simple follicular cyst.

procedure is also advantageous in patients with pelvic adhesions, since laparoscopic access to the ovary may be hampered (15). Most importantly, acceptance of the procedure by patients is high (16–18).

There are several methods for follicular aspiration that involve sonographic

guidance (Fig. 12.10) (16–21). These include transvaginal sonography for guidance of transvaginal aspiration, transabdominal sonography for guidance of transvaginal aspiration, transabdominal sonography for guidance of transvesical aspiration, and transabdominal sonographic guidance for transurethral aspi-

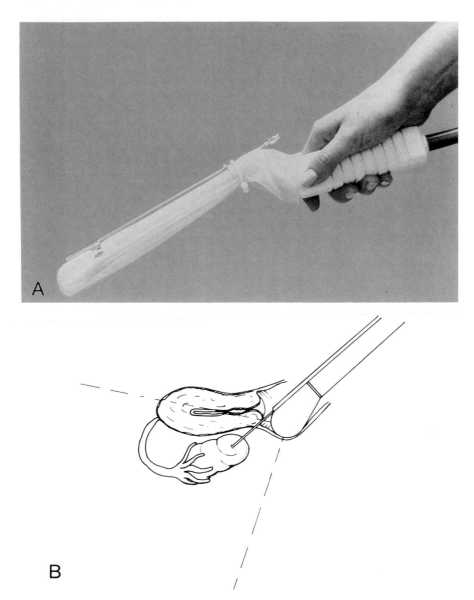

Figure 12.10.   Guided procedures. **A,** Draped probe with needle guide attached. **B,** Diagram of guided transvaginal follicle aspiration. **C,** Display of needle path on monitor. Needle will be displayed along the line of centimeter markers, depending on an entrance angle of either 15 (*short arrow*) or 30 (*long arrow*). **D,** Aspiration needle with scored tip, which enhances visualization of the tip.

ration. Although transvaginal sonography with transvaginal aspiration is most frequently utilized, the actual method that is used may be tailored to each patient, according to the anatomic position of the ovary and other structures. For example, transvaginal aspiration is the preferred route when the ovaries are in the cul-de-sac, whereas the periurethral approach may be used for aspiration of follicles in ovaries that are located near the dome of the bladder.

With all of these aspiration techniques, a long (30 cm) 16- or 18-gauge

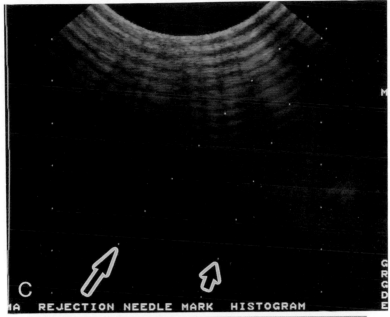

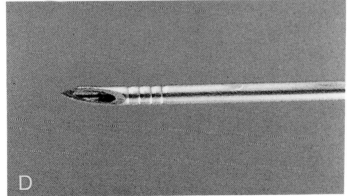

Figure 12.10. C and D.

Table 12.1. Results of Ovum Pickup by Three Methods[a]

	Laparoscopic	Transvesical	Transvaginal
Oocytes recovered per patient	6.4 ± 0.9	6.2 ± 0.3	5.7 ± 0.6
Oocytes recovered per follicle (%)	93.0	86.0	82.0
Fertilization rate (%)	73.6	72.3	70.9
Cleavage rate (%)	82.6	79.4	81.6
Number of embryos transferred	3.9 ± 0.6	3.2 ± 6.4	3.6 ± 0.3
Pregnancy rate per pickup (%)	23.7	22.3	21.6
Pregnancy rate per transfer (%)	26.6	26.7	25.9
Pregnancy rate per cycle (%)	20.2	22.6	21.1

[a]*From Feldberg D, Goldman JA, Ashkenazi J, et al.: Transvaginal oocyte retrieval controlled by vaginal probe for in vitro fertilization: A comparative study.* J Ultrasound Med 7:339, 1988.

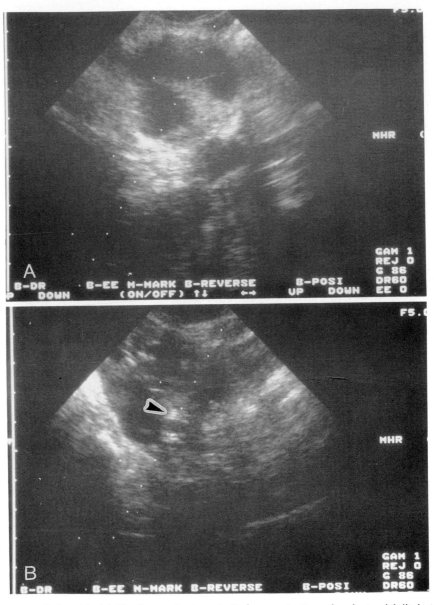

Figure 12.11. TVS-guided follicular aspiration. **A,** Before aspiration, the desired follicle is aligned with the needle path. **B,** After aspiration, the needle tip (*arrowhead*) can be seen within the deflated follicle. **C,** Needle guided into a mature follicle (*arrowhead*) adjacent to a hydrosalpinx.

needle is used that is scored at the tip, which results in enhanced sonographic visualization (Fig. 12.10D). The aspiration procedure is performed under local anesthesia and with supplemental intravenous or intramuscular medication.

For transvaginal aspiration with transvaginal transducers, a needle guide is attached to the transducer probe (Fig. 12.10). This allows the needle to traverse in the beam path of the transducer (Fig. 12.10). The cursor is displayed on the scanner screen, which indicates the path of the needle. After a condom containing sterile gel is placed over the transducer and the sterile needle guide is attached,

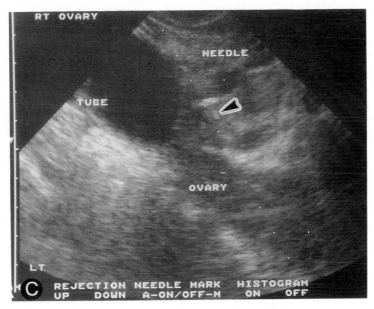

Figure 12.11.   C.

the operator manipulates the transducer to optimally delineate the ovary (Fig. 12.11). The desired follicle is brought into the line of sight and the needle is introduced into the needle guide. While some investigators flush the follicle with buffered media after the initial aspiration, our experience is that in most cases this is not required and only prolongs the procedure.

This aspiration technique has been associated with a low complication rate. One complication that has been described is accidental introduction of the needle into a vessel (usually the internal iliac vein) in the pelvis (14). This problem can be avoided if the operator carefully examines any round structure in both the long and the short axis to differentiate a vascular structure from a follicle.

The use of gonadotropin-releasing hormone (GnRH) analogs (e.g., Lupron) may be associated with the development of follicular cysts. It is thought that the presence of the cysts may impair folliculogenesis due to the elaboration of hormones or have a direct effect on reducing perfusion by parenchymal compression by the cyst itself. In these cases, TVS-guided aspiration affords direct visualization and monitoring of guidance for aspiration of these physiologic cysts (Fig. 12.12).

Guided Tubal Cannulation

TVS is now being utilized for transcervical cannulization of the uterine and tubal lumen (22). A technique for sonographic guidance of the placement of a catheter into the fallopian tubes for the gamete intrafallopian transfer (GIFT) procedure has been described (Fig. 12.13) (22) and has several advantages over hysteroscopically guided tubal cannulation. For this procedure, a catheter is placed transcervically and manipulated into the area of the uterine cornu. A coaxial technique is used and a smaller catheter containing the gametes or embryos is slowly introduced, under sonographic guidance, through the tubal ostia and into the proximal fallopian tube. Once the catheter is in the distal isthmic portion of the fallopian tube, the gametes or em-

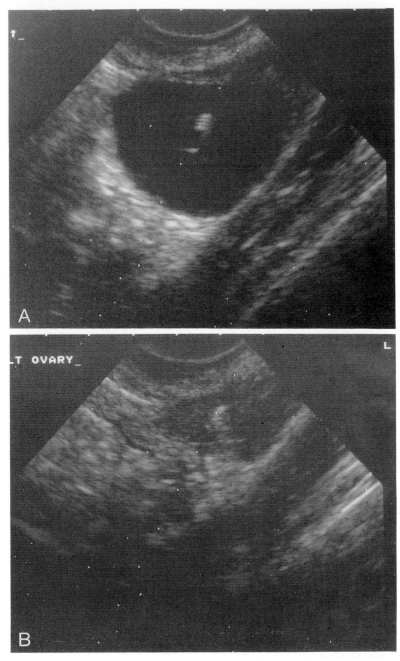

Figure 12.12.   TVS-guided cyst aspiration associated with Lupron cycle. **A,** Needle tip within cyst. **B,** After aspiration with complete collapse of the cyst.

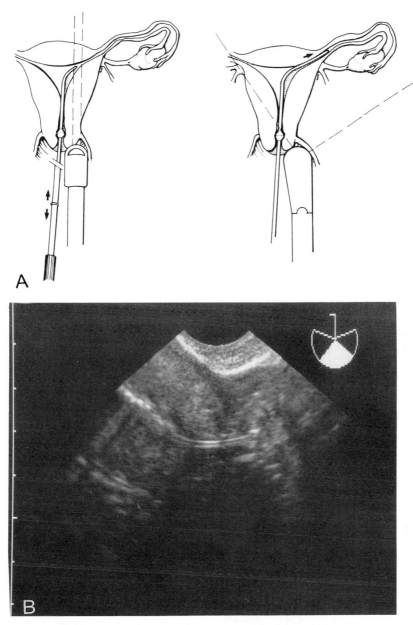

Figure 12.13.   TVS-guided tubal cannulation. **A,** Diagram of TVS guidance. **B,** Cannula through the ostia. **C,** Inner catheter advanced into the isthmic portion of the tube.

bryos may be introduced through the cannula directly into the tube.

ENDOMETRIAL ASSESSMENT

Besides the factors involved in obtaining a fertilized ovum, the develop-

mental state of the endometrium may also be a factor that influences the probability that conception will occur (23). Since the endometrium can also be delineated during examinations performed for follicular monitoring, several investigators have evaluated this specialized mucous mem-

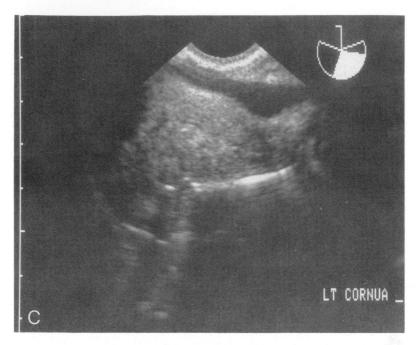

Figure 12.13.   C.

brane in an attempt to study whether there is an optimal thickness or texture (24–27). Clearly, there is an association of the sonographic texture of the endometrium and the circulating levels of estrogen and progesterone (23).

In spontaneous and induced cycles, the sonographic appearance of the endometrium varies according to its specific phases of development. In the menstrual phase, the endometrium appears as a thin, broken echogenic interface. In the proliferative phase, it thickens and becomes isoechoic, measuring 3 to 5 mm in anteroposterior width. Its relative hypoechogenicity is related to the relatively orderly organization of the glandular elements within the endometrium. As ovulation approaches, the endometrium becomes more echogenic—probably related to development of secretions within the endometrial glands and the numerous interfaces that arise from distended and tortuous glands. In the periovulatory period, there is usually a hypoechoic area within the inner endometrium that most likely represents edema of the compactum layer. This finding has been described as a means of confirming that ovulation has occurred. However, with TVS we have observed this finding both prior to and immediately following ovulation. During the secretory phase, the endometrium achieves its greatest thickness (between 6 and 12 mm) and echogenicity. In addition to the echogenic endometrium, a hypoechoic band beneath the endometrium can be identified—probably arising from the inner layer of the myometrium.

The fact that medications being used for ovulation induction may alter the development of the endometrium has been shown by both sonographic and histologic studies (27). However, the relative importance of these changes relative to success or failure of achieving pregnancy is only speculative. One study, which evaluated the endometrial thickness (including both layers) in the secretory phase, has shown that conception was unlikely in endometria that mea-

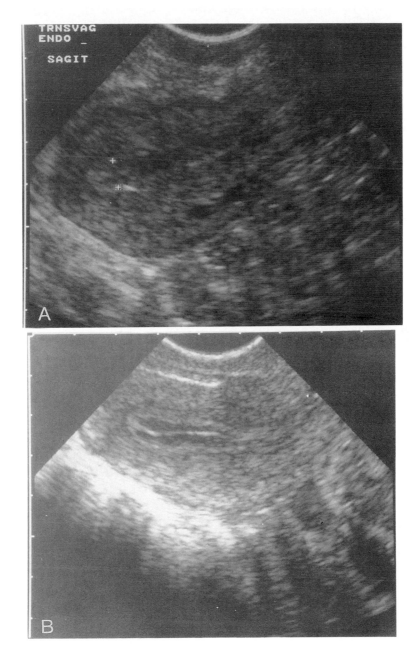

Figure 12.14. Endometrial development; uterus shown in sagittal plane, long axis. **A,** Proliferative phase; endometrium isoechoic to myometrium (between *cursors*). **B,** Late proliferative, postovulatory phase showing multiple layers. **C,** Semi-coronal TVS showing secretory-phase endometrium depicted as uniformly echogenic and thick (between *arrowheads*). **D,** Gray-scale photograph of a transvaginal color Doppler sonogram showing superficial arterial flow within arcuate arteries.

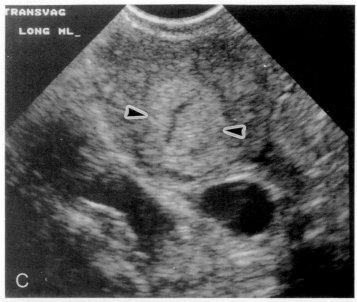

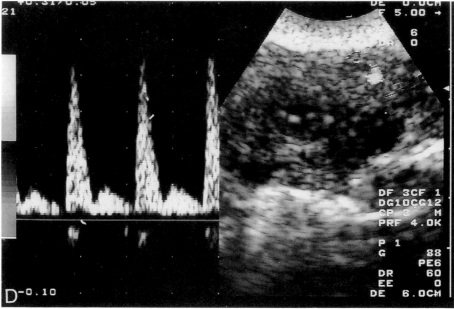

Figure 12.14.   C and D.

sured less than 13 mm 11 days postovulation (25). Other studies have indicated that the texture of the endometrium may be related to the success or failure of pregnancy, but no statistical predictive value could be obtained from these various patterns (23, 26). Other studies involved in sonographic evaluation of endometrium during ovulation induction have failed to demonstrate any specific changes in its thickness associated with success or failure to achieve pregnancy (23, 26). Our studies that utilized TVS have indicated that there is a statistically significant difference in the pregnancy rate when the endometrium has a multi-

Table 12.2. Conception versus Nonconception IVF Groups

	Endometrial Width (mm) (mean ± SD)	4 d (mm)	% Multilayered	No. of Mature Follicles > 1.5 cm	E₂ (pg/ml)	No. of Retrieved Ova	No. of Embryos Transferred
Nonconception	9.5 ± 1.0	3.1	27	3.1	1157	3.3	2.3
Conception	9.8 ± 0.9	1.6	74	3.1	1137	4.1	2.1
P value	NS[a]	0.05	0.0001	NS[a]	NS[a]	0.05	NS[a]

[a]NS, not significant.

layered appearance (Fig. 12.14). In two groups of 20 patients that underwent similar but not identical stimulations, 27% of the nonconception group showed a multilayered endometrium versus 79% of the group that conceived. This was statistically different even though the number of mature follicles, E₂ values, and number of transferred embryos were not (Table 12.2, Fig. 12.14) (28).

TVS may have a role in the further evaluation of patients who have luteal phase inadequacy. It is conceivable that these patients would have underdeveloped endometria that could be characterized sonographically as thinner and less echogenic than expected. Further study is needed to define the role of TVS of the endometrium in this disorder.

OTHER APPLICATIONS

TVS has a secondary role to hysterosalpingography in the evaluation of certain uterine malformations and tubal disorders. Malformed uteri can be characterized sonographically by delineation of the echogenic secretory-phase endometrium within the uterine lumen. Hematometra may result from cervical or lower uterine malformations. A bicornuate uterus may be difficult to distinguish from a septate uterus in the nongravid state (Fig. 12.15A). However, uterine septa are readily apparent as a thick intraluminal interface in a gravid uterus, sometimes separating the fetus and placenta.

The precise location of an intrauter-

ine contraceptive device (IUD) relative to the uterine lumen can also be determined sonographically, particularly with the use of transvaginal sonography (Fig. 12.15B). The location of the IUD relative to a gestational sac may figure in decisions of whether or not to attempt removal of the IUD. If an IUD is inferior to the sac, attempts at removal may be feasible.

Transvaginal sonography can be used to delineate enlarged and dilated fallopian tubes and establish their relationship to the ovary (Fig. 12.9A). The non-distended fallopian tube can only occasionally be recognized. On transvaginal sonography, the area of the proximal tube can be identified by the endometrium that projects into the area of the uterine cornu. An injectable contrast medium has recently been developed that clearly demonstrates tubal patency, especially when monitored with color Doppler sonography.

Sonography also has an important role in evaluating women with infertility who eventually become pregnant. These women have a higher incidence of ectopic pregnancy, anembryonic pregnancy, and spontaneous abortion. Clinical suspicion of these conditions is clearly an indication for TVS evaluation.

FUTURE APPLICATIONS

The transducer used for TVS can be made capable of simultaneous imaging and pulsed Doppler assessment of uterine and adnexal vasculature. Specifically,

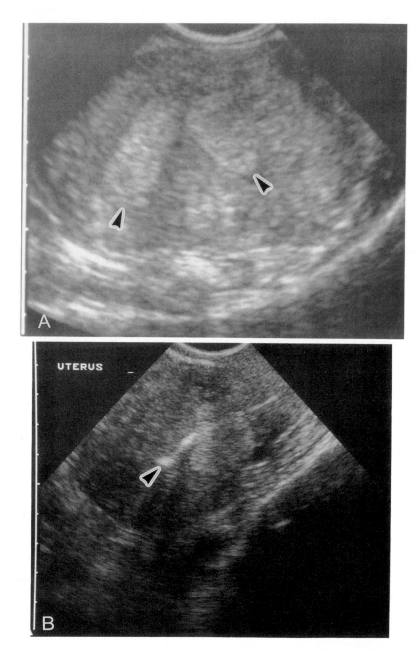

Figure 12.15.   Miscellaneous applications. **A,** Bicornuate uterus with two endometria (*arrow-heads*). **B,** Cu-7 IUD in good position. **C,** Cu-7 (*arrowhead*) posteroinferior to the gestational sac.

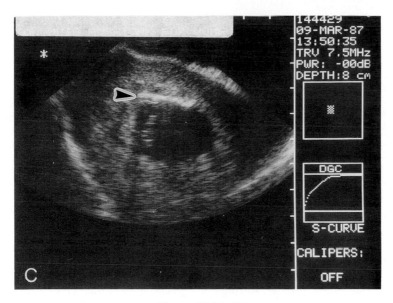

Figure 12.15. C.

the ascending branch of the uterine artery can be assessed with pulsed Doppler. The information obtained can reveal uterine and adnexal perfusion and is extremely important in excluding the possibility of adnexal torsion (Fig. 12.8E) (29). As in other parenchymal organs, the waveform and resistance can be related to physiologic activity. For example, corpus luteum function is characterized by diastolic flow as opposed to the sharp systolic peaks and no diastolic flow characteristic of ovaries in the quiescent state (Fig. 12.3C). The adequacy of corpus luteum development, for example, may be assessed using this method. Similarly, pulsed Doppler capabilities within the vaginal probe may allow assessment of uterine perfusion, which may be related to the relative chance of conception (Fig. 12.14D).

Fingertip probes may allow enhanced visualization of the uterus and ovary over that afforded by conventional TVS imaging.

SUMMARY

TVS affords accurate follicular monitoring and guidance for follicular aspira-

tion. It can also assess endometrial development and provide a means for physiologic assessment of adnexal and uterine blood flow. TVS is an important adjunct in the evaluation and management of the gynecologic patient.

REFERENCES

1. Winfield AC, Fleischer AC, Moore DE: Diagnostic imaging of infertility disorders. *Curr Probl Diagn Radiol* 19:1, 1990.
2. Fleischer AC, Pittaway DE, Wentz AC, et al.: The uses of sonography for monitoring ovarian follicular development, in Sanders RC, Hill M (eds): *Ultrasound Annual.* New York, Raven Press, 1983, pp 163–205.
3. Ritchie WGM: Sonographic evaluation of normal and induced ovulation. *Radiology* 161:1, 1986.
4. Tarlatizis BC, Laufer N, DeCherney AH: The use of ovarian ultrasonography in monitoring ovulation induction. *J In Vitro Fertil Embryo Transfer* 1:226, 1984.
5. McArdle CR, Seibel M, Weinstein F, et al.: Induction of ovulation monitored by ultrasound. *Radiology* 148:809, 1983.
6. Geisthovel F, Skubsch U, Zabel G, et al.: Ultrasonographic and hormonal studies in physiologic and insufficient menstrual cycles. *Fertil Steril* 39:277, 1983.

7. Hann LE, Hall DA, McArdle CR, et al.: Polycystic ovarian disease: Sonographic spectrum. *Radiology* 150:531, 1984.

8. Liukkonen S, Koskimies AI, Tenhunen A, et al.: Diagnosis of luteinized unruptured follicle (LUF) syndrome by ultrasound. *Fertil Steril* 41:26, 1984 (Abstract).

9. Hilgers TW, Dvorak AD, Tamisiea DF, et al.: Sonographic definition of the empty follicle syndrome. *J Ultrasound Med* 8:411, 1989.

10. Fleischer AC, Daniell JF, Rodier J, et al.: Sonographic monitoring of ovarian follicular development. *JCU* 9:275, 1981.

11. Marrs RP, Vargyas JM, March CM: Correlation of ultrasonic and endocrinologic measurements in human menopausal gonadotropin therapy. *Am J Obstet Gynecol* 145:417, 1983.

12. Mendelson EB, Friedman H, Neiman HL, et al.: The role of imaging in infertility management. *AJR* 144:415, 1985.

13. Blankstein J, Shalev J, Saadon T, et al.: Ovarian hyper-stimulation syndrome: Prediction by number and size of preovulatory ovarian follicles. *Fertil Steril* 47:597, 1987.

14. Feldberg D, Goldman JA, Ashkenazi J, et al.: Transvaginal oocyte retrieval controlled by vaginal probe for in vitro fertilization: A comparative study. *J Ultrasound Med* 7:339, 1988.

15. Taylor PJ, Wiseman D, Mahadevan M, et al.: "Ultrasound rescue": A successful alternative form of oocyte recovery in patients with periovarian adhesions. *Am J Obstet Gynecol* 154:240, 1986.

16. Schulman JD, Dorfmann AD, Jones SL, et al.: Outpatient in vitro fertilization using transvaginal ultrasound-guided oocyte retrieval. *Obstet Gynecol* 69:665, 1987.

17. Feichtinger W, Kemeter P: Ultrasound-guided aspiration of human ovarian follicles for in vitro fertilization, in Sanders RC, Hill M (eds): *Ultrasound Annual.* New York, Raven Press, 1986, pp 25–39.

18. Hammarberg K, Enk L, Nilsson L, et al.: Oocyte retrieval under the guidance of a vaginal transducer: Evaluation of patient acceptance. *Hum Reprod* 2:487, 1987.

19. Dellenbach P, Nisand I, Moreau L, et al.: Transvaginal sonographically controlled follicle puncture for oocyte retrieval. *Fertil Steril* 44:656, 1985.

20. Parsons J, Booker M, Goswamy R, et al.: Oocyte retrieval for in-vitro fertilisation by ultrasonically guided needle aspiration via the urethra. *Lancet* 1:1076, 1985.

21. Marrs RP: Does the method of oocyte collection have a major influence on in vitro fertilization? *Fertil Steril* 46:193, 1986.

22. Jansen RPS, Anderson JC: Catheterisation of the fallopian tubes from the vagina. *Lancet* 2:309, 1987.

23. Rabinowitz R, Laufer N, Lewin A, et al.: The value of ultrasonographic endometrial measurement in the prediction of pregnancy following in vitro fertilization. *Fertil Steril* 45:824, 1986.

24. Fleischer AC, Herbert CM, Sacks GA, et al.: Sonography of the endometrium during conception and nonconception cycles of in vitro fertilization and embryo transfer. *Fertil Steril* 46:442, 1986.

25. Thickman D, Arger P, Tureck R, et al.: Sonographic assessment of the endometrium in patients undergoing in vitro fertilization. *J Ultrasound Med* 5:197, 1986.

26. Glissant A, de Mouzon J, Frydman R: Ultrasound study of the endometrium during in vitro fertilization cycles. *Fertil Steril* 44:786, 1985.

27. Fleischer AC, Pittaway DE, Beard LA, et al.: Sonographic depiction of endometrial changes occurring with ovulation induction. *J Ultrasound Med* 3:341, 1984.

28. Fleischer A, Herbert C, Kepple D. Difference in endometrial texture in conception vs. non-conception IVF-ET: depiction with transvaginal sonography, in Henner H (ed): *Ultrascholl-Diagnostic 88.* Berlin, Springer-Verlag, 1989, p 124.

29. Fleischer A, Kepple D, Rao BK. Transvaginal color Doppler sonography: preliminary experience. *Dyn Card Imaging* 3:52, 1990.

13

Transvaginal Sonography in Normal and Abnormal Early Pregnancy

Arthur C. Fleischer
Donna M. Kepple

NORMAL EARLY INTRAUTERINE PREGNANCY

Transvaginal sonography (TVS) affords detailed delineation of the anatomic changes that occur in the first trimester of pregnancy. In general, definitive sonographic findings such as the presence or absence of a gestational sac and the presence or absence of an embryo or fetus with or without heart motion can be established 1 week before these could be confirmed by conventional transabdominal sonographic (TAS) techniques (1, 2). Certain anatomic "milestones" can predictably be seen with TVS (Table 13.1).

The use of TVS is particularly pertinent in women with a history of infertility, since these patients have a higher incidence of nonviable or ectopic pregnancies. Fetal malformation may also be encountered, and TVS offers an opportunity for earlier detection than is possible with conventional TAS.

TVS "Milestones" of Normal Early Intrauterine Pregnancy

One of the earliest sonographic findings in intrauterine pregnancy is thickening of the decidua, which occurs at approximately 3 to 4 weeks (Fig. 13.1). After 4 weeks, a small (3 to 5 mm) hypoechoic area surrounded by an echogenic rim can be seen within the choriodecidual tissue representing the chorionic sac (Fig. 13.2). The sac usually then en- larges from 3 to 10 mm in average dimension. At approximately 5 to 6 weeks, a yolk sac-embryo complex can be seen within the chorionic sac (Fig. 13.3). The embryo can be identified as an echogenic focus immediately adjacent to a pole of the yolk sac (Fig. 13.4). When the embryo measures 5 mm or more, heart motion can consistently be identified, but only if scanners with a high frame rate (over 30 frames per second) are utilized (Fig. 13.5). Measurement of the crown-rump length of the embryo provides an accurate determination of gestational age (3).

The chorionic sac can be seen in most intrauterine pregnancies when the β-human chorionic gonadotropin (β-hCG) is above 500 mIU/ml (2nd International Standard) (4) (Table 13.2). This has particular importance when examining a patient in whom there is a clinical suspicion of ectopic pregnancy (5).

Punctate hypoechoic areas representing blood pools or vascular lacunae can be seen surrounding the developing chorion. When these are large (approximating the size of the gestational sac) and hypoechoic, they are termed retrochorionic hemorrhage. As documented in one study, these hemorrhages are usually associated with a good prognosis for completion of pregnancy (6). If they are over one-fourth of the volume of the gestational sac size, they may be associated with spontaneous abortion. Follow-up sonography is recommended in these patients. The embryo is seen consistently when it measures over 5 mm, which corresponds to approximately 5 to 6 weeks gestational age. Heart contractions begin at this time and usually can be estimated to be about 80 to 90 beats per minute (7). This rate occurs when the heart is forming; there is a slow increase in heart rate up to approximately 10 weeks, when the heart rate is usually between 140 and 180 beats per minute (8). Abnormally slow heart rates (less than 80 beats/min) seen in embryos between 6 and 9 weeks have been associated with spontaneous abortion (9). However, a pregnancy should not be terminated based on this finding,

Table 13.1.   TVS "Landmarks"

4 weeks	Choriodecidual thickening; chorionic sac
5 weeks	Chorionic sac (5–15 mm); yolk sac
6 weeks	Yolk sac/embryo; detectable heart motion
7 weeks	Embryo/fetal movement; prominent rhombencephalon
8 weeks	Physiologic bowel herniation; arms, legs

and another scan in 3 to 5 days is recommended to assess whether or not the embryonic heart rate has normalized.

Certain anatomic features of the embryo/fetus can be seen in detail with TVS (Figs. 13.6 and 13.7). Similarly, some of the normal developmental features delineated by TVS may be mistaken for abnormal. For example, an extra yolk sac or allantoic cysts of the developing umbilical cord may be seen in early fetal development and require follow-up scans (10). The rhombencephalon appears as a hypoechoic area within the posterior aspect of the fetal head corresponding to development of the fourth ventricle and posterior fossa structures (Fig. 13.8). Physiologic herniation of the bowel at the base of the umbilical cord can be identified at 8 to 9 weeks, but should spontaneously regress by 12 weeks (Fig. 13.7).

From 8 weeks onward, several anatomic structures of the developing fetus can be delineated in detail with TVS. These include the arms/hands and legs/feet, the facial structures, the ventricular system and choroid plexus, as well as the

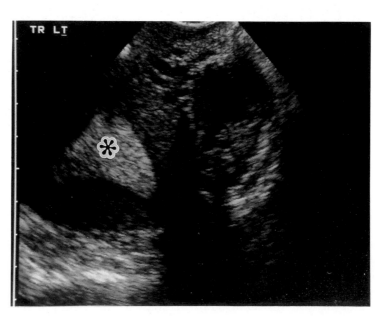

Figure 13.1.   Coronal TVS showing thickened decidua (*asterisk*) at 2$\frac{5}{7}$ weeks after a successful IVF-ER procedure.

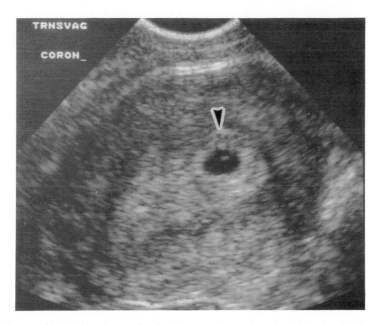

Figure 13.2. Coronal TVS showing a chorionic mass (*arrowhead*) within the thickened choriodecidua in a 5-week intrauterine pregnancy.

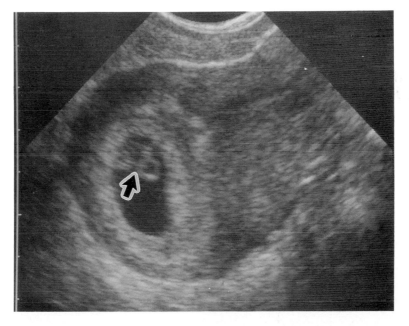

Figure 13.3. TVS of yolk sac/embryo within the gestational sac of a 6-week intrauterine pregnancy.

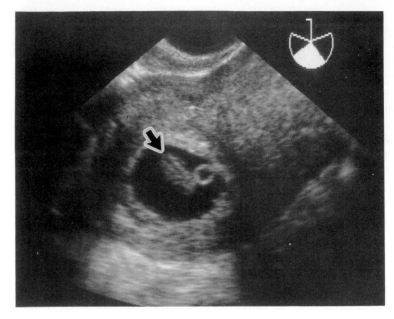

Figure 13.4.   TVS of embryo (*arrow*) and yolk sac of 7-week intrauterine pregnancy.

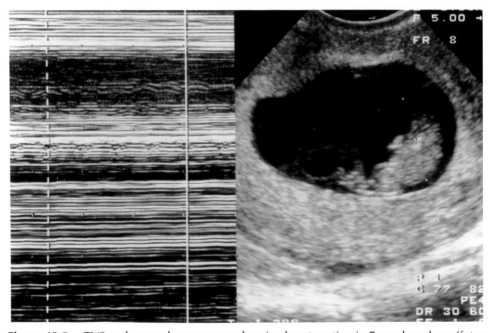

Figure 13.5.   TVS and m-mode sonogram showing heart motion in 7-week embryo/fetus.

spine (Fig. 13.7). Extrafetal structures that can be seen include the amnion, which appears as a thin membrane surrounding the fetus. It separates the amniotic cavity from the extraembryonic celom or chorionic cavity. Fetal body activity can be identified as early as 6 to 8 weeks and usually consists of flexion and extension of the fetal body and movement of the fetal extremities.

With the improved resolution of fetal structures afforded by TVS comes the ability to diagnose some fetal gross anomalies, such as anencephaly, in the first trimester. Equally, however, comes the problem of misdiagnosing as abnormal any unusual features observed during embryonic and fetal development!

Multifetal pregnancy is readily evaluated with TVS. During the first trimester one can distinguish dichorionic from monochorionic twins by examining the chorioamnion surrounding the embryos (Figs. 13.9 to 13.12). The embryonic demise of a twin can also be established with TVS (Fig 13.11).

Table 13.2. TVS "Milestones" versus β-hCGª

	β-hCG	Days	Weeks
	mIU/ml (IRPᵇ)		
Gestational sac	1,000	32	4+
Yolk sac	7,200	36–40	5–6
Embryo with heart motion	10,800	<40	6+

ªFrom Bree RL, Edwards M, Bohm-Velez M, Beyler S, Roberts J, Mendelson EB: Transvaginal sonography in the evaluation of normal early pregnancy: Correlation with HCG level. AJR 153:75, 1989.
ᵇIRP, International Reference Preparation.

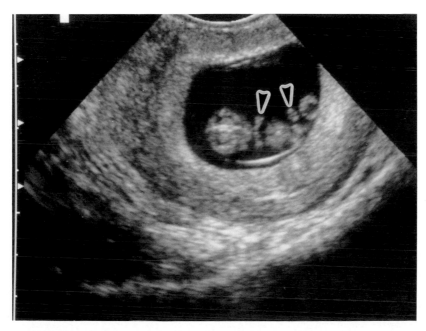

Figure 13.6. TVS showing developing limbs (*arrowheads*) of a 9-week fetus. The fetus is surrounded by the amnion, which is clearly depicted adjacent to the anterior surface of the fetus.

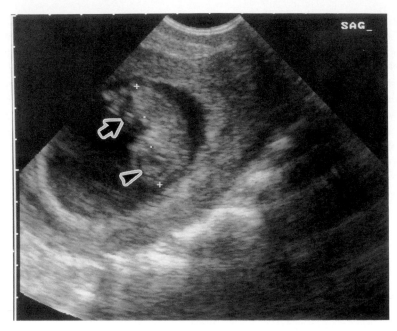

Figure 13.7.   TVS of a 9-week fetus showing developing choroid (*arrowhead*) within the lateral ventricles and physiologic herniation of bowel (*large arrow*).

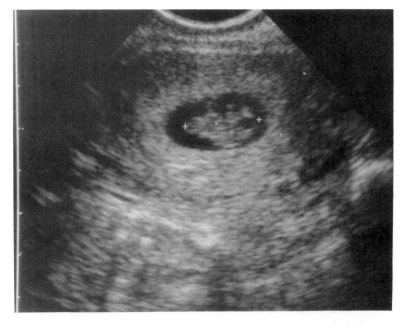

Figure 13.8.   TVS showing a cystic area in the posterior portion of the cranium representing the rhombencephalon of an 8-week embryo.

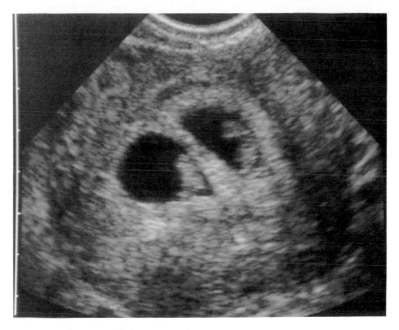

Figure 13.9.   TVS of normal dichorionic, diamniotic twin intrauterine pregnancy at 7 weeks.

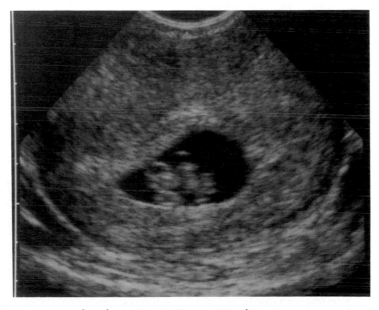

Figure 13.10.   As opposed to the patient in Figure 13.9, this twin pregnancy is monochorionic.

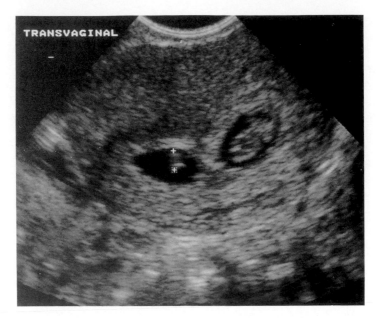

Figure 13.11. Twin intrauterine pregnancy with embryonic demise (between *cursors*).

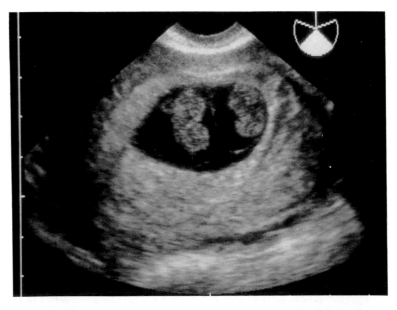

Figure 13.12. Monochorionic, diamniotic twin intrauterine pregnancy at 8 weeks with embryonic demise of both twins. The embryos were morphologically normal.

COMPLICATED EARLY PREGNANCY

Transvaginal sonography depicts detailed anatomic structures as well as revealing some functional aspects, such as heart motion, of early pregnancies. The assessment of a complicated pregnancy obtained by TVS provides important clinical information so that the patient can be optimally managed. Specifically, TVS reveals important information concerning the presence or absence of an embryo-fetus and whether there is heart motion, the intactness of the choriodecidua, and the location (intra- or extrauterine) of the pregnancy (Figs. 13.13 to 13.15).

Embryonic or Fetal Demise

In a normal pregnancy, heart motion should be demonstrated by TVS in embryos that are over 5 mm or 5 to 6 weeks gestation. The actual rate is relatively slow during early heart development (70 to 90 beats/min) but increases at approximately 8 weeks to approxi-

mately 120 beats/min (7, 8). Some authors have observed that embryos between 6 and 9 weeks with slow heart rates (less than 80 beats/min) have a tendency to abort spontaneously (9). However, the embryo with a slow heart rate should always be given the benefit of the doubt and be re-examined in 3 to 5 days for signs of conversion back to a normal heart rate.

Embryonic loss is thought to occur in approximately 20 to 30% of all developing early pregnancies (11). It is more likely in the patient with a history of abortion (habitual aborter) or of a previous fetus with chromosomal abnormality.

Early embryonic demise has a variety of appearances, ranging from a gestational sac devoid of a yolk sac or embryo to a yolk sac-embryo complex without embryonic heart motion (Fig. 13.14). Clearly, embryonic demise should be suspected when there is a lack of enlargement of the embryo on serial scans coupled with deflation of the sac or yolk sac. In some cases of embryonic demise, there is deflation of the yolk sac coupled with

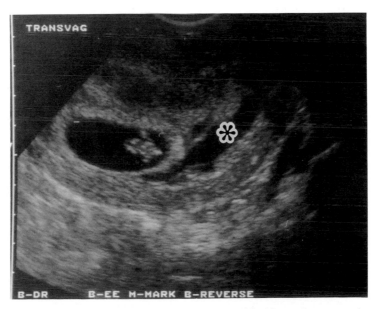

Figure 13.13. TVS of patient presenting with first-trimester bleeding. There is a relatively large area of retrochorionic hemorrhage (*asterisk*) inferior to the gestational sac.

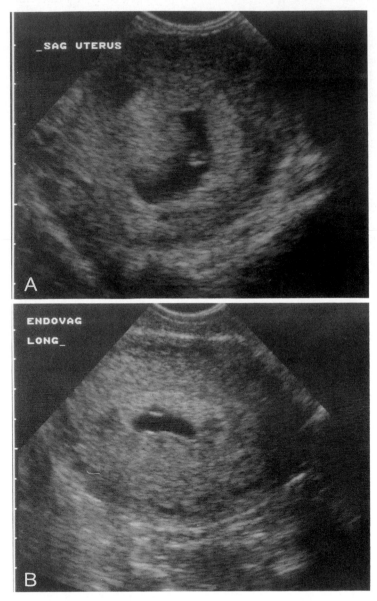

Figure 13.14.   Initial TVS (**A**) and TVS performed 5 days later (**B**) showing resorption of yolk sac/embryo secondary to embryonic demise.

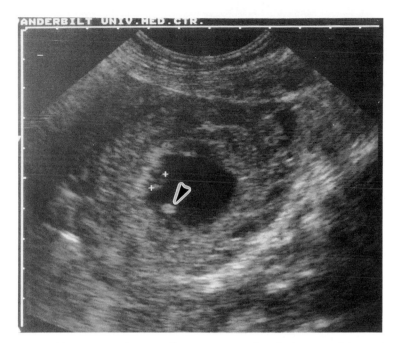

Figure 13.15. TVS showing a "white" yolk sac associated with demise of the embryo (between *cursors*).

an increase in its internal echogenicity (Fig. 13.15).

Of course, one should not terminate the pregnancy based on a single sonographic examination that demonstrates a lack of heart motion during the embryonic stage of development (3 to 5 mm crown-rump length). A follow-up scan is usually indicated to confirm the lack of embryonic or fetal viability. In general, an embryo should be seen in a sac of greater than 6 to 9 mm; embryonic heart motion should be seen when the sac is 10 to 14 mm in size (4).

Abortion

Incomplete spontaneous abortion demonstrates echogenic tissue within the uterine lumen arising from retained choriodecidua (Fig. 13.16A). Completed abortion may be diagnosed occasionally when there is no echogenic tissue (decidualized endometrium or blood) within the uterine lumen and when the cervical os is closed (Fig. 13.16B). The relative amount of remaining choriodecidua can be estimated using a prolate ellipsoid formula (volume [cc] = length [cm] × height [cm] × width [cm] × 0.5). Early trophoblastic disease demonstrates a pattern similar to retained choriodecidua, and hydropic villi are usually not present before 14 weeks (Fig. 13.17).

Ectopic Pregnancy

TVS is a very accurate means of diagnosing an ectopic pregnancy (5, 12, 13). First, an intrauterine gestational sac can be excluded earlier (1.2 weeks) with TVS than with transabdominal scanning. Second, the ability to detect the adnexal mass that represents an ectopic pregnancy itself is significantly enhanced with TVS.

Rarely, intraluminal fluid or blood surrounding the thin decidual reaction in

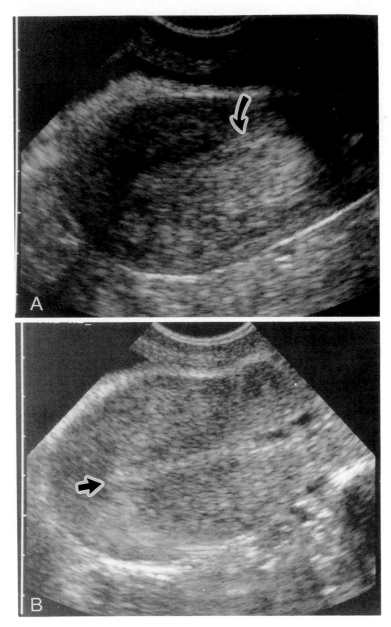

Figure 13.16. TVS findings in abortion. **A,** Incomplete abortion showing echogenic tissue (*arrow*) within the lower uterine segment. **B,** As opposed to the patient shown in **A**, this patient has a completed abortion as evidenced by the closely opposed thin endometrial interfaces (*arrow*).

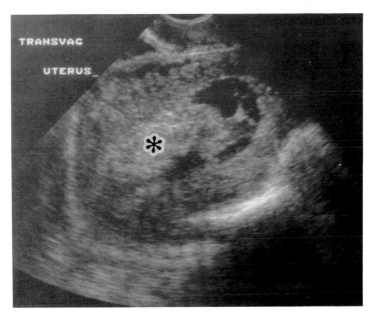

Figure 13.17.   TVS of early molar pregnancy showing echogenic tissue (*asterisk*) within the uterine lumen.

an ectopic pregnancy simulates the appearance of a malformed gestational sac. The thickened decidual reaction that surrounds intraluminal fluid or blood ("pseudosac") seen in some advanced ectopic pregnancies can be distinguished from a normal gestational sac because the choriodecidual thickening at the decidua basalis is not present (Fig. 13.18).

In the adnexa, TVS demonstrates the presence of a "tubal ring," which consists of an echogenic rim and a hypoechoic center (Fig. 13.19). This structure is typically seen in the adnexal regions adjacent to but separate from the uterus and ovary. An embryo may or may not be seen within the gestational sac, since a large number of ectopic gestations have chromosomal abnormalities with resultant embryonic demise and failure to develop a sonographically detectable embryo. One can usually distinguish the tubal ring from a corpus luteum in that the corpus luteum is eccentrically located within the displaced rim of ovarian tissue. In some

cases of a centrally located corpus luteum, the TVS appearance of a tubal ring can be mimicked. Some corpora lutea appear as hypoechoic masses with broken linear interfaces within probably arising synechiae. Most hematoma that are associated with ectopic pregnancy appear as solid, rounded masses that displace the uterus and bowel out of the cul-de-sac. In unruptured tubal ectopic pregnancies, the tubal ring is distinct. The walls of distended tube may be identified as linear structures that surround the tubal mass.

If rupture has occurred, the fallopian tube is enlarged and fusiform and contains irregularly echogenic material. Intraperitoneal blood may be the result of blood oozing out the fimbriated end of the tube due to detachment of the chorionic reaction from the tubal wall (Fig. 13.19). It may also result from attempts at tubal abortion, where the gestational sac is passed out through the fimbriated end of the tube. Usually, the intraperitoneal fluid associated with a ruptured ectopic

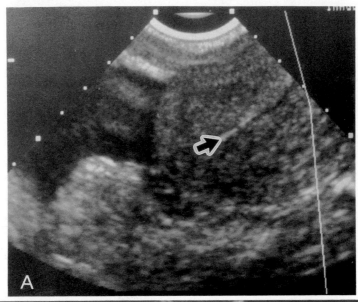

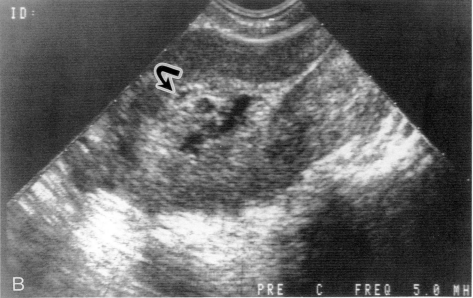

Figure 13.18.   TVS of ectopic pregnancy—uterine findings. **A,** Minimal decidual thickening (*arrow*). **B,** Necrotic decidua (*curved arrow*). **C,** Pseudosac (between *cursors*).

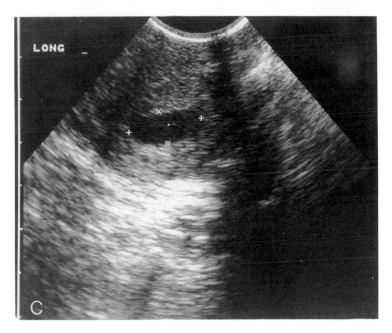

Figure 13.18. C.

pregnancy has echoes within it, reflecting a predominance of clotted blood rather than serous fluid. The low-level echoes arising from blood elements suspended within intraperitoneal fluid can be seen to move in a swirling pattern when the bowel peristalses around them.

Unusual types of ectopic pregnancy can be recognized with TVS (Fig. 13.20). These include cornual, cervical, and ovarian ectopic pregnancies. Cornual ectopic pregnancies form eccentric to the endometrial lumen and extend within 3 to 5 mm of the uterine serosa. Hypoechoic blood lacunae may be seen surrounding the gestation. Cervical ectopic pregnancies form proximal to the endometrial tissue and distend the cervix. They can be distinguished from cervical inclusion cysts in that a relatively thick choriodecidual layer surrounds the hypoechoic lumen. This appearance is similar to choriodecidua in the process of being aborted except that cervical ectopic pregnancies are usually better defined and remote from the endometrial lumen. Ovarian ectopic pregnancies are

extremely rare. The examples that have been seen appear as hypoechoic areas within the ovary with a solid component if an embryo is present.

TVS can be used as a dynamic means to guide needles into the ectopic gestation for injecting methotrexate or potassium chloride (14). Recently the treatment of ectopic pregnancies with systemic or locally administered methotrexate has been investigated. Although the ectopic pregnancy itself can be treated with this regimen, the effects on the treated tube are unknown. In fact, animal work suggests an adverse effect on the tubal epithelium of locally injected methotrexate (15). Further clinical trials are needed to assess the efficacy of this treatment of ectopic gestations before it can be incorporated into routine clinical use.

SUMMARY

In summary, the role of TVS in early pregnancy is to confirm the presence of an intrauterine pregnancy or contrarily

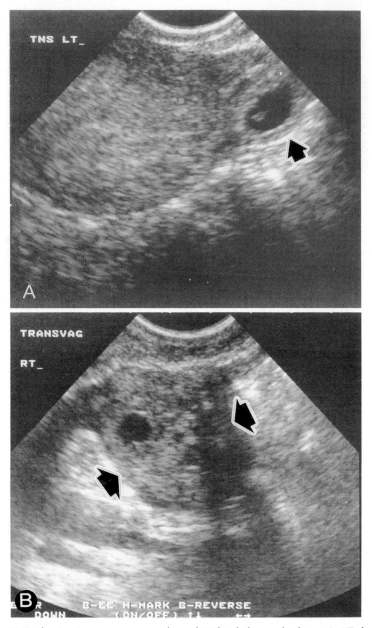

Figure 13.19.   TVS of ectopic pregnancy—adnexal and cul-de-sac findings. **A,** "Tubal ring" (*arrow*) representing an unruptured ectopic pregnancy. **B,** Ruptured ectopic pregnancy associated with hematosalpinx and hemoperitoneum. **C,** Corpus luteum containing a thin septation adjacent to an unruptured ectopic pregnancy (*arrowhead*). **D,** Living 7-week embryo within the tubal sac.

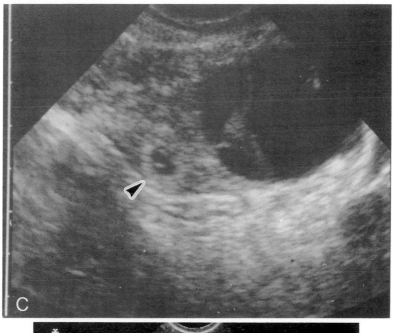

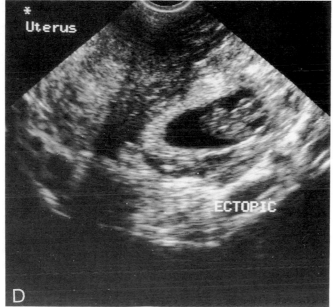

Figure 13.19.   C and D.

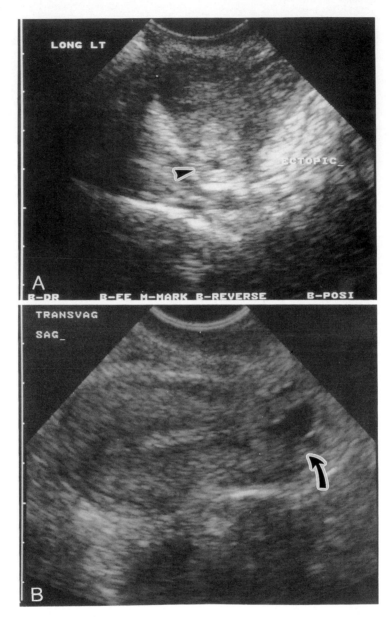

Figure 13.20.   TVS of unusual ectopic pregnancies. **A,** Cornual ectopic pregnancy (*arrowhead*) appearing as an eccentrically located sac. **B,** Cervical ectopic pregnancy (*arrow*) with an intact gestational sac distending the cervix. **C,** Ovarian ectopic pregnancy with a dead embryo (between *cursors*). (Courtesy of Larry Needleman, M.D., Philadelphia, PA.)

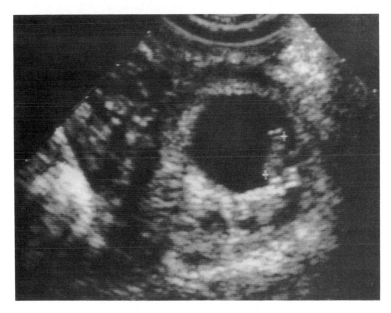

Figure 13.20. C.

provide definitive diagnosis of an ectopic pregnancy by demonstration of an adnexal mass and no intrauterine gestational sac (5). TVS should be carefully applied, and misdiagnosis due to lack of experience with unusual developmental anatomy should be avoided by adopting a conservative approach. TVS has an important role in the evaluation of a complicated early pregnancy. Specifically, incomplete abortion, embryonic demise, and ectopic pregnancy are readily diagnosed with this method.

REFERENCES

1. Pennell RG, Baltarowich OH, Kurtz AB, et al.: Complicated first-trimester pregnancies: evaluation with endovaginal US versus transabdominal technique. *Radiology* 165:79, 1987.
2. Jain KA, Hamper UM, Sanders RC: Comparison of transvaginal and transabdominal sonography in the detection of early pregnancy and its complications. *AJR* 151:1139, 1988.
3. Degenhardt F, Böhmer S, Behrens O, Müjlaus K: Transvaginale Ultraschallbiometrie der Scheitel-Steiss-Länge im ersten Trimenon. *Z Geburtshilfe Perinatol* 192:249, 1988.
4. Bree RL, Edwards M, Bohm-Velez M, Beyler S, Roberts J, Mendelson EB: Transvaginal sonography in the evaluation of normal early pregnancy: Correlation with HCG level. *AJR* 153:75, 1989.
5. Fleischer AC, Pennell RG, McKee MS, et al.: Sonographic features of ectopic pregnancies as depicted by transvaginal scanning. *Radiology* 174:375, 1990.
6. Stabile I, Campbell S, Grudzinskas JG: Threatened miscarriage and intrauterine hematomas: Sonographic and biochemical studies. *J Ultrasound Med* 8:289, 1989.
7. DuBose TJ, Dickey D, Butschek CM, Porter L, Hill LW, Poole EK: The opinion that the fetal heart rate (FHR) is an indicator of the baby's sex (letter). *J Ultrasound Med* 7:237, 1988.
8. Hertzberg BS, Mahony BS, Bowie JD: First trimester fetal cardiac activity: sonographic documentation of a progressive early rise in heart rate. *J Ultrasound Med* 7:573, 1988.
9. Laboda LA, Estroff JA, Benacerraf BR: First trimester bradycardia. *J Ultrasound Med* 8:561, 1989.
10. Barzilai M, Lyons EA, Levi CS, Lindsay DJ: Vitelline duct cyst or double yolk sac. *J Ultrasound Med* 8:523, 1989.
11. Biggers S: In vitro fertilization and embryo transfer in human beings. *N Engl J Med* 304:336, 1982.

12. Dashefsky SM, Lyons EA, Levi CS, Lindsay DJ. Suspected ectopic pregnancy: endovaginal and transvesical US. *Radiology* 169:181, 1988.

13. Nyberg DA, Mack LA, Jeffrey RB, Laing FC: Endovaginal sonographic evaluation of ectopic pregnancy: A prospective study. *AJR* 149:1181, 1987.

14. Fernandez H, Baton C, Frydman R: Prospective randomized study of combined intratubal-IM administration of methotrexate (MTX) or prostaglandins sulprostone (SUL) for conservative management of ectopic pregnancies (EP). Presented at American Fertility Society, October 1990.

15. Leach RE, Ory SJ: The effect of the local injection of methotrexate and potassium chloride on rat fallopian tube epithelium. Presented at American Fertility Society, October 1990.

14

Male Infertility

Fred K. Kirchner Jr.
Murray J. Mazer

When evaluating large numbers of couples for infertility, a male factor alone will be found in approximately 30% of the cases. In another 20%, abnormalities will be found in both partners. Therefore, it is vitally important to screen the male partner even if abnormalities are initially suspected in the woman.

CLINICAL EVALUATION OF THE INFERTILE MALE

A brief summary of the evaluation of the infertile male is in order so that the role of radiologic procedures can be put into perspective. Central to the evaluation is the semen analysis.

Semen Analysis

In general, the minimal parameters that are considered acceptable for potential fertility are an ejaculate volume of 1.5 to 5 ml containing a sperm density of greater than 20 million/ml. The sperm should show at least 60% motility with reasonable forward progression and a morphology of at least 60% normal forms. Additionally, there should be no significant sperm agglutination, pyospermia, or hyperviscosity. If the patient is azoospermic, the semen specimen is evaluated for the presence or absence of fructose. Fructose is produced in the seminal vesicles, and its absence in the semen implies either congenital absence of the seminal vesicles or obstruction of the ejaculatory ducts.

The semen analysis can occasionally be quite variable on different occasions in any one individual; therefore, a minimum of two semen analyses should be obtained to define the parameters of any individual patient. Also, because spermatogenesis takes approximately 72 days, any potential toxic influence, such as a fever, may result in a suboptimal semen analysis 2 to 3 months after the episode. Therefore, in a man with such a history who has a suboptimal semen analysis, the study should be repeated 2 to 3 months later.

If it is determined that the man does indeed have a suboptimal semen analysis, then a careful history and physical examination is indicated. The following is a brief overview of the evaluation of the subfertile male. For a more detailed account, the reader is referred to any standard text of infertility, such as Lipshultz and Howards' *Infertility in the Male* (1).

History

The past history should include inquiries with respect to childhood events. Unilateral cryptorchidism has an adverse effect on a man's potential fertility even if orchiopexy is performed at an early age. Postpubertal mumps may lead to mumps orchitis with devastating testicular damage. Any history of bladder neck surgery, either open or endoscopic, may be a clue to possible retrograde ejaculation.

A history of exposure to toxic substances or radiation should also be elicited, as well as a medication history. Certain medications such as sulfasalazine, cimetidine, and nitrofurantoin have all been implicated as potential spermatotoxic agents.

Men with a history of testicular cancer have been known for some time to have special problems with relation to fertility. These problems have centered around patients who have had retroperitoneal lymph node dissections with subsequent risk of decreased transport of sperm and, in some instances, retrograde ejaculation due to surgical interruption of neural pathways. Also, these patients are at risk from the toxic effects of either radiotherapy or chemotherapy.

More recently, it has become appreciated that many of these men are subfertile prior to the initiation of any therapy (2). Whether this is a bilateral phenomenon representing subnormal testicles with respect to both fertility potential and risk of tumor or simply represents a toxic effect of the tumor on the contralateral testis is not known.

Along similar lines, it has recently been shown in animal studies that testicular torsion that is not rapidly surgically corrected may have a noxious effect on the contralateral testicle. There is experimental evidence to show that early (within less than 8 hr) detorsion or orchiectomy can lessen the chance of damage to the opposite testicle (3). Whether these observations apply to the human situation is not known.

Even a slight increase in temperature can have an adverse effect on spermatogenesis, and therefore a history of the patient's work environment should be elicited. Occasionally, patients who are in the habit of taking long, hot tub baths on a daily basis can improve their semen analysis parameters by switching their bathing habits to cool showers.

Physical Examination

A general physical examination with emphasis on evaluation of the genitalia should be carried out. The general body habitus should be noted, and if eunuchoid proportions are suspected then the arm span should be measured. The arm span should not exceed the patient's height by more than 2 inches. The presence and distribution of body hair should also be noted as well as the presence or absence of gynecomastia.

With respect to the genitalia, adequate size of the penis, retractability of the prepuce, and location of the urethral meatus should be noted. The scrotal examination should be performed with the patient standing, to better assess the presence or absence of a varicocele. Testicles can be measured in a variety of ways, and their size is important with respect to fertility. Approximately 85% of the testicular volume is involved with sperm production, and any decrease in volume will probably be reflected by reduced sperm production. The testicles can be measured with either a tape or calipers, but most urologists find it handy to have a set of graded prostheses that they can hold up near the testicle for assessment of the volume. The normal testicular volume should be greater than 15 ml. Evidence of acute or chronic inflammatory disease in the epididymis is also important to evaluate. Any nodularity or tenderness may indicate problems in this area. Careful palpation of the prostate completes the examination.

Other Tests

At this point in the evaluation, further tests are done depending on the history and the findings of the physical examination. If the patient is azoospermatic, a determination of semen fructose should be carried out. As mentioned above, if fructose is present, then obstruction of the ejaculatory duct or maldevelopment of the seminal vesicles is essentially ruled out. Blood is often drawn for follicle-stimulating hormone (FSH), luteinizing hormone (LH), and testosterone determinations. Usually the latter two will be normal. If the FSH is greater than twice normal, this is indicative of end-organ (testicular) failure and the evaluation can be terminated. If, on the other hand, these values are normal, then testicular biopsy and seminal vesiculograms or ultrasound are indicated.

A large number of patients will fall into the category of "idiopathic oligospermia." These patients should have an endocrine evaluation, although in virtually all cases the findings will be normal. In recent years, the sperm penetration assay has been used to aid in prognosis (4). Occasionally, evaluation for the presence or absence of antisperm antibodies may be indicated, although their exact role in infertility has yet to be completely elucidated.

RADIOGRAPHIC PROCEDURES

As can be seen above, radiographic procedures do not play as central a role in the evaluation of male infertility as they do in female infertility. However, in selected patients, spermatic venography, ultrasound, or seminal vesiculography can be quite helpful in the diagnostic process. In the former instance, therapy (occlusion of the spermatic vein) may be instituted at the time of the diagnostic study.

Spermatic Venography

A varicocele is a scrotal venous tumefaction caused by variceal dilatation of the veins of the pampiniform plexus secondary to obstruction of venous drainage or valve incompetence and is the most common diagnosis made in male patients attending an infertility clinic. The presence of a varicocele appears to be virtually nonexistent in the prepubertal years, and the incidence increases through the teens (5, 6). An incidence of approximately 15% has been described in groups of teenaged boys. On the other hand, in the infertility setting, the number of men found to have varicoceles ranges from 21 to 41%. (7–10). If these individuals undergo ligation of their spermatic vein, the majority, but not all, will show an improved semen quality, although in most series the resulting impregnation rate is less than in those showing improvement in semen parameters (10–13).

Men who fail to improve their semen analysis after spermatic vein ligation may represent either failure of the procedure itself or a subpopulation of men whose infertility is secondary to other unknown causes but who also happen to have a varicocele.

There is recent evidence, in an experimental setting, that varicoceles may act as a cofactor in conjunction with noxious stimuli to cause male infertility. When male rats were given known gonadotoxins, the effect appeared to be accentuated in the presence of a varicocele (14).

The diagnosis of a varicocele is often straightforward. When the patient is examined in the upright position, a characteristic "bag of worms" can be felt above the testicle. Sometimes the varicocele is large enough to be seen on visual examination. The significance of the so-called subclinical varicocele has yet to be demonstrated by any prospective study. Some urologists feel that a more diligent search for a very small, impalpable varicocele should be carried out in a man with abnormal semen parameters. The diagnostic maneuvers include having the patient perform a Valsalva maneuver in the upright position while palpating the spermatic cord, Doppler stethoscope examination (15, 16), scrotal thermography (17–19), scrotal ultrasound (20), isotopic studies (21), and venography. Renal venography (on the left) or cavography (for assessment of the right gonadal vein) should not produce significant filling of the gonadal veins if the valves are competent. Retrograde flow down the go-

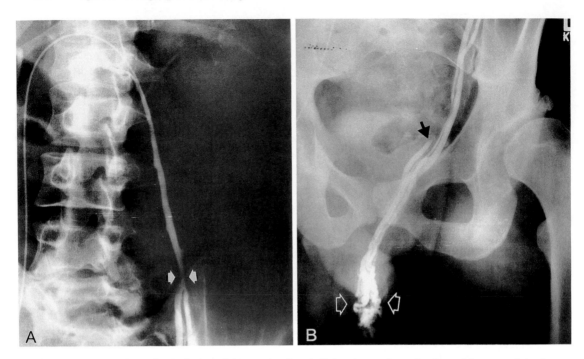

Figure 14.1.   Varicocele: Left gonadal venography. **A,** Selective catheterization of the gonadal vein with injection of contrast medium results in retrograde filling of the spermatic vein and its tributaries, reflecting absent or incompetent valves. Collateral venous pathways are exemplified by the demonstration of two large venous channels that unite at the L5 level into a single major vein (*paired arrows*). **B,** Lower segment of same venogram as in **A.** Numerous venous channels (*large arrow*) are seen draining an engorged and dilated pampiniform plexus (*open arrows*).

nadal veins is a sign of incompetent valves from congenital or acquired causes. If a varicocele is present, the gonadal vein is distended and the pampiniform plexus engorged (Fig. 14.1).

The pathophysiology of the deleterious effect of a varicocele on fertility has yet to be fully elucidated. Numerous hypotheses, including reflux of adrenal or renal metabolites, hormonal imbalance, and hypoxia secondary to venous stasis have all been proposed but not definitely proved. It has been appreciated for a long time that even a slight increase in testicular temperature will have an adverse effect on spermatogenesis. Animal studies have demonstrated that elevated testicular temperature in an experimentally induced varicocele may be secondary to elevated testicular arterial flow. Both of these abnormalities return to normal after ligation of the varicocele (22).

The finding of an incidental varicocele in the noninfertility setting poses a dilemma to both the physician and the patient. There is no way to predict prospectively whether a varicocele has adverse fertility implications. If, in addition to the varicocele, the associated testicle is smaller and softer, then prophylactic spermatic vein ligation can be recommended. It is often not feasible to ask a teenaged boy to produce a semen specimen for analysis, and so the physician is left with counseling the patient and possibly his parents with these facts and letting them help make the decision whether or not an elective spermatic varicocele ligation should be done.

As stated above, varicoceles are much more common on the left side, presumably because the left internal spermatic vein has a longer course than its counterpart on the right. Also, the left internal spermatic vein enters the left renal vein at a right angle. This is in contradistinction to the oblique entrance of the right vein into the vena cava. Increased hydrostatic pressure in the left internal spermatic vein may also result from the so-called nutcracker phenomenon. The left renal vein passes between the superior mesenteric artery and aorta, and an area of narrowing at this point with proximal venous dilatation can often be seen in patients examined with ultrasound or computerized tomography (23).

It has been stated that in 90% of varicocele patients, only a left varicocele is found at clinical examination. However, 8 to 9% of patients are found to have bilateral varicoceles, and in a few patients (1 to 2%) only a right varicocele is detected (24). Some authors have claimed that as many as 25 to 66% of patients with only a palpable left varicocele also have an incompetent right internal spermatic vein (25, 26). However, a cadaver study (27) has shown that valves in the right internal spermatic vein commonly occur at or within 0.5 cm of the orifice. The act of inserting the catheter tip into this orifice may bypass these very proximal valves, leading to a false-positive diagnosis of varicocele.

The traditional therapy for the symptomatic varicocele is high ligation of the internal spermatic vein. Recently, spermatic venography has been popularized because this procedure is not only diagnostic but can be therapeutic. Using a femoral or jugular venous catheter approach, if a varicocele is demonstrated, the internal spermatic vein can be occluded by a variety of techniques such as insertion of coils (28) (Fig. 14.2), a sclerosing agent (29–32), or a detachable balloon (33). Vital to the complete success of this procedure is a meticulous evaluation of collateral veins that often parallel the main spermatic vein above or below the iliac crest to re-enter the upper spermatic vein or the renal vein separately or drain

into the retroperitoneum, renal capsular veins, iliac veins, or the contralateral scrotal spermatic system. By placing the embolizing agent as peripheral as possible in the spermatic vein close to the inguinal ligament, and occasionally, when necessary, more central in the spermatic vein close to the renal vein, the chance of varicocele recurrence is diminished (34). The use of the detachable balloon technique is felt to be particularly successful in thoroughly evaluating the smallest of collateral veins that could become clinical problems if not recognized. The balloon can be inflated as far down the course of the spermatic vein as possible without being detached, while the more proximal introducer catheter is used to inject contrast material without inducing spasm. Contrast material is thus diverted into the most subtle collateral pathways at their upper ends while the balloon is occluding the main spermatic vein channel in the lowermost position. After this more thorough evaluation of all potential collaterals, the balloon is detached in an optimal position along the course of the spermatic vein.

Whether the technique described above will supplant traditional surgical ligation of the internal spermatic vein remains to be seen. Both procedures can be performed on an outpatient basis. Usually the surgical procedure is done under light general anesthesia but can be done with local anesthesia, while the radiologic procedure is generally done under local anesthesia with or without sedation. Success rates with regard to achievement of pregnancy appear to be comparable for both procedures. The cost of the surgical procedure is, in general, slightly higher and the patient will miss a few days of work, whereas after the radiologic procedure he should be able to return to full activity the next day. Except in the most experienced hands, the time of the radiologic procedure is longer. Surgery also obviates the need for radiation ex-

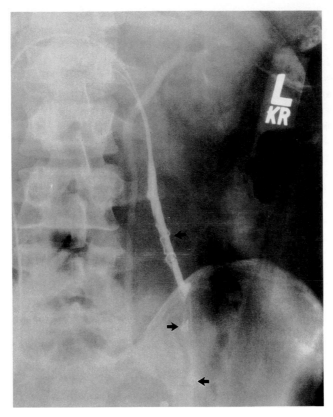

Figure 14.2.   Same patient as in Figure 14.1. Several Gianturco coils (*arrows*) are now seen in the gonadal vein.

posure to the patient. Finally, there is a small but definite risk of wire or balloon embolization with the percutaneous approach.

Recurrence rates for the two procedures appear to be comparable. In a large series from Johns Hopkins Hospital, a 6-year evaluation of outpatient balloon embolotherapy in 300 varicoceles (left-sided in 78%, right-sided in 4%, bilateral in 18%) was conducted (35). Of these, 86% were performed for infertility and 14% performed for scrotal discomfort. Long-term follow-up demonstrated a decrease in varicocele recurrence rate from 11% in the first 70 patients to 4% in the last 230 patients, thus emphasizing that experience with this procedure and careful evaluation of potential collaterals is necessary to achieve optimal results.

Approximately 5% of men treated with spermatic vein ligation will have recurrent varicocele (36), and it is perhaps in this clinical situation that venography assumes a more important role. Other patients who might be candidates for venography are those whose semen analysis fails to improve after spermatic vein ligation. The pattern of collaterals seen on venography after an obliterative procedure may vary depending on the method used to occlude the vein (surgery or percutaneous venous occlusion) (37).

Two particular and unusual anatomic variations are worth mentioning separately. Three percent of men have transscrotal collaterals (25). Two confirmed cases of disappearance of the left varicocele after right internal spermatic vein embolizations in the Johns Hopkins series emphasize the importance of this pathway (38).

There is also a proposed theoretical mechanism for varicocele formation in which an obstruction of the left common iliac vein (probably due to pressure by the right common iliac artery as it crosses the vein) would produce collateral flow via the ductus deferens vein, a branch of the internal iliac vein, through the varicocele and up the internal spermatic vein to the renal vein (39). In this situation, occlusion of the internal spermatic vein might actually result in worsening of the varicocele. Left internal iliac venography and measurement of a pressure gradient across the left iliac vein could be performed in patients with recurrence if no other sources of collateralization are visualized. Embolization of the branch of the internal iliac vein that leads to the varicocele could potentially obliterate the varicocele in this theoretical situation.

Finally, the clinical significance and management of the so-called subclinical varicocele remains controversial. A retrospective evaluation of venographic findings and improvement of fertility after embolization in 46 clinical and 38 subclinical varicoceles is available (40). A major difference between the two groups was the greater degree of reflux in the clinical varicocele patients. However, in terms of semen analysis improvement and pregnancy rates, embolization treatment appeared to be equally effective in clinical and subclinical varicoceles (40).

In a recent study, 22 patients underwent either radiographic occlusion of the varicocele or surgical ligation of the internal spermatic vein for radiographically determined subclinical varicoceles. Although most of these patients showed increases in sperm numbers, there were no significant changes in motility or morphology, and the effect on pregnancy rates has yet to be determined (41).

The issue of patient selection for evaluation of subclinical right internal spermatic vein varicocele also remains controversial. Because incompetence of the right internal spermatic vein is an uncommon finding, some choose to perform venography on the right only in patients who have palpable right varicoceles or who have left varicoceles but no evidence of reflux on the left (38).

Seminal Vesiculograms

Seminal vesiculography is reserved for men who have azoospermia or severe oligospermia (sperm density less than 1 million/ml) and who have no evidence of pituitary insufficiency (hypogonadotrophic hypogonadism) or "end-organ failure" as reflected by an elevated FSH level. Generally, testicular biopsy with frozen section evaluation is done at the same time as the proposed radiographic study. If the biopsy shows severe germinal hypoplasia or aplasia, then the seminal vesiculogram is not done. The procedure is generally done on an outpatient basis under general anesthesia, although local anesthesia can be used. Concerns have been raised that this study may induce an inflammatory response and subsequent obstruction at the injection site; however, it is felt that with meticulous technique, using a fine needle (23-gauge butterfly), this should be of minimal concern (41). Techniques of injection that involve incising the vas probably should not be done. After injection of 2.5 to 5 ml of dilute water-soluble iodinated contrast material, the vas, ampulla of the vas, seminal vesicles, and ejaculatory ducts should be easily visualized (Figs. 14.3 and 14.4). Patency of the duct as it enters the prostatic urethra is confirmed by seeing the contrast in either the urethra or the bladder. This is an important observation, and the study can be supplemented by mixing a small amount of methylene blue with the contrast agent. By placing a urethral catheter during the

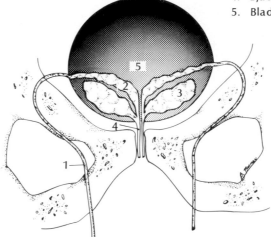

1. Vas deferens
2. Ampulla of vas
3. Seminal vesicle
4. Ejaculatory duct
5. Bladder

Figure 14.3.   A diagrammatic representation of a bilateral seminal vesiculogram and the anatomy that should be visualized.

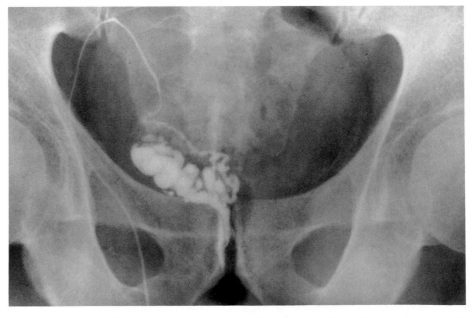

Figure 14.4.   A normal right seminal vesiculogram. In most cases, it is only necessary to perform a unilateral seminal vesiculogram. (Courtesy of R. Dunnick, Durham, NC.)

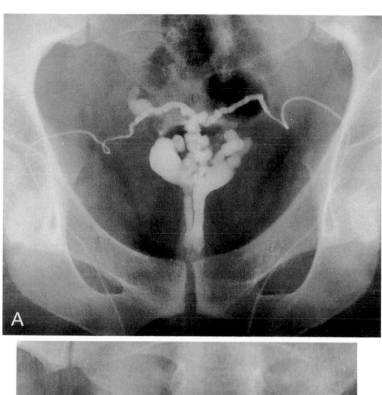

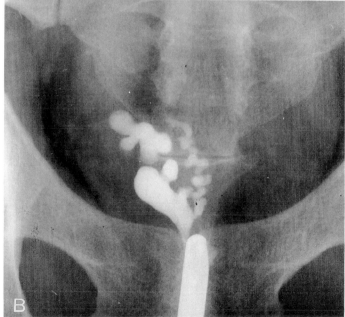

Figure 14.5. **A,** Operative vasogram showing dilated ejaculatory ducts and nonfilling of prostatic urethra or bladder. **B,** Right ejaculatory duct catheterized following transurethral resection and demonstrating patency. (From Porch PP Jr: Aspermia owing to obstruction of distal ejaculatory duct and treatment by transurethral resection. *J Urol* 119:141, 1978.)

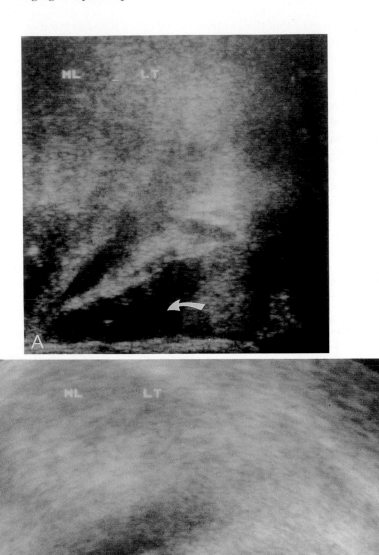

Figure 14.6. **A,** Transrectal ultrasound showing a sagittal view of the prostate with a dilated ejaculatory duct (*arrow*). **B,** Transverse view of the prostate in the same patient, again showing dilated ejaculatory ducts (*arrow*).

study, it can be observed that the contrast material has reached the urethra.

This study is often normal, an especially frustrating finding if the patient should also have a normal testicular biopsy (42). Perhaps the most easily reparable problem that is found is obstruction of the distal ejaculatory ducts, which can be treated by judicious transurethral resection of the area of the prostate where the ejaculatory duct enters (43) (Fig. 14.5). The finding of diverticula-like structures in the ampulla of the vas may be a normal variant (44) or may represent inflammatory changes (45).

Finally, if at the time of the scrotal exploration the biopsy shows spermatogenesis and the seminal vesiculograms show no obstruction, the epididymis should be carefully inspected and palpated, looking for evidence of dilated epididymal tubules. If obstruction of the epididymis is encountered, then an epididymovasostomy should be performed at the same sitting.

Transrectal Ultrasound

In the authors' opinion, transrectal ultrasound of the prostate and seminal vesicles will rapidly take the place of seminal vesiculography. In general, the indications for such a study are the same as for seminal vesiculograms. Specifically, in the azoospermic patient who has an absence of fructose in his ejaculate, the possibilities are absence or atrophy of the seminal vesicles or obstruction of the ejaculatory ducts. Transrectal ultrasound is an ideal modality to demonstrate either of these conditions. One of the authors recently treated a young man with scant ejaculate volume and absent fructose in the ejaculate who on ultrasound evaluation of the prostate and seminal vesicles was found to have markedly dilated ejaculatory ducts (Fig. 14.6). Transurethral resection of the distal ejaculatory duct resulted in a normal semen analysis 1 month

later with conception occurring approximately 6 weeks after the surgery.

On the other hand, if the examiner feels that the vas deferens may not be developed, this can also be confirmed on ultrasonography with the finding of absent or atretic seminal vesicles.

EXPERIMENTAL MODALITIES

A method of assessing testicular metabolic integrity using P-31 magnetic resonance spectroscopy has been described (46). This promising area of investigation may enable us in the future to assess testicular function noninvasively and relatively expeditiously.

SUMMARY

The evaluation of the infertile male requires a systematic and thorough investigation carried out in a logical and expeditious manner. It should be stressed that infertility is a "couple problem" even if the primary pathophysiology appears to reside in one individual. Careful explanations of the rationale for the various tests and procedures should be made not only to the patient but also to his spouse. Such words as "abnormal" should be avoided, and the physician caring for such couples must be aware of the great amount of stress that this condition engenders and be prepared to offer sympathetic counseling.

REFERENCES

1. Lipschultz LI, Howards SS: *Infertility in the Male.* New York, Churchill Livingstone, 1983.
2. Bracken RB, Smith KD: Is semen cryopreservation helpful in testicular cancer? *Urology* 15:581, 1980.
3. Nagler HM, deVere White R: The effect of testicular torsion on the contralateral testis. *J Urol* 128:1343, 1982.
4. Rogers BJ: The sperm penetration assay: Its usefulness reevaluated. *Fertil Steril* 43:821, 1985.
5. Oster J: Varicocele in children and ado-

lescents. *Scand J Urol Nephrol* 5:27, 1971.

6. Steeno O, Knops J, Declerck A, Adimoelja A, Van de Voorde H: Prevention of fertility disorders by detection and treatment of varicocele at school and college age. *Andrologia* 8:47, 1976.

7. Hendry WF, Sommerville IF, Hall RR, Pugh RCB: Investigation and treatment of the subfertile male. *Br J Urol* 45:684, 1973.

8. Dubin L, Amelar RD: Etiologic factors in 1294 consecutive cases of male infertility. *Fertil Steril* 22:469, 1971.

9. Stewart BH: Varicocele in infertility: Incidence and results of surgical therapy. *J Urol* 112:222, 1974.

10. Cockett ATK, Urry RL, Dougherty KA: The varicocele and semen characteristics. *J Urol* 121:435, 1979.

11. MacLeod J: Further observations on the role of varicocele in human male infertility. *Fertil Steril* 20:545, 1969.

12. Brown JS: Varicocelectomy in the subfertile male: A ten-year experience with 295 cases. *Fertil Steril* 27:1046, 1976.

13. Dubin L, Amelar RD: Varicocelectomy: 986 cases in a twelve-year study. *Urology* 10:446, 1977.

14. Peng BCH, Tomashefsky P, Nagler HM: The cofactor effect: varicocele and infertility. *Fertil Steril* 54:143, 1990.

15. Greenberg SH, Lipschultz LI, Morganroth J, Wein AJ: The use of the Doppler stethoscope in the evaluation of varicoceles. *J Urol* 117:296, 1977.

16. Dhabuwala CB, Kumar AB, Kerkar PD, Bhutawala A, Pierce J: Patterns of Doppler recordings and its relationship to varicocele in infertile men. *Int J Androl* 12:430, 1989.

17. Lewis RW, Harrison RM: Contact scrotal thermography: Application to problems of infertility. *J Urol* 122:40, 1979.

18. Ali JI, Weaver DJ, Weinstein SH, Grimes EM: Scrotal temperature and semen quality in men with and without varicocele. *Arch Androl* 24:215, 1990.

19. Goldstein M, Eid JF: Elevation of intratesticular and scrotal skin surface temperature in men with varicocele. *J Urol* 142:743, 1989.

20. McClure RD, Hricak H: Scrotal ultrasound in the infertile man: Detection of subclinical unilateral and bilateral varicoceles. *J Urol* 135:711, 1986.

21. Wheatley JK, Fajman WA, Witten FR: Clinical experience with the radioisotopic varicocele scan as a screening method for detection of subclinical varicoceles. *J Urol* 128:57, 1982.

22. Green KF, Turner TT, Howards SS: Varicocele: Reversal of the testicular blood flow and temperature effects by varicocele repair. *J Urol* 131:1208, 1984.

23. Buschi AJ, Harrison RB, Brenbridge ANAG, Williamson BRJ, Gentry RR, Cole R: Distended left renal vein: CT/sonographic normal variant. *AJR* 135:339, 1980.

24. Tjia TT, Rumping WJM, Landman GHM, et al.: Phlebography of the internal spermatic vein (and the ovarian vein). *Diagn Imaging* 51:8, 1982.

25. Bigot JM, Chatel A: The value of retrograde spermatic phlebography in varicocele. *Eur Urol* 6:301, 1980.

26. Comhaire F, Kunnen M, Nahoum C: Radiological anatomy of the internal spermatic vein(s) in 200 retrograde venograms. *Int J Androl* 4:379, 1981.

27. Nadel SN, Hutchins GM, Albertson PC, et al: Valves of the internal spermatic vein: Potential for mis-diagnosis of varicocele by venography. *Fertil Steril* 4:479, 1984.

28. Gonzales R, Narayan P, Castaneda-Zuniga WR, Amplatz K: Transvenous embolization of the internal spermatic veins for the treatment of varicocele scroti. *Urol Clin North Am* 9:177, 1982.

29. Lima SS, Castro MP, Costa OF: A new method for the treatment of varicocele. *Andrologia* 10:103, 1978.

30. Seyferth W, Jecht E, Zeitler E: Percutaneous sclerotherapy of varicocele. *Radiology* 139:335, 1981.

31. Hunter DW, Bildsoe MC, Amplatz K: Aid for safer sclerotherapy of the internal spermatic vein. *Radiology* 173:282, 1989.

32. Thon WF, Gall H, Danz B, Bahren W, Sigmund G: Percutaneous sclerotherapy of idiopathic varicocele in childhood: A preliminary report. *J Urol* 141:913, 1989.

33. White RI Jr, Kaufman SL, Barth KH, Kadir S, Smyth JW, Walsh PC: Occlusion of varicoceles with detachable balloons. *Radiology* 139:327, 1981.

34. Kaufman SL, Kadir S, Barth KH, et al.: Mechanisms of recurrent varicocele after balloon occlusion or surgical ligation of the internal spermatic vein. *Radiology* 147:435, 1983.

35. Mitchell SE, White RI Jr, Chang R, et al.:

Long-term results of outpatient balloon embolotherapy in 300 varicoceles. Abstract #216, 71st Scientific Assembly of the RSNA, November 1985.

36. Sayfan J, Adam YG, Soffer Y: A natural "venous bypass" causing postoperative recurrence of a varicocele. *J Androl* 2:108, 1981.

37. Murray RR Jr, Mitchell SE, Kadir S, et al.: Comparison of recurrent varicocele anatomy following surgery and percutaneous balloon occlusion. *J Urol* 135:286, 1986.

38. Shuman L, White RI Jr, Mitchell SE, et al.: Right-sided varicocele technique and clinical results of balloon embolotherapy from the femoral approach. *Radiology* 158:787, 1986.

39. Coolsaet BLRA: The varicocele syndrome: Venography determining the optimal level of surgical treatment. *J Urol* 124:833, 1980.

40. Marsman JWP: Clinical vs. subclinical varicocele: Venographic findings and improvement of fertility after embolization. *Radiology* 155:635, 1985.

41. Gordon JA, Clahassey EB: Evaluation of stricture formation as a complication of vasopuncture and vasography in the guinea pig. *Fertil Steril* 29:180, 1978.

42. Ford K, Carson CC III, Dunnick NR, Osborne D, Paulson DF: The role of seminal vesiculography in the evaluation of male infertility. *Fertil Steril* 37:552, 1982.

43. Porch PP Jr: Aspermia owing to obstruction of distal ejaculatory duct and treatment by transurethral resection. *J Urol* 119:141, 1978.

44. Banner MP, Hassler R: The normal seminal vesiculogram. *Radiology* 128:339, 1978.

45. Dunnick NR, Ford K, Osborne D, Carson CC III, Paulson DF: Seminal vesiculography: Limited value in vesiculitis. *Urology* 20:454, 1982.

46. Chew WM, Hricak H, McClure RD, Wendland MF: In vivo human testicular function assessed with P-31 MR spectroscopy. *Radiology* 177:743, 1990.

Index

Page numbers followed by "t" denote tables; those followed by "f" denote figures.

sonographic techniques, 36
sonographic assessment of, 265
Tubal spasm, temporary tubal obstruction due
to, 193, 194f–195f
Tubal sterilization
hysterographic follow-up of, 213–226,
226f–231f
laparoscopic techniques, 217
reversal, pre- and postoperative
hysterosalpingography with, 226–238,
227f, 232f–238f
techniques, 213, 225f
Tuberculosis
genital, 151
hysterosalpingographic diagnosis of,
185–189, 188f
peritubal adhesive disease secondary to, 185
proximal tubal obstruction secondary to, 196
tubal, 172
Twin pregnancy
embryonic demise in, transvaginal
ultrasound of, 273, 276f
transvaginal ultrasound in, 273, 275f–276f

Uchida technique, of tubal occlusion, 213
hysterographic follow-up, 213, 226f–227f
Ulcerative colitis, tubal occlusion in, 172
Ultrasonography
guidance of transcervical fallopian tube
catheterization, 204–205
transabdominal, of ovarian hyperstimulation,
251–252, 252f–254f
transrectal, or prostate and seminal vesicles,
298f, 299
transvaginal
of abortion, 279, 280f
applications of, 242
of bicornuate uterus, 265, 266f
Doppler techniques in, 246f–247f,
252–253, 252f–253f, 263f–264f,
265–266
in early pregnancy, 265, 269–287
abnormal findings in, 277–283
milestones of, 269–273, 270t, 270f–276f,
273t
normal findings in, 269–273
of ectopic pregnancy, 279–283, 282f–287f
of embryonic demise, 276f, 277–279,
278f–279f
endometrial assessment using, 261–265,
263f–264f
of fallopian tubes, 265
follicular aspiration guided by, 254–259,
256f–260f
for follicular monitoring, 244–254,
246f–254f
future applications, 265–267
in gynecologic infertility, 242–267

instrumentation, 242–244, 243f–244f
of intrauterine device, 265, 266f–267f
in multifetal pregnancy, 273, 275f–276f
of septate uterus, 265
of trophoblastic disease, 279, 281f
tubal cannulation guided by, 259–261,
261f–262f
of uterine malformations, 265, 266f
of uterovaginal anomalies, 61
of uterus, 117
Unexplained infertility, 10
hysteroscopic evaluation and treatment of,
133–136, 137f
incidence of, 133
Ureter, ectopic insertion into vagina, 69f
Urinary tract
congenital malformations of, 59
in DES-exposed patient, 89
Urogenital sinus, 58, 63, 85
Uterine cavity, 39, 40f, 96–115. *See also*
Endometrial cavity
abnormalities, 117
after cesarean section, 39, 44f, 115
contribution to infertility, 118t
in DES-exposed patient, 86–88
estimated prevalence of, 118t
adenomyoma in, 112f, 112–115
adenomyosis, 49, 49f–50f, 112–115,
113f–114f
air bubble in, 96–97, 97f
benign neoplasms, 100–106, 102f–106f
filling defects, 96–112
foreign bodies in, 109–111, 110f–111f
hysteroscopic evaluation and treatment of,
136, 145f
hysteroscopic view of, 119f–122f, 137
IUD in, 109–111, 110f–111f
malignant neoplasms, 99–100, 101f–102f
marginal irregularities, 112–115
neoplastic filling defects, 156
normal, 48–50, 48f–53f
polyps, 97, 98f–100f
post-abortion fetal parts in, 111–112
postsurgical abnormalities of, 115
retained conception products in, 108f–109f,
109, 156
size, 96
wedge-like deformity, with solitary myoma,
103, 105f
Uterine dehiscence, 165
Uterine factors
incidence of, 117
in infertility, 117, 118t
Uterine perforation, in hysterosalpingography,
33, 213, 225f
Uterine perfusion, assessment of, 265–167
Uterine rupture, in pregnancy, after treatment
of intrauterine adhesions, 165